Psychiatry
FOR MEDICAL STUDENTS

BY ROBERT J. WALDINGER, M.D.

American
Psychiatric
Press, Inc.

1400 K STREET, N.W.
WASHINGTON, D.C. 20005

Note: The author has worked to ensure that all information in this book concerning drug dosages, schedules, and routes of administration is accurate at the time of publication and consistent with standards set by the United States Food and Drug Administration and the general medical community. As medical research and practice advance, however, therapeutic standards may change. For this reason, and because human and mechanical errors sometimes occur, we recommend that readers follow the advice of a physician directly involved in their care or the care of a member of their family.

Library of Congress Cataloging in Publication data.
Main entry under title:

Waldinger, Robert J.
  Psychiatry for medical students.

  Includes bibliographies and index.
  1. Psychiatry.   I. Title.
RC454.W28   1984   616.89   83-25692
ISBN 0-88048-003-3

Printed in the U.S.A.

Contents

Introduction

THIS IS A BOOK FOR BEGINNERS. It was written not only for medical students who are doing their first clinical clerkship in psychiatry, but also for nurses, social workers, psychologists, and others who are trying to make sense out of their first encounters with people who are emotionally disturbed. The book assumes no prior knowledge of psychiatry.

I wrote this book because I wished it had been written for me. When I was a medical student, I was skeptical of psychiatry with all of its jargon, and I was bewildered by the complicated illnesses and profound emotional distress that I encountered among psychiatric patients during my first experience in mental health care. At the local bookstore, I found quite a few massive comprehensive textbooks, and many excellent books devoted to particular areas of psychopathology. But what I wanted was one short book that would give me the basics— that would provide me with an introduction to topics like schizophrenia and ECT, transference and tranquilizers—and would do so in plain English.

That is what this book is meant to do. My aim has been to write chapters that can be read and referred to quickly while you are in the midst of a busy student rotation. Then, when you have time, you can do further reading to pursue in more detail those areas that particularly interest you.

A second goal of this book is to help you make sense of your own reactions to what you see clinically—because your feelings about patients and their problems often provide you with crucial diagnostic information. And the experience of working with people who are in severe emotional distress can be grueling, particularly when you are new at it. In order to take care of other people, you have to take care of yourself—and that means paying attention to your own reactions to clinical work and knowing when to get emotional support from friends, colleagues, and teachers. Throughout these chapters, I have tried to help you focus on yourself as well as on your patients.

The book is laid out in four major sections. Chapters 1 through 4 are designed to give you the basic skills with which to carry out a diagnostic evaluation. Chapters 5 through 9 cover particular mental disorders, while Chapters 10 through 13 address some areas that are of clinical concern to everyone who works in mental health care. Finally, Chapters 14 and 15 describe psychotherapies and somatic therapies, respectively.

Because this text is *not* encyclopedic, much is left out. But it will provide you with a place to start. And if these chapters help make psychiatry more accessible to you and prompt you to delve further into the field, then the book will have accomplished its purpose.

Acknowledgments

MANY GENEROUS AND CAPABLE PEOPLE contributed to the writing of this book. I am indebted to my teachers and colleagues at McLean Hospital, who commented on the early drafts of this manuscript:

Jonathan O. Cole, M.D.
Robert Fein, Ph.D.
Arlene Frank, Ph.D.
Cynthia N. Kettyle, M.D.
Benjamin Liptzin, M.D.
Margaret McKenna, M.D.
Alan F. Schatzberg, M.D.
Sharon R. Weinstein, M.D.
Roger Weiss, M.D.

Carolyn B. Robinowitz, M.D., Deputy Medical Director of the American Psychiatric Association, offered valuable perspectives on medical student education. I owe special thanks to Diane Mosbacher, M.D., Ph.D., who somehow found the time and energy during her fourth year of medical school to examine the entire text from a student's vantage point. She heightened my awareness of many social and political issues relevant to the care of patients, and helped me to free the text of some of its cumbersome jargon.

John G. Gunderson, M.D., provided me with a place to work and secretarial support in the Psychotherapy Department at McLean. He also prodded me when my pace slowed, and brought his considerable clinical expertise to bear on many parts of the manuscript. Philip Isenberg, M.D., Director of Residency Education at McLean, helped me to conceptualize the textbook and to maintain its focus on needs of beginning students. Evelyn Stone shepherded the book through each stage of production. Without her knowledge of psychiatric publications and her constant willingness to listen and advise, the book would not have been realized.

Frances MacNeil did the lion's share of the typing of the manuscript, and remained helpful and supportive through many long and choppy drafts. Finally, Amy Shaughnessy and David Andrews of the American Psychiatric Press, Inc., worked tirelessly to make the book more comprehensible to those with no background in the field, and managed to take some of the rough edges off my prose.

For all of their assistance and encouragement, I am very grateful.

Part I

INTRODUCTION

The problems that people bring to the psychiatrist run the gamut from memory loss to marital difficulties, from palpitations to hallucinations. The first section of this book is designed to offer you basic tools with which to approach this vast array of problems.

The primary diagnostic tool available to the psychiatrist is the interview. Chapter 1 discusses interviewing technique, highlighting how good interviewing differs from everyday conversation, and reviews some of the more common problems encountered by inexperienced interviewers.

Chapter 2 is a brief description of psychodynamic psychology. It is an attempt to demystify such basic psychodynamic concepts as the id/ego/superego and the unconscious mind. It is also designed to acquaint you with the stages of human development and the ideas of psychological conflict and defense that can be invaluable to you in understanding what patients tell you about themselves and their past.

Chapter 3 focuses specifically on how to do a psychiatric evaluation, because that is usually the first task confronting the student in a mental health care setting. It outlines the aspects of a patient's life that you need to explore as part of an initial evaluation, and provides examples of interview questions that will help you gather this information.

Chapter 4 complements Chapter 3 in that it describes the mental status examination, which is part of every psychiatric evaluation. But in addition to describing the exam and offering ideas about how best to conduct it, the chapter is designed to serve as a glossary, defining many of the terms used to label psychiatric symptoms. It is important that you become familiar with these so that you use them correctly in your work.

These four chapters serve as a prelude to the rest of the book. Once you have grasped the essentials of interviewing, psychodynamics, and the process of doing an evaluation, you will be prepared to take a closer look at specific mental disorders and the methods we have for diagnosing and treating them.

1

The Psychiatric Interview

An INTERVIEW IS, in essence, a conversation. So a chapter in interviewing technique may seem a waste of time. After all, most of us are well practiced in everyday conversation.

However, the clinical interview is a very particular kind of conversation and differs from daily discourse in many crucial respects. These differences are subtle, and interviewing is a skill that takes time to master. Good clinicians are good interviewers, regardless of specialty, and the principles discussed below are important tools in all branches of medicine. The basic principles of interviewing apply equally to evaluating congestive heart failure, conducting an emergency-room psychiatric consultation, or embarking on long-term psychotherapy. This chapter places particular emphasis on how to interview a new patient as part of a diagnostic evaluation, because that is usually your first task as a student in a mental health care setting.

The aim of interviewing is not simply to gather information on the patient's past, but to arrive at an empathic understanding of how the patient feels. Such understanding is essential to accurate diagnosis and effective treatment, and the success of the interview hinges on its development. The more sensitive you are as an interviewer, the greater will be your grasp of your patient's problems. And the easier it will be

3

for patients to elaborate on the nature of their pain. Emotional distress is often quite isolating, and the experience of sharing one's problems with a concerned listener can be enormously relieving. In a sense, the initial interview is actually the start of treatment.

To evaluate effectively, you must discover as much as you can about how your patient's mind works. During the interview, patients will offer many clues, both in *what* they tell you (the *content* of the interview) and in *how* they tell it (the *process* of the interview).

The process of the interview is crucial to understanding the patient's problems. But process is much more difficult to focus on than content, because most of us are not accustomed to doing so. Attending to process means listening with a "third ear," mentally stepping back from a conversation and watching it even as you participate. It means taking note of how people speak, what topics they bring up and in what order, which subjects they emphasize and which they avoid, how they sit or gesture, what responses they elicit from you, and how they make you feel. This style of listening does not come naturally to most of us, because in everyday conversation we focus on the content of what is said, and think about process only when there is some obvious discrepancy between the two (e.g., when a friend screams at you, "I am not angry!"). Paying attention to process is hard work, but it is a skill worth developing. Through process, patients will give you a glimpse of how they cope with their world and how they approach new relationships. Consider the following:

> A young man has just been fired from his most recent job, and complains to you that he is "depressed" because he cannot get along with a series of "difficult" employers. He also notes that his romantic relationships have never worked out "because women just don't understand me." In your interview, you find that he drones on and on about minute details of his work as an actuary. He becomes frustrated and momentarily angry whenever you attempt to introduce a new topic, saying, "I'll get to that, doctor—but first let me finish my story." When you ask about his feelings of depression, he invariably changes the subject back to his work. At the end of the interview, you find that you have gathered little information about his life, or about the specific problems that brought him to see you. You also find yourself feeling angry and impatient with him. The content of the interview is of little help to you. However, your attention to the process of the interview provides you with a glimpse of this man's difficulties. He has rigidly insisted on imposing his own order on your meeting, and has avoided any subject that might arouse unpleasant feelings. You might infer that his inflexibility and need to flee from emotion hamper both his relationships with women and his ability to work with employers. You might also infer that he makes other people feel angry and impatient with him, just as he has done with you.

Clearly, patients must be given the opportunity to show you the processes by which they form a relationship. They will do this in even a single interview, provided that you give them the freedom to do so. The interviewer who subjects the patient to an endless stream of specific questions will never gather this kind of information. He or she will not learn, for example, how the patient handles silences or sadness. What's more, the interviewer who tends to talk a lot leaves less time to listen, and will likely lose touch with his or her own feelings about the patient. You should, therefore, be as nondirective as possible. Guide patients only when they seem to stray from the themes relevant to the interview. Obviously, this is not always an easy task, especially for the neophyte interviewer.

Your first goal is to stay out of the way, so that the patient can talk, and you can listen. You must begin by taking steps to create an atmosphere that is conducive to free-flowing conversation.

SETTING THE TONE

Place. In order to devote your full attention to the work at hand, you and your patient must be physically at ease. Choose a quiet place for the interview where you are likely to have as few interruptions as possible. Ideally, this will be a place where you cannot be overheard, so that the patient will feel free to discuss confidential matters, and noises will not distract either of you.

Meeting the patient. You may be the first person to whom your patient has come for help. Patients almost certainly will be anxious about talking to a stranger. They are likely to be worried by their symptoms and apprehensive about what your assessment will be. They may feel embarrassed about personal matters that must be discussed in the interview. Thus, patients are made vulnerable not only by their illnesses, but also by the very nature of the encounter with you. So you must put the new patient at ease and treat him or her with particular courtesy.

Upon meeting the patient, shake hands and introduce yourself. It is always proper to use formal address (i.e., Mr., Ms., Mrs.) both as a courtesy to the patient and as part of professional decorum. Initially, you may be tempted to put yourself and your patients on a first-name basis, but this usually hinders, rather than helps. After all, the patient has not granted you the privilege of using his or her first name, and your doing so may seem presumptuous. Moreover, in using familiar forms of address, you convey the idea that the interview is something other than a professional encounter. As patients reveal intimate information about themselves, your professional attitude will be reassuring. You can convey warmth and concern without using terms that imply that you are close friends. Of course, children and adolescents are exceptions to this rule, as it is customary to call them by their first names in business as well as in social settings.

Invite your patient to sit down. If the patient is offered a choice of seats, note whether he or she sits near to or far from you. Chairs should be arranged comfortably for conversation. And you should sit so as to feel physically relaxed. If you are comfortable, you will be better able to listen and your relaxed appearance will help put the patient more at ease.

Initiate and maintain eye contact with the patient, but don't overdo it. A fixed stare is bound to disquiet your patient. You will find that varied eye contact will be most effective in establishing rapport. Take notes if you feel comfortable doing so. Should the patient ask about your note taking, you should explore his or her concerns about the confidentiality of your meetings, and you can use the opportunity to reassure the patient that privacy will be respected.

Time. Let the patient know at the outset how much time there is to talk. Traditionally, psychiatric interviews last 45 to 50 minutes. Of course, some evaluation interviews require more than this (e.g., an emergency room consultation), while very agitated patients may not tolerate a meeting lasting longer than a few minutes.

Be prompt for any arranged meeting with a patient. If you must be late for a first meeting, an apology is in order. If you are late for subsequent meetings, you should listen for the patient's reaction (e.g., anger, hurt, relief). You should also examine your own feelings if you are repeatedly late for meetings with one patient (e.g., when a patient makes you feel helpless or incompetent).

Note how the patient uses time. For example, some patients will arrive far in advance of their appointments. Others will arrive late, and you will want to pay close attention to lateness as a possible indication that the patient has some feeling about meeting with you that he or she is not directly expressing (e.g., anger at you, or fear of discussing a painful subject in the interview). When patients arrive late and apologize, do not reassure them that the lateness is "ok." Instead, inquire about the circumstances. Obviously, lateness is sometimes unavoidable, especially for someone trying to find the way to an unfamiliar location. But often excuses will be vague ("I forgot to set my alarm clock," "I was engrossed in work and forgot the time") and indicate a lack of attention on the patient's part or ambivalence about seeing you. So you may want to ask, "How did you feel about coming today?" to elicit the patient's feelings about the interview. Remember: if people truly want to be on time, they can almost always manage it. Be sure to end the session on time, so that your patients will see that it is not in their interest to arrive late.

Defining the goals of the interview. A simple statement at the beginning about the length and purpose of the interview will set the stage for your evaluation. Be sure your patient understands from the outset the reason for your meeting (e.g., to evaluate the problems brought to you by the patient and to determine what treatments, if any, would be of help). Discuss how many meetings the patient will have with you, and whether you are likely to continue seeing the patient when the evaluation is finished, or refer the patient to someone else for treatment. This is especially important if you are spending a short period of time in a hospital or outpatient clinic as part of a student clerkship. Your patients will develop feelings for you (often, feelings of attachment and trust) as they tell you about their lives and problems. They must be prepared to lose their relationship with you when your work together is finished or when you leave this particular assignment.

YOUR INTERVIEWING STYLE: HELPING YOUR PATIENT TELL YOU WHAT IS WRONG

We all have preconceived notions about psychiatry. Stereotypically, the psychiatrist is a cold and distant person who never speaks except to ask a question and who remains unmoved by patients' distress. Yet working with people who are in pain can be a very moving experience. In your first few interviews, you may feel as if you are having an intimate discussion with a close friend.

A good psychiatric interview is not a cold interrogation, nor is it a friendly chat, for neither style offers the patient the security and the freedom to speak openly about intimate problems. Effective interviewing is not stilted or artificial; in fact, it may even sound like everyday conversation. But interviewing differs from daily discourse in that it is specifically designed to give the patient as many opportunities as possible to tell you what is wrong. The specific techniques discussed below can help you to do just that.

Interviewing Techniques

Opening the Interview. Once you have introduced yourself and agreed upon the purpose of the meeting, ask a general question that allows the patient to begin wherever he or she chooses. You might begin with

"What brings you to see me today?" or

"Can you tell me what has been troubling you?"

If a patient seems very anxious at the start of your interview, and has difficulty responding to an open-ended question, you might ask some specific neutral questions concerning age, marital status, and living situation, to allow the patient some time to get more comfortable.

Allow the interview to flow freely. Let patients describe the events of their lives in any order they choose. Your comments and questions should flow naturally from what the patient says. Rather than jump from one topic to another, stay with the patient—encourage him or her to elaborate on thoughts and feelings. As the interview proceeds, you can guide the patient to fill in gaps in his or her story without abruptly changing the subject. For example, if a patient has spent the first half of the interview reviewing recent events, you might turn the conversation to the patient's past with "You mentioned your family, could you tell me more about your background?" If you keep in mind an outline of what needs to be covered, you can later rearrange what the patient has said in an orderly form for your written report.

The inexperienced interviewer is often tempted to ask a prepared list of questions and follow a prescribed order in gathering information (as in a standard medical "review of systems"). However, this will simply restrict the patient's options to tell you what is wrong, and will give the impression that you are not really listening.

Provide structure for patients who have trouble ordering their thoughts. Some patients—e.g., those suffering from severe anxiety or psychosis—may be confused by open-ended questions and may respond to them by rambling incoherently. In such cases, you must more actively structure the interview, both so that you can gather information about the patient and so that the patient does

Table 1-1. Some interviewing principles.

Allow the interview to flow freely rather than jumping from one topic to another.
Provide structure for patients who have trouble ordering their thoughts.
Phrase your questions to invite the patient to talk.
Avoid leading questions.
Help patients to elaborate on thoughts and feelings.
Avoid jargon.
Use the patient's words whenever possible.
Avoid asking questions that begin with "why?"
Take note of the patient's strengths.

---

not become increasingly anxious and disorganized. A general question like "Tell me about your background" will not evoke a cogent response from such a patient. Instead, you must show the patient precisely where you want the interview to go, with specific questions such as "What was your father's occupation?" and "How old were you when he died?" You may shift back and forth from a more-structured to a less-structured interviewing style as the interview proceeds; tailor the specificity of your questions to your patient's needs.

Phrase your questions to invite the patient to talk. How you phrase questions will have an enormous impact on the information you gather. *Open questions* allow the patient to elaborate; *closed questions*, which require short answers (often "yes" or "no"), leave little room for detail. Some examples:

Closed: Have you felt depressed for a long time?
Open: Can you tell me how you feel when you are depressed?

Closed: Are you from a large family?
Open: Tell me about your family.

Open questions help patients reveal relationships between their symptoms and events in their lives. Closed questions keep the patient quiet and make *you* do all the work. This leaves you with the impossible task of knowing which out of possibly hundreds of closed questions will get to the root of the patient's problems. And unless you prepare these questions ahead of the interview, you'll be compelled to concentrate so hard on thinking them up as you go that you will lose touch with what the patient is saying.

Avoid leading questions. Like closed questions, leading questions are conversation-stoppers. They imply that you already know how the patient feels. In the case of a man whose brother had just died, a typical leading question would be

"Did you feel sad when your brother died?"

This question sends a clear message that you expect the patient to feel sad. In fact, the patient may have hated his brother, and must then confront the choice of challenging your expectation or concealing his real feelings. The obvious nonleading question in this instance would be

"How did you feel when your brother died?"

In short, don't assume that patients will react to events as you do. Leave them ample opportunity to explain how they really feel.

Help patients to elaborate. When patients seem to run out of steam or come to a stopping point, a nod may suffice to show them that you are eager to hear more. Or you may offer an encouraging comment like

"Tell me more about that."

"Please go on."

"Oh?"

"And?"

You may also echo a key word or phrase from the patient's statement. For example, if the patient said, "My wife Irma thinks I'm impossible to live with," you could say "Impossible to live with?"

You may want to help the patient focus on feelings. For example, you could ask "How did you feel about that?" or "How did you feel when that happened?"

And to get the patient to be more specific when he or she is speaking in generalities:

"Can you give me a specific example?"

"What do you mean when you say 'crazy'?"

Reflect your patients' feelings back to them. This technique involves echoing the *tone* the patient has conveyed. This helps in two ways. First, when you show patients that you are trying to understand how they feel, you communicate your concern and thereby encourage them to open up. Second, reflecting patients' feelings in this way serves to test your own perceptions, i.e., to confirm or deny that you have understood. Here are some examples:

Patient: I can't seem to accomplish anything. Nothing has worked out for me in my life. Why should I expect the future to be any different?

Interviewer: You seem discouraged.

Patient: It just isn't fair. Frank walked out and left me—flat. He had no right.

Interviewer: You sound pretty angry with him.

When you correctly verbalize patients' feelings, they will confirm it by elaborating further. You may help them in this way to see their feelings more clearly. But if you have *not* understood your patients, they will then have a chance to correct you.

Remember: reflecting the patient's tone does not involve *sympathy*. Avoid statements like "Your story makes me feel sad," or "That's absolutely awful!" Your goal is *empathy*, which means *understanding* how the other person feels, and not necessarily sharing those feelings.

Paraphrase the patient's thoughts. This technique is similar to reflecting the patient's feelings, but focuses on ideas more than emotions. Like reflecting feelings, paraphrasing the patient's thoughts lets the patient know that you are listening and trying to understand. It provides a check on your perceptions, and helps the patient clarify his or her comments. Examples of paraphrasing might include the following:

Patient: Your medicine is no good.

Interviewer: You mean, when you took it you did not feel better?

Patient: I come in here and talk to you, but what good is it doing me?

Interviewer: You're wondering whether our talks have helped you.

Another useful technique is *summarization*, i.e., recapitulating and condensing what the patient has said. Summarization encompasses both thoughts and feelings. It is similar to reflecting feelings and paraphrasing, but summarizing allows you to cover more material or a longer time span. The following are a few instances in which summarizing may help clarify what the patient has said:

- When the patient's discussion has been long-winded, rambling or confusing.
- When the patient appears to have talked about everything important on a specific subject.
- When you want to ensure that you and the patient have a mutual understanding of what has been discussed so far, so you may move on to other matters.
- When you want to highlight certain ideas or events that you believe to be particularly important.

Here are some examples of summarization:

Interviewer: So for the past three months you have been hearing your dead mother's voice tell you that you should kill yourself. Since this began, you have been unable to go to work and have refused to leave your bedroom.

Interviewer: So you have felt depressed ever since your brother became ill, and for the past several days you have had trouble falling asleep and have not felt like eating.

Additional Tips on Interviewing

Avoid jargon. Our daily language has become increasingly "psychologized" in recent years, but psychological jargon usually confuses rather than clarifies. Also, your using jargon may make the patient feel dehumanized. Patients themselves sometimes use jargon to avoid genuine feelings. For example, the patient who "explains" his recent suicide attempt as "a temporary decompensation due to a reactive depression" has told you absolutely nothing about what prompted him to try to kill himself, or how he feels about it. Therefore, take care not to use jargon, and when patients (or colleagues) use it, be sure to ask them what they mean. Inexperienced interviewers are often reluctant to ask patients to explain such terms as "depression" or "psychosis." However, if you ask for such explanations, you will be surprised at the many meanings offered. And you will begin to understand more about your patient's particular language.

Be careful, too, about offering the patient a tentative diagnosis. Diagnostic labels can be confusing and frightening if presented before you and your patient have a clear understanding of the problem at hand.

Use the patient's words as frequently as possible, rather than your own. This is particularly important, for example, in dealing with sexual matters, where the ways people describe their experiences are practically infinite. If a patient says that he or she is "gay," be sure to use the patient's term rather than a word like "homosexual," which may have different connotations for the patient. This principle applies to virtually all subjects, but particularly to matters about which the patient is likely to be sensitive.

Avoid asking questions that begin with "why." Patients do not usually know "why," and asking implies that you expect them to produce facile explanations. With your help, patients will discover more about the roots of their problems as they reflect upon their lives in the sessions. When you are tempted to ask "why," rephrase your question so that it elicits a detailed response, e.g., "What happened?" or "How did that come about?" or "What thoughts do you have about that?"

Thoughts versus feelings. In the interview, most people will use a mixture of ideas and emotions to paint a picture of their lives. However, some people keep a tight rein on their emotions and will dwell exclusively on ideas and explanations—i.e., they will intellectualize to protect themselves from uncomfortable feelings. With such people, it is very helpful to emphasize emotion in your interview by asking patients how they *feel*. Conversely, other people deal with problems and anxiety almost exclusively in emotional terms, e.g., "Oh, doctor, I get so upset I just can't think straight." For them, it helps to emphasize their capacity to think by asking questions like "What do you think about that?"

Often, the patient's immediate response to a difficult or anxiety-provoking question is "I don't know." Rather than immediately asking another question, you may get more information if you just sit quietly after an "I don't know" response, or ask the patient, "What comes to mind?" and see what happens.

Sensitive subjects should be approached tactfully but not avoided. After initially refusing, the patient may discuss difficult or embarrassing material if you rephrase your question and/or return to the topic at a later time.

Take note of the patient's strengths. People seek psychiatric help because they have problems, and these often obscure positive personality traits and accomplishments. If you listen for strengths and show interest in them, you will convey to your patients a sense that you want to get a balanced view of their situation. If patients do not offer any examples of how they feel good about themselves, you might ask "What are you proud of?" or "What do you like about yourself?" The reply will give you information about self-esteem.

Humor. Humor can be a wonderful tool in building an alliance with your patient. Be careful, though, for it can backfire. Patients may use humor defensively to avoid unpleasant feelings or to keep you amused. Your own use of humor may be misunderstood as ridicule. The key is to stay in tune with how your patient is feeling—and when you're not sure of those feelings, ask.

Keep track of where the interview is going. While

it is important to allow patients to tell their stories as they choose, the time in which you must complete the evaluation is usually limited. Thus, you should not hesitate to guide patients onto more relevant matters if they ramble or repeat themselves. Keep track of time, so that you have a chance at the end of the interview to ask about topics that may have been ignored or that need to be explored further.

YOUR REACTIONS TO THE PATIENT

In the psychiatric interview, you are your own best and most important diagnostic instrument. Thus, your emotional reactions to the patient constitute invaluable data. Your reactions not only tell you how the patient makes others feel, but may tell you how the *patient* feels behind all of his or her defenses (e.g., the helplessness you feel in talking with a woman who intends to commit suicide may reflect *her* sense of helplessness in the face of intolerable emotional pain). If the patient awakens in you strong feelings of anger, depression, sexual arousal, or anxiety that you do not acknowledge, you may be rendered incapable of effective listening and may miss key aspects of the patient's problem.

Anxiety is probably the most common obstacle to effective listening. It is only natural to be somewhat anxious as a beginning interviewer. But sometimes particular patients (e.g., threatening ones) or particular topics (e.g., suicide) arouse so much anxiety that the interviewer screens out anxiety-provoking information. For example, when a depressed patient speaks casually of having a loaded gun in the house, the interviewer may become so frightened that he or she does not hear what has been said, or minimizes the seriousness of the situation. The anxious interviewer may even unwittingly change the subject and leave the patient's suicidal thoughts unexplored. If you allow yourself to *be aware of your anxiety* and examine its source, you will be much less likely to retreat from difficult subjects during the interview. (For more detailed discussion of anxiety in dealing with violent patients, see Chapter 13.)

Identifying with the patient is another common occurrence among inexperienced interviewers, and can hinder an accurate assessment of the patient's problems. You may mistakenly assume that you share certain feelings or experiences with your patient. This assumption could distort the facts and hamper your work, as in the following:

A young man seeks a psychiatric evaluation at his college health service, con.plaining that he can never complete his term papers on time, and that he is in jeopardy of flunking out of college. The psychiatrist, a first-year resident, comments to the patient that she, too, had difficulty completing assignments on time during college and medical school. She assumes that she and her patient are alike in this respect; that his symptom, like hers, is confined to his school work; that he will "grow out of it"; and that his fears of academic failure are exaggerated. The resident reassures him that the problem is not serious and sends him home.

In this case, the resident has failed to learn that her patient procrastinates in every area of his life: He is routinely late for appointments, never pays bills on time, and always keeps his dates waiting (apologizing profusely for his lateness when he finally arrives). His problem is much more pervasive than hers, and causes him to be much more dysfunctional.

In addition, the resident does not recognize that their respective symptoms have very different roots. The resident struggles with her concerns about surpassing her mother in terms of professional education and advancement, and her trouble meeting deadlines in her work reflects a conflict between her wish to excel and her fear of losing her mother's love if she does. The undergraduate, by contrast, is caught in a more global struggle to exert control over all aspects of his life, and he stubbornly refuses to submit to what he sees as other people's demands. Because she has mistakenly equated her patient's situation with her own, the resident does not get an accurate picture of this man's problem, and she intervenes in a way that is not likely to be helpful.

When you start to feel that you and your patient are in some way alike, tread carefully. Make sure you differentiate what you know about yourself from what you know about your patient. And as a general rule, avoid talking about your own life. Doing so usually diverts the focus from the patient's problems.

Avoid premature reassurance. You may be tempted to allay the patient's fears with such assurances as "Everything will be fine" or "There is nothing seriously wrong with you." However, reassurance is only genuine when (1) you have explored the precise nature and extent of the patient's fears, and (2) you are certain of what you are telling the patient. Premature reassurance can actually heighten the patient's anxiety, by giving the impression that you have jumped to a conclusion without doing a thorough evaluation, or that you are just saying what you think the patient wants to hear. It also leaves the patient alone with his or her fears about what is "really" wrong. Instead of minimizing these fears, try to find out more about them. When, for example, the patient expresses fears of being incurable, you might explore this area with an open-ended question: "What do you mean by incurable?" Or you might say, "You seem quite worried about this. Tell me more about it."

Address what is going on in the room. If the patient speaks incoherently, for example, or is actively hallucinating in your office, it will most likely be a relief to both of you if you acknowledge the patient's distress and try to clarify what you do not understand. Even the most disorganized patients often know when they are not making sense. If you are confused, say so.

Set limits on inappropriate behavior. Although understanding is your goal in the interview, there are times when you must simply put a stop to what the patient is doing. This includes threats and menacing behavior, refusal to leave office, and disruptive behavior in the office or waiting area. When, for example, a manic patient wants to remove his clothing, or an angry patient threatens to throw an ashtray through your office window, you must put a stop to such behavior before you can go on with the interview. You might acknowledge the patient's distress with a comment like "You seem to be having difficulty controlling yourself. We'll have to stop our meeting until you are able to sit quietly again." As is discussed in more detail in Chapter 13 (Violence), you should never continue an interview when you feel you or the patient is in danger of being physically harmed. In general, if a patient's behavior becomes unmanageable, do not hesitate to stop what you are doing and summon help.

CLOSING THE INTERVIEW

As the interview comes to a close, leave a few minutes for any comments or questions that the patient has yet to voice. Often, patients will save critical information or profound concerns for the end of the session.

You might signal the close of the interview with a question such as "In the minutes remaining, is there anything you'd like to add?" or "Is there anything else you think I should know?"

Also, ask your patient if he or she has questions for you. Patients are understandably anxious about their problems, and may ask you such questions as "What do you think, doc?" or "So tell me, can you help me?"

Obviously, there are no pat answers to such questions, in part because the feelings and fears that prompt them are unique to each patient. Your job is to provide as straightforward a reply as possible. And don't be afraid to admit that you do not yet know the answer, and that it may take more time to fully understand your patient's problems. In the long run, a relationship built on honesty will be much more beneficial than one based on false reassurance.

This chapter has focused on basic principles of conducting a psychiatric interview. Chapter 2 is designed to give you an overview of psychodynamic principles of mental functioning and normal human development. You can then use this psychological framework to begin to make sense of what your patients tell you about their lives.

REFERENCES

MacKinnon RA, Michaels R: The Psychiatric Interview in Clinical Practice. Philadelphia, WB Saunders, 1971.

Nicholi AM Jr (ed): The Harvard Guide to Modern Psychiatry. Cambridge, MA, Harvard University Press, 1978, pp 3-40. (Chapter 1 contains a general discussion of interviewing technique and the doctor-patient relationship.)

Sullivan HS: The Psychiatric Interview. New York, WW Norton, 1954.

2

Psychodynamics—
Some Basic Concepts

PSYCHODYNAMICS REFERS TO the study of mental forces and how they motivate behavior. For thousands of years, human beings have struggled to elucidate and schematize the nature of mental life, and a great many models of the mind have been put forward.

Modern psychodynamic psychiatry is founded on the work of Sigmund Freud (1856-1939). His theories of mental structure and functioning have been widely applied clinically to help understand and relieve many of the symptoms of the mentally ill.

Freud has been a controversial figure in Western culture for nearly a century, and his ideas continue to be closely scrutinized and hotly debated among thinkers in virtually all areas of the social and biological sciences. But Freud's work did not arise out of a vacuum, and was in many respects evolutionary rather than revolutionary. Specifically, Freud incorporated the concepts of many important eighteenth and nineteenth century theorists into his schemata of mental life. There is much that remains controversial in Freud's work, and as he himself was quick to point out, much that is in need of revision. Nevertheless, Freud's ideas have profoundly influenced our way of thinking about the human mind and behavior. His concepts have permeated every aspect of our culture including the arts, politics, philosophy, and education.

This chapter does not attempt to teach Freudian psychology, but only to define some of the "household words" in the language of psychodynamics that you are bound to encounter in your clinical work. To the student who has had no prior clinical experience in psychiatry, psychodynamic theories will likely seem confusing and even nonsensical. Phrases like "the unconscious mind" and "oedipal rivalries" may seem, to the uninitiated, abstract and removed from real experience. Psychodynamic concepts are best learned not from books, but by talking with patients, watching others perform psychiatric interviews, and discussing your clinical experiences with colleagues and supervisors. Once you have developed a curiosity about the forces that cause your patients emotional distress, you will be much more likely to find the psychodynamic theories of Freud and others to be intelligible, helpful, and even exciting.

MAPS OF THE MIND

Freud put forth two major models for understanding mental life: the topographic model and the tripartite model. Modern psychodynamic theory rests on both of these.

The Topographic Model— Conscious/Preconscious/Unconscious

The discovery of the unconscious may well be Freud's most important contribution to modern thought. The idea that each of us has an ongoing mental life that operates *without our awareness* is an astounding concept. Freud first presented this idea in 1900, in *The Interpretation of Dreams*, in order to explain such phenomena as the forgetting of dreams and our ability in dreams to recall hitherto forgotten events from early life.

His topographic model divides the mind into three "agencies," based on the extent to which the thoughts, feelings, and perceptions in each agency are accessible to our awareness. These agencies of the mind are not tangible—they don't occupy physical space in the brain—but are simply metaphors; that is, they are theoretical constructs that help us organize our clinical observations.

The **conscious** includes all thoughts and feelings we are aware of, including sensory input from the environment as well as input from "within"—i.e., from the preconscious.

The **preconscious** contains all those ideas, feelings, and memories available to us when we choose to focus attention on them. For example, most of us do not maintain the threat of nuclear war in the forefront of consciousness, but the thought is available when we choose to focus on it. A primary function of the preconscious is to censor—to police our psyche and to prevent unconscious thoughts that might generate anxiety from reaching consciousness. The censor operates either by completely blocking access of unconscious material to consciousness, or by disguising unconscious material so that the conscious mind cannot recognize it.

For example, a young girl's unconscious sexual longing for her father would arouse considerable anxiety if she became aware of it, so her censor represses her incestuous impulses. The censor may block these sexual feelings entirely, or disguise them as their opposite—i.e., hatred. In the latter case, the girl would be using the defense of *reaction formation* (see below), and would be aware only of an aversion for her father. Her sexual yearnings would remain buried in the unconscious.

The **unconscious** contains ideas, impulses, feelings, and fantasies that lie out of reach of the conscious mind and cannot be made conscious by focusing one's attention. This material has been banished from awareness—i.e., it has been repressed because it is in some way unacceptable, as in the example noted above. Unconscious material may reach consciousness when the censor is relaxed, as in dreams, or when it is overpowered and neurotic symptoms result. (For example, if the young girl's repressed incestuous impulses toward her father intensified, she could develop a conscious reaction against these impulses that might take the form of a snake phobia.)

Along with these three aspects of the mind, Freud's topographic model includes two types of thought processes—primary process and secondary process.

Secondary process is the mode of thinking with which we are most familiar. Our conscious and preconscious mental activities are carried out in secondary process thought, which makes sense to us and to the people with whom we communicate. It is logical, it is not filled with gross inconsistencies, and it is relatively well organized. Secondary process thought is governed by the *reality principle*—i.e., it respects the constraints of the real world. Thus, for example, the rules of secondary process dictate that today cannot be yesterday or tomorrow, and one cannot be in two places at once. These are, of course, statements of the obvious, and secondary process seems obvious because it appears to most of us that this is the only type of thinking we do. But there is another type—primary process—that is strikingly different.

Primary process is unorganized mental activity that seems foreign to us because it operates primarily in the *unconscious*. Primary process thinking does not respect logic, contains no sense of time, allows for blatant contradictions and inconsistencies, and aims at immediate gratification without regard for the demands of the real world. Dreams are the best examples of primary process thinking. (For example, in a dream you may be five years old but also a medical student, the year may be 1993, and your professor may look exactly like your mother.) The rules of logic do not apply in primary process thinking, but certain other mechanisms operate to make primary process seem bizarre to our conscious minds. The most important of these mechanisms are

> *Symbolization:* an object or idea comes to signify something else based on a resemblance between the original and its substitute (e.g., a banana may symbolize a penis).
>
> *Condensation:* several concepts or objects become fused in a single symbol (e.g., one's father, boss, and minister may become the same person in a dream).
>
> *Displacement:* emotions, ideas, or wishes are transferred from their original substitute (e.g., anger might be displaced from a parent to a teacher).

Dreams exhibit all of these characteristics, and this is why a dream often seems like nonsense after you wake up. Also, in your clinical work you will likely be able to detect primary process in the speech of severely psychotic patients, whose ability to censor unconscious material is impaired.

Primary process is a normal part of conscious mental activity in children below the age of five. For example, young children commonly use *magical thinking*, i.e., they equate thinking with doing, and believe that their wishes actually define what is real. Hence, a child may believe that wishing someone dead will make it happen. As children grow, they become increasingly aware of the relationship between fantasy and reality, and cease to use magical thinking. Other primary process modes of thought (e.g., denial) also gradually disappear under the pressures of the child's expanding knowledge of the real world.

The Tripartite Model—Id/Ego/Superego

Freud's topographic model categorized mental *content* according to whether or not it was available to consciousness, but this scheme did not account for the different types of mental *functions* that he encountered in his work with patients. Dividing the mind according to functions and forces, he devised the tripartite model of id, ego, and superego. Like the divisions of the topographic model, the id, ego, and superego are not concrete entities but metaphors that clinicians have found useful in differentiating one type of mental function from another.

Id. The *id* is the name given to our most basic biological drives and our most primitive impulses. The guiding force of the id is the *pleasure principle*—i.e., the tendency to demand immediate satisfaction of desires, seek immediate pleasure, and avoid pain. The id encompasses states of pain and rage; cravings of sexual longing, hunger, and thirst; and the drive for self-preservation.

Id impulses and instincts are for the most part unconscious. The aspects of instinctual drives that do reach our awareness have usually been censored—i.e., "laundered" to look more respectable to our conscious adult selves.

Ego. In everyday language, the word *ego* has come to refer to self-love or self-esteem. The psychiatric usage of the term, though, is quite different from this. The ego is the part of the personality that mediates between inner strivings and the realities of the world. It comprises all of those faculties of thought, feeling, perception, and action we use to harmonize the urges of the id with the requirements of the external environment and the inhibitions and aspirations of the superego (see below).

The ego strives to maintain mastery over the drives of the id, and it is the ego that delays gratification and substitutes more acceptable pleasures for less acceptable ones. The ego contains the compromising, evaluating, puzzle-solving, and defense-creating aspects of the personality. Ego functions are largely, but not entirely, conscious.

The ego develops as the growing infant interacts with the environment—especially with parents and other caregivers. Ego development includes the acquisition of defensive maneuvers for self-protection, as well as intellectual functions like comprehension, judgment, and language. The mature individual with a healthy ego is someone who is flexible in handling various life stresses, rather than one who must repeatedly resort to inflexible, maladaptive behaviors under pressure.

Superego. The superego, like the ego and the id, is a metaphor. The fictional character who most closely personifies the superego is

Jiminy Cricket, who sat on Pinocchio's shoulder and acted as his guardian of moral standards and promoter of personal ideals. Freud conceived of the self-critical faculties of the mind as constituting a separate psychic agency that observes and evaluates our thoughts, feelings, and actions, comparing actual ego functioning with ideal standards. The superego consists of what we commonly call the "conscience," as well as the standards known as the *ego ideal*.

Each of us develops an image of the person he or she would like to become. This "ideal image" is derived from the standards of behavior that we perceive in parents, teachers, and other important people in our childhood. The ego ideal is highly individual. It provides our inspiration to achieve and directs our strivings for gratification.

Children also adopt many of the prohibitions and obligations of parents and other important figures, by accepting parental dictates as demands of absolute obedience. This process by which parental standards and morality are incorporated into one's personality is central to superego formation and is thought to begin around the age of four to six years, and continue throughout life. As the child's social sphere expands, parental morality no longer seems absolute, while the standards of peer groups, teachers, and other admired figures take on new importance. Many, though not all, aspects of superego are conscious.

People who develop harsh and strict superegos are their own cruelest taskmasters. They are often rigid, inhibited, anxious, and very unhappy. Those with more tolerant superegos can be flexible and accept their limitations without giving in to impulses that violate their own or society's fundamental moral ideals.

The id, ego, and superego exist in a constantly changing relationship. A disturbance in the checks and balances of these three agencies often results in mental discomfort, unacceptable behavior, or both. The id and superego largely remain out of our awareness until they cause trouble—e.g., when an unacceptable instinctual impulse becomes conscious and arouses anxiety, or when criticism by the superego prompts feelings of guilt. The well-adjusted individual makes compromises intuitively that resolve conflicts among id, ego, and superego.

PSYCHOSEXUAL DEVELOPMENT

Freud postulated the existence of two basic human drives: libidinal instincts and aggressive instincts. *Libido* refers to sexual energy, though the term is also used more broadly to refer to all strivings for pleasurable experience. He put forth the idea that the child's strivings for pleasure are organized and modified in a series of developmental stages. In each stage, the child has particular needs to be met and problems to be solved.

According to Freud, the way we negotiate each of these stages is crucial, for "unfinished business" from any one stage is carried with us as development proceeds, and can become a source of psychopathology in adult life. The stages of psychosexual development are briefly outlined in Table 2-1 and described below. The timetable for these stages is only a crude approximation, since each child develops at his or her unique pace.

Oral stage (age 0 to 18 months). The newborn infant needs total care, and so must immediately begin to form relationships with other human beings. The mouth is the part of the body through which pleasure is secured and hunger satisfied. The mouth thus becomes the focus for a variety of the infant's sensations, interests, and activities. Because of its pleasure-giving potential at this stage, the mouth is spoken of as an *erogenous zone*. The infant's primary relationship is, in most cases, with the mother, although "good mothering" at this stage may actually come from any caregiver(s), male or female, whose attention to the infant is warm and consistent. Such caring lays the foundation for a sense of security and basic trust in others that the infant will carry into later life, while a lack of caring may establish a deeply rooted sense of mistrust and insecurity.

The infant must learn to tolerate frustration when his or her urgent demands are not instantly met. Contact with the mother cannot ever be as immediately or constantly gratifying as the infant would wish, and the child must cry in order to make certain needs known. This frustration, if not unduly prolonged, prompts the infant to develop healthy self-soothing techniques and defense mechanisms that protect against overwhelming excitement and rage. It also helps the infant differentiate between self and others, as it becomes clear that mother is a separate being who is not always present when the infant wants her.

We often label adult emotional states *infantile* if they are reminiscent of behavior at the oral stage of development, i.e., states characterized by urgent demands, extreme dependence, lack of responsibility for or consideration of others, and a very low tolerance for frustration. People with such characteristics are said to have *oral personalities*, and they are commonly preoccupied with fantasies and needs that focus on the mouth.

Table 2-1. The stages of psychosexual development.

Stage	Age	Description
Oral	0 to 18 months	The mouth is the focus for sensations and activities. "Good mothering" now lays the foundation for a sense of security and basic trust in others.
Anal	1½ to 2½ years	The child finds pleasure in experiencing control over bodily needs. This period ideally fosters self-control, independence, the ability to give, and personal pride.
Phallic	2½ to 4 years	The focus of attention shifts to the genitals. The child begins to explore the world more autonomously and learns to take pride in his or her abilities. This stage is crucial in developing a stable sense of self-worth.
Oedipal	4 to 6 years	The child longs for a special relationship with the parent of the opposite sex and has feelings of jealousy and hostility for the parent of the same sex. Resolution requires development of a special relationship with the same-sex parent.
Latency	6 to 12 years	The child masters physical, intellectual, and social skills; identifies with those of the same sex; and learns mastery of impulses.
Adolescence	Teen years	Physical maturation heightens interest in sexual activities. The adolescent is preoccupied with personal identity and how others perceive him or her. The adolescent ideally assumes more responsibilities for self-control and self-direction.

Anal stage (age 1½ to 2½ years). As the infant's nervous system matures, it becomes possible to recognize and control the need to eliminate. This is a pleasurable experience for the child, both because of a growing awareness of the sensations involved in the excretory functions, and because of the new experience of control over bodily needs. During toilet training, the child and the parent interact around the child's control of bowel and bladder function, and this interaction is thought to influence later personality traits.

The child must make compromises between primitive wishes to do whatever he or she pleases, and the rewards obtained by conforming to the demands of important caregivers. Ideally, this period fosters the beginnings of self-control, independence, the ability to give, and a sense of personal pride. However, if toilet training is harsh and the parents are punitive, the child may develop strong attitudes of shame and disgust, and be both fearful of and enraged at controlling caregivers. In later life, these unresolved problems of self-control may manifest themselves as rigid behavior patterns. The four classic traits of the *anal character* are aptly described by the following mnemonic:

Parsimony,

Orderliness,

Obstinacy, and

Punctuality.

Obviously, toilet training is only one of the areas of childhood experience in which issues of self-control and societal expectation emerge. It has become a symbol in our culture for a developmental step that all children must take in the process of becoming social beings.

Phallic stage (age 2½ to 4 years). The focus of the child's attention gradually shifts from the mouth to the anus to the genitals. At this stage, the penis or clitoris is a "new" discovery and a source of pleasure. The differences between the sexes become more discernible to children at this age, promoting the beginnings of identification as male or female. In addition, the child's increasing motor and intellectual capacities make it possible to explore, to be curious, and to take initiative and pride in solving simple problems. Ideally, parents greet such initiatives with pleasure—which mirrors the child's own sense of accomplishment—while setting realistic limits on the child's sense of his or her unlimited power (e.g., not letting the toddler run into the street). This stage is thought to be crucial in developing a stable sense of self-worth—i.e., that one is an attractive and lovable human being.

Psychoanalytic theorists trace many of the origins of narcissistic personality disturbance to problems in the phallic stage of development. They posit that children whose self-esteem does not consolidate during this stage develop into adults who are plagued by persistent feelings of inferiority, extreme sensitivity to perceived slights or insults, and constant reliance on the responses of others as measures of their worth.

Oedipal stage (age 4 to 6 years). Oedipus, you will recall, was the tragic hero of Sophocles' drama about a man who unwittingly murdered his father and married his mother. According to Freud, this Greek classic has remained compelling to audiences for centuries because it recaptures a fantasy that children experience and subsequently repress.

The *Oedipus complex* refers to the child's increasing longings for a special relationship with the parent of the opposite sex. Along with these longings go feelings of jealousy and rivalous hostility toward the "competition"—i.e., the parent of the same sex. Thus, little boys feel as if they are competing with father for mother's love, and little girls see mother as a rival for father's affections.

Children at this stage both hope and fear that their murderous and incestuous wishes will come true. Because they cannot yet differentiate clearly between fact and fantasy, children develop the concern that their wishes will hurt their rival, and that the rival will retaliate. This is the fear that psychoanalytic theorists refer to as *castration anxiety*.

How does the child resolve this romantic dilemma? The normal resolution to the Oedipus complex involves recognizing that this incestuous pursuit is futile, and giving it up in favor of a special relationship with the same-sex parent. The child identifies with the rival and adopts many of the same-sex parent's goals, standards, and behaviors. Instead of wanting to marry mother, the little boy settles for growing up to be like father and marrying a woman who is like mother. For little girls, the process is similar, but at present there is great controversy among psychological theorists about how little girls deal with the Oedipus complex.

Resolving the Oedipus complex requires that the child, to some extent, begin to identify with the parent of the *opposite* sex. Thus, the little girl who cannot "have" Daddy can be partly satisfied by becoming like Daddy in some respects—e.g., by adopting certain of her father's interests or attitudes. Children normally emerge from the oedipal stage having identifications with both parents.

People who develop neurotic symptoms are thought to have been unable to successfully resolve the Oedipus complex. Thus, you will often hear the term "oedipal" used synonymously with "neurotic." By contrast, the term *pre-oedipal* (or *pre-genital*) is reserved for more severe illnesses like personality disorders and psychosis, implying that these more severe disturbances originate in the oral, anal, or phallic stages of development.

Latency stage (age 6 to 12 years). The term *latency* refers to Freud's observation that sexual curiosity seemed to become dormant or latent during this period, to re-emerge in adolescence with renewed force. However, the term is something of a misnomer in that sexual interests do not disappear during this phase, but remain present throughout childhood.

Latency is a time for mastering a host of physical, intellectual, and social skills. The child's world enlarges beyond the nuclear family to include school and other activities outside the home. This affords the opportunity to identify with new role models— e.g., teachers, peers— and to modify or solidify behavior patterns learned in the family. In this period, the child normally identifies strongly with those of the same sex. The emphasis is on learning social skills and mastering one's own impulses—hence the latency-age child's fascination with games that have elaborate rules and rituals (e.g., hopscotch, "tag"). The child learns about the pleasures and pains inherent in dealing with peers. Failure to conform to peer-group standards can result in ostracism and a sense of inferiority, but successful mastery of age-appropriate skills can foster a sense of pride and social acceptance.

Adolescence. The onset of puberty, with the rapid maturation of the genitals, stimulates a heightened interest in sexual activities. However, the adolescent's drive toward maturation is not confined to sexuality. Adolescents become preoccupied with personal identity and how they are perceived by others—hence the adolescent's concern that he or she dress, speak, and act "cool."

Standing on the threshold of independence from parents, adolescents identify strongly with groups of peers as a means of separating themselves from their families. They try out emancipatory behaviors (e.g., smoking, drinking, staying out late with friends), often rejecting many of the values and demands of their parents in favor of peer group mores. Courtship and first sexual activities normally occur during this phase. Ideally, the adolescent becomes freed from parental controls, while assuming more responsibility for self-control and self-direction. Adolescence lays the groundwork for mature sexual relationships based on mutual respect.

Development does not end with adolescence, of course, but continues throughout life. The preceding discussion is a very crude sketch of Freudian developmental theory. The process by which human beings mature is infinitely complex, and our understanding of it is far from complete.

MECHANISMS OF DEFENSE

Each of us uses a variety of techniques to relieve tension and shield ourselves from painful experiences. However, not all of our self-protective maneuvers are carried out consciously. Those techniques that we employ unconsciously to alleviate anxiety and eliminate conflict are termed *defense mechanisms*. The defenses listed in Table 2-2 and described below are among those most commonly encountered in clinical practice. The first 12 defense mechanisms are "immature" in that they may work to protect the person who uses them from distress but they do so at a significant cost (e.g., by grossly distorting reality). The "mature" defenses do not require such distortions.

Repression, the fundamental mechanism of defense that underlies all others, is akin to forgetting. It involves forcing thoughts, memories, and feelings into the unconscious and actively keeping them out of awareness. Repression is responsible for lapses of memory (e.g., forgetting the hour of a dreaded examination) or seemingly inexplicable

Table 2-2. Some common defense mechanisms.

Immature	**Mature**
Repression	Altruism
Denial	Humor
Retroflexion	Suppression
Acting out	Anticipation
Projection	Sublimation
Splitting	
Reaction formation	
Conversion	
Dissociation	
Displacement	
Intellectualization	
Isolation of affect	

naiveté. The "forgetting" of repression is often accompanied by symbolic behavior that suggests that the repressed material is not really forgotten (e.g., the woman who is unaware of her sexual attraction to her therapist, but who dresses seductively for her appointments). Repression prevents us from recognizing our own thoughts and feelings, while *denial* prevents the recognition of external reality.

Denial involves disbelieving a fact of external reality in order to avoid pain or anxiety. Denial often results in grossly distorted thinking and behavior, as in the case of the patient who refuses to accept the death of her husband and goes on "communicating" with him as if he were still alive. People commonly use denial to avoid recognizing the presence of serious physical illness, and may delay consulting a physician about ominous symptoms until it is too late (e.g., the woman who denies the growing lump in her breast for many months). Denial is not conscious—i.e., it involves more than simply pretending that something is not so. Unacceptable facts are banished from awareness entirely, and the individual has no access to them.

Retroflexion (turning against the self) is an unacceptable impulse or feeling (usually hostile) made acceptable by deflecting it from its original object back upon the self. This is most commonly seen among people who are labeled "depressive" or "masochistic" (e.g., the woman who berates herself for being a bad wife after she is abandoned by a physically abusive husband). *Hypochondriasis* is related to retroflexion, and involves transforming a reproach toward others into somatic complaints. It allows the individual to bemoan his or her condition in lieu of complaining about others.

Acting out is a term used too often and too loosely to describe any patient behavior of which mental health professionals do not approve. When used correctly, the term *acting out* refers specifically to the process of acting on an unconscious wish or impulse in order to avoid being aware of the emotion that accompanies it. In other words, action is used in the service of remaining unaware of intolerable feelings—e.g., a man who behaves with uncharacteristic promiscuity and who has no awareness of sexual longings for his therapist.

Projection is a process by which motives and feelings unacceptable to the self are unconsciously attributed to others instead. For example, a man who struggles to fend off his own unconscious homosexual impulses may complain, "Every man on the street makes homosexual advances toward me." Projection is used both by people whose thinking is grossly out of touch with reality (as in the example above), and by healthier individuals as well. Racial and other forms of prejudice are based on the use of projection.

Splitting involves dissociating positive and negative aspects of oneself and others, and compartmentalizing them into "all good" or "all bad" images. People who use splitting see themselves and others in black-and-white terms, dividing the world into "good guys" and "bad guys." This relieves the anxiety that comes with recognizing ambivalence—e.g., that one can be mad at someone one loves.

Reaction formation occurs when unacceptable unconscious impulses are disavowed and *opposite* conscious attitudes and behaviors are adopted. For example, a man whose strong sexual urges are severely repressed may lead a campaign for censorship of "salacious" literature in school libraries; a woman who unconsciously despises her children may smother them with undue affection.

Conversion takes the unconscious conflicts that would otherwise give rise to anxiety and instead gives them symbolic external expression through some bodily symptom—such as hysterical blindness or paralysis (e.g., a woman whose arm suddenly becomes paralyzed due to her unacceptable impulse to stab her unfaithful husband). Conversion is a major defense used in hysterical neurosis.

Dissociation involves a temporary but drastic modification of one's character or of one's sense of personal identity to avoid emotional distress. Examples of dissociation include such states as sleepwalking, amnesia, and multiple personality. Even acting in a play may involve dissociation, when it allows the actor a "safe" way to express instinctual wishes that would be unacceptable in real life.

Displacement redirects feelings from an original object to a more acceptable or less dangerous substitute. This defense is commonly found in everyday life—as when a man who is angry at his boss takes it out on his family.

Intellectualization involves thinking about instinctual wishes in affectively bland terms in order to avoid experiencing strong emotions.

Isolation of affect involves separating an idea from the feelings associated with it and generally banishing these feelings from consciousness. This defense is closely related to intellectualization. It is characteristic of people with obsessive-compulsive personality styles. People use isolation to protect themselves from emotions they find threatening or unacceptable—e.g., sexual or angry feelings. Thus, a man who is enraged at his wife may be totally unable to feel his anger, but finds himself preoccupied with emotionless, matter-of-fact thoughts about hurting her. While extensive reliance on isolation can hamper one's ability to form satisfying relationships and to experience life fully, isolation can be useful in certain situations. For example, health care professionals who routinely deal with people who are in pain usually need to isolate thoughts from feelings to prevent being overwhelmed and rendered incapable of performing their jobs.

All of us, when under stress, occasionally fall back on some of the defenses listed above. However, healthier individuals do not rely heavily on any of these, but instead allay anxiety and diminish intrapsychic conflict by using the following, more adaptive defenses.

Altruism involves constructive and instinctually gratifying service to others, including philanthropy and other activities from which one derives vicarious or more direct pleasure. Unlike reaction formation, altruism is gratifying to the person who uses the defense.

Humor facilitates our ability to express feelings and focus on anxiety-provoking thoughts without causing distress to ourselves or others. Forbidden wishes can be expressed in comic fashion and not acted upon.

Suppression, unlike repression, which operates unconsciously, involves a conscious decision to postpone paying attention to an unpleasant subject. This includes minimizing misfortunes, "keeping a stiff upper lip," and postponing *but not avoiding* difficult experiences.

Anticipation involves planning for future discomfort in a realistic fashion to effectively decrease anxiety, e.g., by carefully planning for an impending separation from a loved one.

Sublimation is essential to civilization. It consists in diverting unacceptable instinctual drives (e.g., sexual and aggressive impulses) into personally and socially acceptable channels. One common example is competitive sports, in which aggression is "tamed" and channeled, but not inhibited. Many artistic endeavors are thought to result from sublimated libidinal energies.

PSYCHODYNAMICS IN CLINICAL PRACTICE

What relevance do these maps of the mind, developmental stages, and mechanisms of defense have to your clinical work? Obviously, you will never be able to get a radiographic image of an ego, or measure an Oedipus complex by blood level, or isolate and culture a defense mechanism. Yet you can use these concepts to help you make sense out of symptoms and behaviors that might otherwise seem nonsensical. Indeed, Freud was among the first to advocate the idea that psychological symptoms (such as obsessions and phobias) have meaning, and that they represent the human mind's complex and often ingenious efforts at easing intrapsychic distress.

You will not often hear your patients talk directly about these concepts—about their defenses or their developmental problems—but you will hear "derivatives" of them. For example, a patient is not likely to tell you about (or even to recall) his difficulties with a rigid and punitive parent around the issue of toilet training at age two. But you may see him replay this traumatic situation by struggling with a series of "unreasonable" bosses over his working conditions, or by struggling with you over whether or not he will take a prescribed medication.

As you hear more about a patient's life, you will discover recurring themes—like strains of music that thread through a symphony—and you can usually relate these themes to problems the patient experienced at particular stages of development. In attempting to master issues not resolved in childhood, people continually recreate infantile problems in many areas of their adult lives. Much of psychotherapy, particularly in treating neuroses and personality disorders, consists of helping patients to discover these "leftover" problems, along with the defenses patients use to keep from recognizing them.

Of course, Freud did not have the last word on concepts about mental functioning. Great advances continue to be made in our understanding of the human psyche. Ego psychology, object relations theory, and self-psychology are among the most important post-Freudian schools of thought that you are likely to encounter as you learn more about psychodynamic concepts. And as your understanding of psychodynamics deepens, your skill as a clinician will increase, regardless of the field of medicine you choose.

Psychodynamic concepts can be invaluable to you in organizing the many details of a patient's life story. Even in a single interview, you can learn enough to relate many of the recurrent problems in patients' adult lives to their childhood experiences, and begin to outline some of the defenses and psychological conflicts that cause or exacerbate their current distress. The next chapter discusses the process of taking a psychiatric history, a process that will be greatly enhanced by your familiarity with the basic ideas about mental functioning discussed above.

REFERENCES

Freud A: The Ego and the Mechanisms of Defense, rev. ed. New York, International Universities Press, 1966.

Gedo JE, Goldberg A: Models of the Mind: A Psychoanalytic Theory. Chicago, University of Chicago Press, 1973. (An excellent review of psychoanalytic theories of mental structure and function, beginning with Freud.)

Kolb LC: Personality development, in Modern Clinical Psychiatry, 10th ed. Philadelphia, WB Saunders, 1983, pp 58-79. (An overview of human development, written from a psychoanalytic perspective.)

Nemiah JC: Foundations of Psychopathology. New York, Oxford University Press, 1961. (A general introduction to psychodynamic concepts, with lively case examples.)

A Psychiatric Glossary, 5th ed. Washington, DC, American Psychiatric Association, 1980.

Vaillant GE: Theoretical hierarchy of adaptive ego mechanisms. Arch Gen Psychiatry 24:107-118, 1971.

The Psychiatric History

THIS CHAPTER DEALS with two separate but related tasks: taking a psychiatric history, and reporting it to someone else. They are related, in that the information you gather in your interviews with the patient provides the material for the case report. But that is the extent of their resemblance.

Taking a psychiatric history. You can almost never adhere strictly to an outline in taking a psychiatric history. People do not talk about themselves in outline form, nor would you be an effective interviewer if you tried to force them to do so. You must keep an outline in your own mind, so that you will know which topics you want to cover in the course of your evaluation. But never use it as a checklist—this will only alienate your patients and limit the amount of information you can gather.

The outline of the psychiatric history presented in this chapter includes a list of subjects to be covered in a psychiatric evaluation and examples of interview questions that may help you explore these topics.

Reporting a psychiatric history. The history must be organized and presented in a way that gives readers (or listeners) a coherent picture of your patient's current condition. Given that virtually any detail of the patient's life may be relevant to his or her emotional state, you are likely to feel overwhelmed by the task of fitting all the information you have collected into a single presentation. It is therefore essential that you (1) pare down the history to include only those details you believe will help others understand your patient's problems, and (2) adhere to an outline when you present a case verbally or in writing.

The psychiatric history is organized much like a standard medical history, as the outline in this chapter shows. In addition to familiarizing yourself with this outline, look at Appendix A, which contains a sample case report. This will give you a general idea of how a written evaluation is prepared. However, many psychiatric facilities have their own specific formats for these reports, and you should be sure that your evaluation summaries are consistent with the record-keeping system of the particular institution in which you work.

The initial evaluation summary is often the portion of the patient's record that is most widely read—e.g., by new staff members coming to a ward or an outpatient clinic. The write-up therefore will be essential in communicating your patient's situation to others. It should be clear, concise, and accurate. Beware of too much detail—after all, no one reads a 50-page case history.

The outline included here is too detailed for most evaluations. You should take care to elaborate on aspects of the psychiatric history that are germane to your patient's current problems, but do not hesitate to cover less relevant categories in a cursory fashion. For example, if your patient has a "negative" family psychiatric history, you need only write, "The patient denies any history of psychiatric illness or substance abuse in family members."

At a minimum, every area of the psychiatric history must be mentioned in every summary that you prepare. When in doubt about what to include in a case report, discuss your write-up with a supervisor—for both your own and the patient's benefit.

Table 3-1. Organization of the psychiatric history.

Identifying data	Medical history
Referral source	Drug and alcohol history
Chief complaint	Mental status examination
History of the present problem	Formulation
Past history	Diagnostic impression
Family psychiatric history	Treatment plan

OUTLINE FOR A PSYCHIATRIC EVALUATION

The psychiatric evaluation begins with a rough sketch of the patient's situation. Identifying data such as age, sex, and occupation; the source of the patient's referral to you; and the patient's chief complaint orient your audience quickly to who the patient is and why he or she has come to see you. Because these statements set the stage for the rest of the case report, they come first.

With this brief introduction, you have prepared your audience to learn about the patient in depth. You begin with a description of the present problem, starting with its onset and proceeding chronologically to the date of your interview. You then place the patient's current difficulties in the context of his or her childhood development and important formative experiences. (The description of the present problem and past history are usually the most detailed sections of the case report.) Information about the patient's physical health, drug and alcohol use, and psychiatric illness in family members completes the history.

The mental status examination—discussed in Chapter 4—is not actually part of the history. Rather, it is your description of the patient as he or she appears and behaves in the interview. It is the psychiatric counterpart of the physical examination.

With all of this information in mind, your audience is then prepared to understand your assessment of the patient's problems (the formulation of the case), your diagnostic impression, and your plan of treatment. By presenting the report in this order, you permit others to follow the thought processes that brought you to your conclusions about the case. Without such an outline, your report can easily become a barrage of disorganized detail in which you and your audience get lost.

IDENTIFYING DATA

Identifying data include:
- Name
- Age
- Marital status
- Sex

- Occupation
- Number of children
- Place of residence
- Number of previous psychiatric admissions (if an inpatient)

This information alone can tell you much about the patient's situation. For example, "This is the sixth psychiatric admission for Mrs.

Petrocelli, a 38-year-old divorced homemaker and mother of six...who lives with her children in a Brooklyn apartment." Also detail the patient's ethnic and religious background if this is particularly relevant to his or her current situation.

REFERRAL SOURCE

Find out why your patient came to you, and you may learn something of his or her expectations. For example: "My brother Erwin says this is the best clinic in the state."

CHIEF COMPLAINT

Ask the question "What brings you to see me?" to elicit the patient's chief complaint. Use the patient's own words in a one-sentence description of what is wrong.

HISTORY OF THE PRESENT PROBLEM (HPP)

Where does the present problem begin? In many cases, the patient will tell you: e.g., "My wife died six months ago and I've been depressed ever since."

Determining when the patient's current difficulties truly began is often difficult and requires some judgment about what may have precipitated his or her emotional distress. You may, for example, choose to date the onset of the present problem from the time a prominent symptom appeared (e.g., a first suicide attempt), from the date of a first psychiatric hospitalization, or from the time of a major personal loss (e.g., abandonment by a spouse). Whatever you decide, though, make sure to arrange the events of the HPP in *chronological* order—that is, bring the reader (or listener) from the onset of the problem right up to the time the patient came for help.

Explore in detail the patient's chief complaint and other problems that hamper his or her life at present (see Table 3-2). Note when these problems began, as well as how persistent they have been. Describe any prominent psychological symptoms (e.g., hallucinations, memory loss, panic attacks), and any mood changes reported by the patient. Be particularly thorough in documenting previous suicidal or homicidal thoughts or acts. Pay attention to any physical symptoms that have been present during the illness. Determine the degree to which these problems have impaired the patient's relationships with others and his or her ability to function at work. Also, note any circumstances in the patient's life that may have precipitated the present crisis.

Map the current problems in the patient's life.

Onset of problems: Time, setting. The time of onset may not be clear (e.g., "I've been depressed all my life").

Duration of problems: Has the problem been present continuously or has it recurred intermittently?

Psychological symptoms: Describe in detail any disturbances of thought or perception that are central to the patient's present problem. While such symptoms are reported in the mental status examination when the patient actually exhibits them during the interview, they are included in the HPP when they are part of the patient's history (for example, "The patient reports that for the last six months he has heard his dead father's voice commanding him to kill himself").

Symptoms of psychosis—e.g., hallucinations, delusions, disassociative states, ideas of reference.

Cognitive problems—e.g., impaired memory or concentration.

Table 3-2. Exploration of current problems in the patient's life.

Onset of problems (time, setting)
Duration and course (chronic vs. episodic)
Psychological symptoms
  Symptoms of psychosis
  Cognitive problems
  Mood changes (irritability, depression, elation)
Somatic symptoms
  Medical conditions
  Vegetative signs (anorexia, weight loss, insomnia, anergy, agitation or
    retardation, decreased sexual energy and interest, diurnal mood
    variation)
  Neurological symptoms
  Somatic complaints without organic basis
Severity of problems—degree of impairment in functioning
Possible precipitants

Mood changes

• *Irritability*—rage, violent thoughts or acts. Techniques for exploring homicidal thoughts and fantasies are outlined in Chapter 13.

• *Depression*—guilt, hopelessness. Recent suicidal thoughts and acts should be reported in the HPP. Techniques for exploring suicidal feelings are outlined in Chapter 12.

• *Elation*—outline extent of hyperactivity (for the symptoms of mania and hypomania, see Chapter 6).

Somatic symptoms. Medical conditions that seem to be an integral part of the present psychiatric problem. Describe course of illness and treatment (past and present).

Vegetative signs—anorexia, weight loss, insomnia, energy, agitation or retardation, decreased sexual energy and interest (see Depression in Chapter 6).

Neurologic symptoms—e.g., seizures, recent head trauma.

Somatic complaints with no known organic basis.

Severity of problems. To what extent have current problems interfered with the patient's ability to work and to participate in relationships? Some patients are totally incapacitated by psychiatric illness, while others function very well at daily tasks despite emotional distress.

Possible precipitants. Pay close attention to what was going on in the patient's life at the time symptoms developed, and pay close attention to changes in

Important relationships (friends, lovers, family)

Job or financial situation

School

Physical health.

Always try to answer the question "Why now?" What prompted the patient to seek help this week rather than last week, this month rather than next month? Many times, the problem has been present for quite a while, but some key event in the patient's life has upset an equilibrium and made life less tolerable.

For example, a woman comes to you seeking help for agoraphobia (a fear of being alone or on her own in public places), from which she has suffered for the past 12 years. During this time, she has been afraid to go out of the house unless accompanied by her husband, and cannot stay alone in the house unless she can speak to him by telephone at regular intervals while he is at work. Why does she seek help now, after 12 years? On close scrutiny, you discover that her husband is about to be promoted to a job that will require him to travel for several days each month, and the patient is enraged that he is "abandoning" her.

Does the patient know anyone who has had similar problems? For example, you may discover that your 30-year-old depressed patient has a mother who also became depressed at age 30. Identification of this kind often exists just outside the patient's awareness. Yet it may be very important in determining the types of symptoms the patient develops as well as when during the patient's life these symptoms first take hold.

How has the patient dealt with these problems to date? (1) Detail any efforts patients have made to cope on their own or get help from others. (2) Mention the patient's previous psychiatric history, if any. This includes psychotherapy, medications, hospitalization, along with the patient's response to these treatments. How the patient felt about previous therapists may give you clues to the kind of relationship he or she is likely to form with a therapist in the future.

PAST HISTORY

The past history summarizes the patient's life, in chronological order, from infancy until the present problem began. Deciding which details of a patient's past are pertinent to his or her current distress is not always easy. But two aspects of your patient's early life are almost always relevant and deserve particular attention.

Relationships with parents, siblings, and other important people during childhood. As is discussed in Chapter 14, our childhood relationships exert a powerful influence on how we deal with people as adults. In the case of the agoraphobic woman described above, you might discover that she had an intense attachment to her mother, that she felt herself to be like her mother in every way, and that she and mother were "inseparable pals" throughout her childhood.

Major "milestones" in growing up—e.g., starting school, puberty, leaving home. How we react as children to times of stress or separation from parents often carries over into our behavior under similar circumstances as adults. For example, it would not be surprising to discover that the agoraphobic woman was terrified of going to kindergarten and missed many days of school during the months it took her to overcome her fear. Nor would it be surprising to learn that at age 18 she turned down a scholarship to a college in another city, and did not leave her parents' home until she married at age 26.

Past history places the patient's current problems in a broader context, helping you to see patterns of behavior that have persisted throughout the patient's life. Thus, although most people seek psychiatric help because they are concerned about the present, it is worth your while to spend some time learning about the past in the course of your evaluation.

The points to be explored in a patient's history are outlined in Table 3-3 and described more fully below. Bear in mind that there is more detail here than will be applicable to any one patient's situation.

Table 3-3. Outline of the past history.

Family constellation (father, mother, siblings, others living at home)—
    important family relationships, major separations or losses

Infancy
    Birth order
    Birth history
    Developmental milestones

Childhood
    Health—hospitalizations
    Preschool years
    Starting school—academic performance
    Friendships

Adolescence
    Onset of puberty
    Early sexual experiences
    Peer relationships
    Experimentation with drugs, alcohol

Adulthood
    Education
    Military experience
    Employment
    Social life/friendship
    Romantic relationships
    Sexual history
    Marriage
    Children

Family Constellation

List age and occupation of the patient's father, mother, siblings, and others living at home—relatives, babysitters, other caretakers. Describe their personalities and relationship with the patient. Include disruptions in this relationship due to illness, death, or separation. Questions that may be helpful in eliciting this information include

Tell me about your family.

Who took care of you when you were small?

Who were you closest to in your family?

Who do you feel you are most like among those in your family?

Infancy

Patient's place in the family. A patient's birth order can provide valuable clues about his or her family role (e.g., the "baby" or the "little mother"). Also inquire about how much attention patients received from parents and others (e.g., a mother with four children all under age six will obviously have less time and energy to devote to individual children than a mother of two). The birth of younger siblings is usually a major event in a child's life.

Patient's birth history. Was the pregnancy planned or unplanned? Note any complications of pregnancy or delivery.

Developmental milestones. Did the patient have difficulty in learning to walk or talk? Was the patient considered by parents to be a "bright" or "slow" child? The patient will not remember the early months of life, but what one has been told about birth and infancy becomes an important part of one's self-concept (e.g., "You were always a fussy, unhappy baby," or "You were smarter than every other kid in the neighborhood").

Childhood

Note any major family event—e.g., illness, death, divorce, separations, moves.

Preschool years. Activities, caregivers, playmates. Helpful questions include "How far back can you remember?" and "What do you recall about your life before you started school?"

Health. Any hospitalizations? Note prolonged separation from family as a result of these.

Starting school. Inquire about the patient's relationships to teachers and peers, school performance, extracurricular activities, what the patient hoped to be when he or she grew up, whether the patient had to change schools due to moves or disciplinary problems. Typical questions include "What do you remember about starting school?" and "What were you like in elementary school?"

Adolescence

Ask about the onset of puberty in the patient's life and accompanying emotional reactions to physical changes. Note where the patient acquired initial information about sex. Detail information about early sexual experiences (heterosexual and homosexual), peer relationships, quality of friendships, and experimentation with drugs and alcohol. Questions might include
  Tell me about junior high school/high school.
  From whom did you learn about sex?
  Did you have any romantic relationships as a teenager?
  Any close friendships?

Adulthood

Information relevant to the present problem should be included in the HPP.
  Education. Note the level achieved, aspirations.
  Military experience (if any).
  Employment. Stability, satisfaction, relationships with peers and authorities, and job performance are all factors that should be included.
  Social life/friendship. Describe leisure activities, religious/moral values.
  Romantic relationships. Characterize lovers, stability of relationships. People commonly choose lovers based on their earliest important relationships—i.e., they seek lovers who remind them in some ways of parents other caregivers.
  Sexual history. Note degree of intimacy and satisfaction, sexual orientation, sexual dysfunction. Many people with psychiatric disorders are troubled by sexual dysfunction, and a simple question may open up an entire area of emotional distress—e.g., "Is there anything about your sex life or sexual feelings that is troubling you now?"

Marriage. Describe relationship with spouse, satisfaction in marriage, separations, divorce.

Children. List their ages and describe the patient's relationship with each. Also describe disruptions in these relationships due to illness, death, separation. Note any miscarriages or abortions, since these often have a major impact on family life.

FAMILY PSYCHIATRIC HISTORY

This is a critical part of every evaluation. Ask about any relatives of the patient (including grandparents, aunts, uncles, cousins) who have had emotional problems, who have seen a psychiatrist, who have been hospitalized for psychiatric reasons, or who have had problems with drug or alcohol abuse. Pursue any "yes" responses to these questions by inquiring about

Symptoms of the illness

Course of the illness (chronic versus episodic)

Types of treatment: medication, psychotherapy,

"shock treatment," hospitalizations, and

Responses to various treatments

In this way you may elicit a family history of affective illness, psychosis, alcoholism, or other conditions that could influence your diagnosis of the patient. You may also learn about your patient's ideas regarding mental illness (e.g., "I'm afraid I'll be locked up in an asylum like my grandfather was.").

MEDICAL HISTORY

Major medical problems should be explored in detail. Note major medical conditions, current treatment for them, disabilities, and any other medical facts pertaining to the patient's psychological state. Pay particular attention to a history of neurologic disorders, especially seizures or head trauma. Be sure to list all current medications—including over-the-counter drugs—since these can profoundly affect your patient's emotional state. Obtain relevant medical records from doctors and other health care facilities. Outpatients who have somatic complaints but have not obtained a recent physical examination should be advised to do so, and inpatients should be examined upon admission.

DRUG AND ALCOHOL HISTORY

Note types of drugs and alcohol used. Also detail how frequently and in what amounts these are taken as well as symptoms of withdrawal and other complications (e.g., hepatitis). If drug use is a major problem, include it in the HPP.

When inquiring about drugs, use terms the patient is familiar with (e.g., "angel dust") if the patient is not likely to know chemical names (e.g., "PCP"); see the table of commonly abused drugs in Appendix B. Also, inquire about so-called "social use" of drugs like alcohol, marijuana, and cocaine. Patients who heavily abuse these substances may rationalize their behavior as "just being sociable" (see Chapter 11).

MENTAL STATUS EXAMINATION

For a detailed discussion of the mental status examination (MSE), see Chapter 4. The results of the mental status examination can usually be summarized in a short paragraph. Each aspect of the MSE (appearance and behavior, speech, emotions, thought, etc.) must be mentioned. Where no abnormalities are present, you may simply say so without elaborating.

FORMULATION

The case formulation is the clinician's attempt to integrate all the data collected during the evaluation and to arrive at a tentative understanding of the factors contributing to the patient's problems. Basically, your formulation assesses the biological and social forces that have fostered the development of the patient's personality style and current illness. This assessment is based on what you have learned from the patient's history and mental status exam. In short, your formulation summarizes the case for the reader. It does not include a diagnosis, but musters evidence in support of your diagnostic impression.

Composing a case formulation need not be an intimidating task; two or three well-organized paragraphs will usually suffice. The outline starting on the next page may help you in organizing your formulation.

Introduction

In one or two sentences, describe your patient, the presenting problem, and your understanding of why the patient seeks help at this particular time. Summarize the patient's symptoms and the extent to which they cause distress to the patient and/or others. Also note how the symptoms impair the patient's ability to function in his or her usual daily tasks and in ongoing relationships.

Biological Factors

Discuss any organic problems present (e.g., seizure disorder, endocrine abnormality) and how these might contribute to the patient's problem. Include drug or alcohol abuse. Also note any predisposition to illness caused by organic factors (e.g., a history of minimal brain dysfunction in childhood) or family history that might suggest a genetic contribution to the problem. If no biologic factors have been noted, state this explicitly.

Psychological Factors

Psychodynamics. Note the patient's major conflicts, defense mechanisms, and personality strengths and weaknesses. Also, describe the type and quality of relationships your patient is capable of forming with men *and* women (see Chapter 2).

Social situation. Comment on your patient's current life situation, including his or her important relationships and occupational status, as well as changes in these.

Mental status. Note any important findings from your own mental status examination of the patient (e.g., delusional thinking, paucity of expressed emotion).

Hypotheses About Causes

Try to link the biologic and social factors in a coherent statement about how the patient's illness came about. Obviously, this statement will be somewhat speculative, but it may provide you with hypotheses that you can test as treatment proceeds. Note any patterns you see in the course of the illness—recurrent decompensations, a slow but constant deterioration, or specific somatic or environmental precipitants (e.g., a patient who becomes psychotic every time his wife gives birth to another child).

DIAGNOSTIC IMPRESSION

You will be called upon to make a tentative diagnosis based on your formulations. Keep in mind that accurate psychiatric diagnosis is difficult and often requires observation of the patient over time. Thus, your initial impression may change as you get to know your patient better and watch how he or she responds to your treatment.

The *Diagnostic and Statistical Manual of Mental Disorders*, 3rd edition (DSM-III) should be available in the health care facility where you are working. You can compare your patient's signs and symptoms with the various sets of diagnostic criteria in DSM-III to see which syndromes most closely fit your patient's condition. Once you have done this, you will probably want to discuss your diagnostic impression with a supervisor.

DSM-III organizes psychiatric diagnosis along a series of five axes (the use of this multiaxial system is explained in detail on pp. 23-32 of DSM-III):

Axis I: Clinical syndromes. This includes all psychiatric disorders except personality disorders and developmental disorders.

Axis II: Personality disorders and specific developmental disorders. The separation of personality disorders from other disorders is clinically useful, because many patients will have a personality disorder underlying another clinical syndrome. In such cases, patients will be assigned both Axis I and Axis II diagnoses (e.g., manic-depressive illness on Axis I, and compulsive personality disorder on Axis II).

Axis III: Physical disorders and conditions. This category is self-explanatory. Your primary concern in arriving at a diagnostic impression should be with Axis I and Axis II, for all patients with psychiatric disorders will have diagnoses in either Axis I or Axis II, or in both. Patients may have more than one diagnosis in any of the first three axes, but where no diagnosis is made (e.g., when no physical or personality disorder is present) it is sufficient to write "no diagnosis" beside the appropriate axis number.

Axis IV: Severity of psychosocial stressors. This axis allows for the identification of specific stresses that seem to have precipitated or exacerbated the patient's current condition. Considered here are interpersonal, family, occupational, financial, legal, developmental, and physical factors.

Axis V: Highest level of adaptive functioning in the past year. This category allows you to judge how well your patient has been able to function at work, in social relations, and during leisure time in the previous year. This information is likely to have some prognostic significance, since patients usually return to their previous levels of functioning after an episode of illness. (For example, a man who is now floridly manic but worked effectively as a corporate executive between manic episodes in the past year is likely to return to this high level of job performance when the current crisis passes.)

You will want to consult DSM-III to see how to evaluate your patients' situations with respect to psychosocial stressors (Axis IV) and highest level of functioning (Axis V). In many health care facilities, the use of Axis IV and Axis V is optional.

An example showing how to use the multiaxial system for diagnosis is included in Appendix A. Further examples can be found in DSM-III, pp. 30 and 31.

Along with your diagnoses, you may want to include one or more diagnoses that have not been ruled out, i.e., diagnoses you feel have not been excluded and that still warrant serious consideration. However, avoid entering unsubstantiated diagnoses into a patient's permanent record, since government agencies and insurance companies may have access to such documents, and could be misled by inappropriate diagnostic labels.

TREATMENT PLAN

The treatment plan is your recommendation on how the patient's problems can best be alleviated. It may include any of the many therapies listed in Chapters 14 and 15. Often, you will recommend more than one treatment. For example, your plan for a depressed outpatient might read as follows: "Trial of tricyclic antidepressants, supportive psychotherapy once weekly, and one or more meetings with the patient and her husband to assess marital difficulties."

The treatment plan is based on many factors, the most important of which is your assessment of what is wrong. In addition to diagnosis, however, you must consider the following.

What is your patient's most pressing problem?
Obviously, you must attend to emergencies first. For example, a severely depressed young man may be an excellent candidate for treatment with antidepressant medication, but his clear suicidal intentions make it impossible to begin any drug treatment until he can be prevented from harming himself. Thus, hospitalization would be the most important recommendation at this time.

How receptive is your patient to various forms of treatment? You might, for example, decide that a woman with anorexia nervosa needs a behavior modification program to help alter her eating patterns, and twice-weekly psychotherapy to work on the severe personality disorder that underlies the eating problem. However, the patient denies that she has any emotional difficulties and vehemently rejects the idea of psychotherapy, despite your emphatic recommendation. She does, however, accept a referral to a behavior therapist, and you list insight-oriented psychotherapy as a possible future treatment in your plan.

What services are available to the patient? To some extent, you must gear your treatment plan to the resources available in your area. Suppose, for example, you are working in a busy urban outpatient clinic when a young man comes to you in acute distress over a failed romance. Although it is apparent that he has persistent difficulties with women and could benefit from long-term insight-oriented psychotherapy, you know that there are no staff members available at this time to provide long-term treatment. However, the clinic can offer short-term psychotherapy that provides the patient with support and helps him weather the current crisis. He may return for long-term therapy at some future time.

What are the patient's financial resources? Ideally, money would never need to be considered in deciding on a treatment plan. But in fact, psychiatric treatment is costly, and patients often need treatment over a period of months or years. Thus, it is imperative that you help patients plan for ongoing care that is financially feasible. For example, a family may be willing to exhaust its life's savings to pay for their schizophrenic son's stay in a private hospital rather than send him to a state-run facility. However, this would not be in the patient's best interest, since he will almost certainly need long-term follow-up care as an outpatient and will require financial assistance from his family for a long time to get the treatment he needs.

In devising a treatment strategy, do not hesitate to recommend further evaluative procedures when you feel that important questions about the patient's condition remain unanswered. This includes consultations by other professionals (e.g., a consultation by a neurologist for a suspected seizure disorder), psychological testing (e.g., an intelligence test to rule out mental retardation), and meetings with rehabilitation specialists (e.g., to assess a patient's ability to work).

The next chapter covers a particular part of the psychiatric evaluation, the mental status examination (MSE). The chapter is designed not only to familiarize you with the structure of this examination, but also to define for you many of the most important terms used to describe the symptoms of psychiatric illness.

REFERENCES

Cameron PM, Kline S, Korenblum M, Seltzer A, Small F: A method of reporting formulation. Can Psychiatr Assoc J 23:43-50, 1978.

Diagnostic and Statistical Manual of Mental Disorders, 3rd ed. Washington, DC American Psychiatric Association, 1980, pp. 23 - 34.

MacKinnon RA, Michels R: The Psychiatric Interview in Clinical Practice. Philadelphia, WB Saunders, 1971.

Nicholi M Jr. (ed.): History and mental status, in The Harvard Guide to Modern Psychiatry. Cambridge, MA, Harvard University Press, 1978, pp 3-40.

4

The Mental Status Examination

THE MENTAL STATUS EXAMINATION (MSE) is an assessment of the patient's current state of mind. Like a physical examination, the MSE evaluates the patient's mental functioning in the here and now; like physical findings, the mental status may change over time.

The term "mental status exam" is used to refer both to (1) the process of gathering information about the patient's state of mind during an interview and (2) the section of the psychiatric case report reserved for this information. The MSE is recorded separately from the history in evaluation summaries and progress notes, as a way of distinguishing what you observe about the patient from what the patient tells you about himself or herself.

The outline of the MSE presented in this chapter is very detailed (see summary in Table 4-1). This may give you the impression that a mental status examination takes four or five hours to complete. Do not be misled. In most cases, you will not need to devote more than a few minutes of an evaluation interview to a formal exam, because most of the necessary information about mental status will come not from asking specific questions but from your observations of the patient's appearance, behavior, and manner of speaking in the course of routine conversation.

When do you do a mental status exam? Actually, you assess a patient's mental status every time you meet but, in most cases, you do this informally. A detailed and careful MSE is usually part of an initial evaluation. This serves as a baseline examination with which to compare your impressions of the patient on subsequent meetings. For

Table 4-1. Summary outline of the mental status examination.

Appearance and behavior
   Dress and grooming
   Posture and gait
   Physical characteristics
   Facial expression
   Eye contact
   Motor activity
   Specific mannerisms
Speech
   Rate
   Pitch, volume, clarity
   Abnormalities
Emotions
   Mood
   Affect (variability, intensity, lability, appropriateness)
Thought
   Process (flow of ideas, quality of associations)
   Content
      Distortions (delusions, ideas of reference, depersonalization)
      Preoccupations (obsession, phobias, somatic concerns)
      Suicidal or homicidal ideation
Perception
   Illusions
   Hallucinations
Sensorium and intellectual functions
   Consciousness
   Orientation
   Concentration
   Memory (immediate, recent, and remote)
   Fund of knowledge
   Abstraction
   Judgment
   Insight
Attitude toward the interviewer

example, you may notice that a patient you have just admitted to the hospital has trouble concentrating on your interview with her, because she hears her grandmother's voice telling her to jump out of your office window. As part of your MSE, you test her other intellectual functions and discover that she also has difficulty remembering recent events (e.g., what she ate for breakfast). In your follow-up interviews, you need not go through an entire formal MSE again, but can simply test those areas where you noted abnormalities on admission—perception, concentration, and recent memory. In this case, as treatment alleviates auditory hallucinations, the patient may recover both her ability to concentrate and her ability to remember recent events.

Do you do a formal mental status exam with every new patient? Clinicians disagree on this issue. Some insist that you can gather all the information you need about a patient's mental state from informal conversation alone. They argue that asking structured questions (e.g., asking the patient to interpret proverbs or do simple arithmetic) alienates you from the patient and destroys any rapport that has developed between you in the course of the interview. Other clinicians warn that abnormalities of mental functioning can be masked by the patient and go unnoticed in an unstructured interview, and that formal questioning is the only way to elicit them.

There is no clear way to resolve this debate. With each patient you see, you must use your judgment about the extent to which formal testing of mental functions is necessary to answer your questions about the patient's condition. Certainly, it is incumbent upon you to learn how to do a complete mental status examination as part of your training in psychiatry.

Often, patients will tell you about abnormalities of mental functioning that are symptoms of their presenting problem and that you need to explore in a formal mental status exam. For example, if an elderly patient tells you that he has trouble remembering to turn off the stove at home, you will want to do a careful evaluation of his memory, along with other intellectual functions. Patients will usually give you clues to important abnormalities, either in what they tell you (e.g., "I keep hearing voices") or in how they tell it to you (e.g., continually losing the train of thought in midsentence). If you pay attention to these clues and explore in depth anything that seems unusual, you are likely to pick up any important abnormalities in the patient's mental state.

Psychosis. One of the most important questions you will need to explore in the mental status examination is whether the patient is currently psychotic. But first you must understand what we mean when we use the term "psychotic."

Surprisingly, there is some debate among clinicians on this point. Many textbooks define *psychosis* as a major mental disorder in which thinking, emotions, communication, and behavior are so severely impaired that they significantly interfere with the individual's capacity to meet the ordinary demands of daily life. Such definitions emphasize loss of functioning.

However, many people who are severely impaired in their daily lives (e.g., those with severe personality disorders) would not be considered psychotic. And some patients who harbor carefully concealed delusions (e.g., that their thoughts are being monitored by foreign spies) may nevertheless function well at jobs and even manage to maintain a family life.

There is no single definition that will satisfy all clinicians. For practical purposes, psychosis may be defined as an inability to distinguish between what is real and what is not, even when evidence of reality is clearly available. We speak of the psychotic individual as having impaired *reality testing*—i.e., being unable to test subjective ideas and experiences against objective facts of the external world.

The loss of the ability to test reality is a crucial aspect of psychosis. Those whose misperceptions of reality can be corrected by evidence are not said to be psychotic.

A hallmark of psychosis is confusion between what comes from one's own mind and what emanates from the outside world. The psychotic person loses a sense of boundaries between inside and outside. Some common psychotic beliefs are that one can control others' thoughts, that external forces have put thoughts into one's own head, and that other people can read one's thoughts—all involving the notion of a "permeable" mind. Hallucinations, which are pathognomonic of psychosis, are internal stimuli (e.g., hearing voices) that are falsely believed to be of external origin.

In the narrow definition given above, psychosis involves false ideas or perceptions about oneself and the world that cannot be altered even when evidence of their falsehood is presented. In reality, there is no precise boundary between psychotic and nonpsychotic thinking, for false ideas and perceptions are held by people with varying degrees of tenacity. You must watch and listen carefully for evidence of psychosis, since it can be well masked in an interview. The most common psychotic symptoms you will see involve disorders of thought content (e.g., delusions) or disorders of perception (e.g., hallucinations); these are described in some detail below. Bizarre forms of speaking and behaving are also commonly associated with psychosis.

Psychosis is not, in and of itself, an illness. It is a symptom of a wide variety of illnesses, ranging from drug overdoses to manic-depressive illness. Some disorders involve psychotic symptoms by definition (e.g., schizophrenia), while others may or may not include psychotic symptoms (e.g., depression). An individual may be psychotic for a period of minutes, or for many years. Psychotic symptoms often wax and wane in their severity, but they may remain unchanged over long periods of time. Thus, each time you interview a patient, you must reassess whether psychosis is present.

Using the MSE. Although specific psychiatric illnesses are associated with particular abnormal findings in the MSE, beware of jumping to diagnostic conclusions based on the MSE alone. Each symptom in this outline can occur in any of several psychiatric disorders. A given symptom provides only a small portion of the evidence required to make a diagnosis. The patient's history and course over time will provide critical data. If you rely only on the MSE, you will often be fooled.

Avoid using this outline for the MSE as a checklist; your exam should vary according to each patient's needs. Let the patient's history and your clinical judgment guide you to explore in detail only those areas of mental functioning about which you have specific questions.

In many cases, you will have more than one meeting with the patient you are evaluating, so you need not gather all the necessary information at one sitting. After a first meeting with a new patient, you may find it helpful to seek the advice of a supervisor in deciding which aspects of the MSE to explore in follow-up interviews.

Do not, however, neglect to ask about suicidal and homicidal ideation in the first interview with *every* new patient you see. Dangerousness to self or others is a psychiatric emergency, and its assessment must not be postponed or overlooked.

APPEARANCE AND BEHAVIOR

The patient provides a wealth of information without saying a word. Take care not to overlook the many things you can learn through nonverbal communication.

Dress and Grooming

Grooming is an important indicator of a patient's ability to care for himself or herself; manner of dress often provides valuable clues to a patient's self-image. Dress may be seductive or slovenly or overly fastidious. Depression or psychosis may prevent normally well-groomed individuals from attending to personal hygiene, and they may become disheveled and disorganized. Any change in appearance should be explored with the patient and family, documenting when the change occurred and under what circumstances.

Posture and Gait

Rigid posture and gait may indicate patient's anxiety. Physical handicaps are almost always of great emotional significance to the patient and should be noted.

Physical Characteristics

Note the patient's apparent versus chronological age (young-looking, old-looking), physical health (vigorous, frail), and weight (obese, emaciated).

Facial Expression

The patient's facial expression often mirrors his or her mental state (e.g., sad, suspicious, angry, silly, bland, mobile).

Eye Contact

Note whether the patient makes frequent eye contact with you, avoids a direct gaze, stares into space, or glances furtively about the room. Eye contact often decreases with increasing anxiety or paranoia. Patients with psychosis or dementia, who cannot concentrate on the interview, may not focus on you visually.

Motor Activity

Observe the patient's physical activity during the interview. Constant restlessness and pacing may signal anxiety, agitated depression, or mania. Slow movements and little reactivity are signs of the psychomotor retardation common in depression, drug reactions (e.g., extrapyramidal side effects), and *catatonia*, a state in which the patient becomes immobile, with muscular rigidity or inflexibility. Catatonia may be accompanied by stupor or excitement, or by a refusal to cooperate with others (negativism).

Specific Mannerisms

Repetitive gestures such as tics or grimacing should be noted. Also, pay attention to agitated behaviors (e.g., hand-wringing, hair-pulling) that may accompany anxiety or depression. Patients on antipsychotic medications should be observed for involuntary movements of the tongue and mouth or the extremities (these are suggestive of tardive dyskinesia), and for the general motor restlessness that is characteristic of akathisia (see Chapter 15).

SPEECH

This category of the MSE is reserved for observations about the way the patient speaks. By contrast, your observations about what the patient says are included under "Thought" (below).

Rate

Pressured speech is very rapid, frenzied speech that may exceed the speaker's physical powers of articulation and/or the listener's ability to comprehend. It is often present in the manic phase of manic-depressive illness.

Rapid speech is found in a variety of other conditions, most commonly in acute anxiety states.

Slowed speech is common among depressed patients who have generalized psychomotor retardation.

Mutism occurs in some severely psychotic patients.

Pitch, Volume, and Clarity

Speech may, for example, be described as high-pitched, infantile, loud, whispered, mumbled, or garbled.

Abnormalities

Stuttering—extent to which this interferes with conversation; circumstances that alleviate or exacerbate stuttering.

Speech impediment—nature of the impediment, and extent to which it interferes with communication.

Aphasia—the loss of facility in language comprehension or production at the level previously possessed. It is commonly found in patients who have cerebral lesions (e.g., secondary to cerebral vascular accidents). *Amnesia* (or *anomic*) *aphasia* is the loss of the ability to name objects. *Broca's aphasia* is a syndrome characterized by the loss of the ability to produce spoken and (usually) written language, although the patient retains the ability to understand language. *Wernicke's aphasia* is a syndrome that involves the loss of the ability to comprehend language, coupled with the production of inappropriate language (e.g., nonsensical speech).

EMOTIONS

The patient's emotional state consists of both mood and affect. *Mood* is a pervasive and sustained emotion experienced by the patient. *Affect* refers to the outward manifestation of mood, i.e., the way the patient shows feelings. Mood and affect are not always the same, and the range of emotions patients report and display is vast—e.g., depression, despair, hopelessness, anger, irritability, tenseness, anxiety, panic, terror, elation, emptiness, guilt, self-loathing.

Mood

Patients often volunteer information about how they feel during an interview, but it may be helpful to ask about mood (e.g., "How would you describe your general mood recently?"). If it is possible, use the patient's own words to report the quality and intensity of mood, and note whether the patient reports a change in mood in the course of the interview.

Affect

Predominant affect. In the course of the interview, note the patient's predominant expression of emotion, e.g., depression, elation.

Variability. Normally, emotional tone varies in the course of conversation, from animated to subdued, from sad to happy, etc. Disturbances of affect often destroy this variability, so a depressed patient may not brighten up even when discussing pleasant subjects, and a manic patient may be incapable of maintaining a calm and sober attitude in the psychiatric interview.

Intensity. Emotional reactivity may be increased or decreased. Increased reactivity is common among histrionic individuals, who show intense disproportionate emotional responses (e.g., rage if you arrive two minutes late). Decreased reactivity is also common: *blunted affect* refers to a generalized decrease in affective intensity, while *flat affect* describes a more extreme situation—the virtual absence of any evidence of emotion. Blunted and flat affect are classically seen in schizophrenia. Blunted affect is also a symptom of Parkinson's disease; among psychiatric patients, it is more commonly a parkinsonian side effect of antipsychotic (neuroleptic) medication.

Lability. Watch for rapidly shifting and unstable emotional reactions, particularly among patients who suffer from affective disorders. Depressed patients are often unable to control sudden tearful outbursts, while manic patients experience uncontrollable bouts of rage or laughter.

Appropriateness. You must judge whether the patient's affective responses are appropriate to his or her thought content and to the interview situation. For example, the patient who speaks with apparent indifference about a recent death in the family or abandonment by a spouse may unconsciously be trying to avoid experiencing emotional pain.

THOUGHT

You evaluate thought processes and thought content based on what the patient says. *Thought process* refers to the way the patient puts ideas together—to the associations between ideas and to the form and flow of thoughts in conversation. *Thought content* refers to ideas the patient communicates. A *thought disorder* is a disturbance of content or process, or of both. A *formal thought disorder* specifically denotes abnormal thought process.

Thought Process

Rate and flow of ideas. Patients frequently use the term *racing thoughts* to describe being flooded with ideas and unable to keep up with them. This condition is often seen in anxiety states, as well as in psychosis (e.g., mania, schizophrenia). If you suspect this condition, you might ask, "Do your thoughts ever go so fast you cannot keep up with them?"

In the case of *retarded or slowed thoughts*, patients experience their thinking as slowed down, and may consider their minds empty of thoughts. This condition is seen in depressed patients.

Circumstantiality involves thinking that is delayed and indirect in reaching a goal or getting to the point. This style is common in obsessional patients and in schizophrenics.

Blocking is a sudden obstruction or interruption in the spontaneous flow of thought, perceived by the patient as an absence or deprivation of thought. It is seen in schizophrenia and in severe anxiety states.

Perseveration is the tendency to emit the same verbal response again and again to varied stimuli. This may range from constant repetition of one phrase (e.g., "night and day, night and day, night and day...") to an inability to shift the focus of conversation away from one particular topic.

Associations are the relationships between ideas. Normally, these relationships are intelligible to the listener; i.e., one idea seems to follow from another. Disturbances in the associative process may be quite subtle and, when one idea does not appear to follow from another, you may erroneously assume that your attention lapsed from what the patient was saying. When something does not appear to make sense, *always* ask for clarification.

Loose associations involve the shifting of ideas from one subject to another in an oblique or unrelated manner; the speaker is generally unaware of the disturbance. Loose associations are commonly seen in psychotic states—e.g., "I'm tired. All people have toes."

Flight of ideas is skipping verbally from one idea to another. Speech is fragmented and associations are determined by chance or by temporal factors. This is commonly seen in manic patients.

Tangentiality is a style of speech in which the patient replies to questions in an oblique or irrelevant way (e.g., when asked about his mother's illness, a patient embarks on a lengthy discussion of the various "get well" cards his mother has received).

Clanging involves using the sound of a word, rather than its meaning, to give direction to the flow of ideas (e.g., "I'm sad, mad, bad.") It is sometimes present in mania.

Punning is used in a similar way, substituting for logic as a means of associating one idea with another; it is seen in mania (e.g., "What's the weather like? Is the sun out? He is out in the yard playing with his new football.").

Other abnormalities of thought process include the following:

Neologisms are new words or condensations of several words that are not readily understood by others. This disturbance is seen in schizophrenia and organic brain syndromes (e.g., a paranoid patient used "plickening" to mean "the plot thickens").

Word salad is a jumble of words and phrases that lacks any comprehensible meaning or logical coherence. It is characteristic of schizophrenia.

Echolalia is a parrot-like repetition of another's speech.

Thought Content

Patients' ideas about themselves and the world are frequently at the core of their presenting problems. Careful exploration of unusual or pervasive thoughts will often assist you in making a diagnosis.

Here are two helpful rules to keep in mind when assessing thought content:

1. *Always* ask for clarification when you do not understand something the patient has said.
2. Begin with general questions and move on to specifics.

Some open-ended questions for assessing abnormal thought content include "Have you had any unusual or troublesome experiences?" "Have you had any strange or disturbing thoughts?" "Have you had thoughts you feel other people would not understand?" If you get positive answers to any of these general questions, explore unusual thoughts in more detail, using the categories below.

Delusions. A *delusion* is a false belief firmly held despite incontrovertible and obvious proof or evidence to the contrary. Further, the belief is not one ordinarily accepted by other members of the person's culture or subculture. Delusions are pathognomonic of psychotic illness, although they do not occur in all psychotic patients.

These beliefs may affect all areas of the patient's thought and functioning, or they may be "encapsulated" and confined to one particular topic. Examples of delusions are shown in Table 4-2.

Delusions of grandeur: Exaggerated ideas of one's importance or identity (e.g., "I am the Messiah"). You may discover these with such questions as "Do you feel you have special knowledge or powers?"

Delusions of persecution: Ideas that one has been singled out for harassment (e.g., "The FBI is out to get me."). Interview questions might include "Do you think anyone wants to hurt you, or has spread lies about you?"

Delusions of control: The idea that one's feelings, thoughts, or actions are imposed by some external source (e.g., "A computer puts these angry thoughts in my head.") or, conversely, that one can control others' feelings, thoughts, or actions. To elicit such thoughts, you might ask, "Have you felt that your thoughts were influenced or controlled by some outside force?" or "Do you feel that you can control the thoughts of others?"

Somatic delusions: False beliefs about body image or body function (e.g., "I don't care what the doctors say; I know that I have cancer".). You might explore somatic delusions with a general question: "Has anything unusual happened to your body?"

Thought broadcasting: The notion that other people can read one's thoughts. Your question could be "Do you feel that others can hear your thoughts or read your mind?"

Table 4-2. Types of delusions.

Delusions of grandeur
  "I am the Messiah."
Delusions of persecution
  "The FBI is out to get me."
Delusions of control
  "A computer puts these angry thoughts in my head."
Somatic delusions
  "I don't care what the doctors say; I know that I have cancer."
Thought broadcasting
  "People always know what I'm thinking."
Ideas of reference
  "The President sends me special messages during his television press
    conferences."

Ideas of reference involve incorrectly interpreting casual incidents and external events as having direct personal reference. These ideas often reach delusional proportions; that is, the person believes them despite evidence that they are false (e.g., "That newspaper headline was a secret signal to me from the President that he needs my help in Washington."). You may elicit such ideas with a question like, "Do you feel you receive special messages that others do not (on television, over the radio, etc.)?"

Depersonalization is a sense of unreality or strangeness concerning the environment, the self, or both. *Derealization* refers to feeling detached from one's environment. A patient may describe feeling "like I have stepped outside of myself and watch myself doing things," or say "I feel as if everything is unreal and those around me are actors in a play." Depersonalization and derealization are common in anxiety states as well as in borderline personality disorder.

Preoccupations. An *obsession* is a persistent, unwanted idea that cannot be eliminated by logic or reasoning. The obsessive thought is usually consciously distasteful to the patient but is often unconsciously desired (e.g., "I'm afraid my father will be hit by a truck."). Obsessive thoughts often occur along with *compulsions*, which are persistent unwanted urges to perform acts that are contrary to one's ordinary wishes (e.g., compulsive hand-washing).

A *phobia* is an obsessive, persistent, unrealistic fear of an object or situation. Some common phobias are *acrophobia* (fear of heights), *agoraphobia* (fear of leaving a familiar home setting, fear of open spaces), *claustrophobia* (fear of closed spaces), and *xenophobia* (fear of strangers). For a detailed discussion of phobias, see Chapter 8.

Morbid preoccupations (e.g., with guilt or death) are often found in depressed people. When these concerns with personal guilt and worthlessness are frankly out of touch with reality, they are said to be of delusional proportions.

Suicidal and homicidal ideation. Assessment of suicidal and homicidal thoughts are part of *every* mental status examination. Actively raise these issues in the first interview with *every new patient*. This includes assessing thoughts, plans, potential for action, deterrents to action, and the patient's feelings about these suicidal and/or homicidal ideas. If you have reason to suspect that a patient may become suicidal or homicidal, you must constantly reassess and monitor these aspects of the patient's mental status. For a discussion of homicidal and suicidal patients, see Chapters 12 and 13.

PERCEPTION

Human beings are continually barraged by a wide range of stimuli from the five senses. Perceptual disorders involve misinterpreting sensory input (an *illusion*) or perceiving sensory input in the absence of any actual external stimulus (a *hallucination*). Thus, hearing one's name in a train whistle is an illusion, while hearing one's name called in a silent room is a hallucination.

Illusions

Illusions may be of pathological or nonpathological origin. Seeing a face in a cloud and hearing voices in the rustle of leaves are common experiences but, in the face of reasonable evidence, the normal person recognizes these as misinterpretations. However, illusions also occur in toxic states (e.g., drug-induced), in acute anxiety states, and in schizophrenia.

Hallucinations

Hallucinations are perceptions the patient believes to be real despite evidence to the contrary; i.e., the patient perceives something that does not exist. Hallucinations are invariably symptoms of psychosis and may be seen in all types of psychotic illness. They may be induced acutely by such factors as drugs, alcohol, and stress. They may involve any of the five senses.

Helpful general questions for eliciting reports of hallucinations include "Do you ever hear voices or see things other people do not hear or see?"; "Does your mind ever play tricks on you?"

Auditory hallucinations are the most common in psychiatric illness, particularly in schizophrenia. It is useful to document what the patient hears and to ask the identity of the speakers (e.g., "I hear my mother's voice telling me to kill myself.").

Visual hallucinations are less common than auditory ones but are often found in toxic psychoses, and less often in schizophrenia and mania (e.g., "I see a devil with red eyes staring at me.").

Olfactory hallucinations (smell) are encountered in schizophrenia and in lesions of the temporal lobe.

Gustatory hallucinations (taste) are rare and are usually associated with olfactory hallucinations.

Tactile hallucinations (touch) occur mainly in toxic states and drug withdrawal syndromes (e.g., the sensation that insects are crawling under the skin occurs in delirium tremens and in cocaine toxicity).

In evaluating hallucinatory experiences, it is important to note the *circumstances* in which hallucinations occur, with an eye to the possible participating factors (e.g., "What was going on when you heard these voices?"), and the *content* of the hallucinations (e.g., threatening, benign, grandiose, accusatory, religious, sexual). Content often provides important clues to the patient's fears and wishes, and may identify general areas of intrapsychic conflict. Your questions might include "Whose face did you see in the dark?" or "Whose voice was it, and what did they say?"

Always try to ascertain whether the patient's consciousness is clear or clouded at the time the hallucinations occur. If consciousness is clouded, look to drugs and organic processes as likely causes. A careful history of drug and alcohol use is critical to understanding hallucinations diagnostically.

Be sure to differentiate pathologic hallucinations from *hypnagogic* hallucinations, which are false sensory perceptions healthy people experience midway between being awake and falling asleep.

Finally, be alert to unreported hallucinatory experiences during the interview, e.g., when the patient does not attend well to you and instead appears to be paying attention and even responding to internal stimuli.

SENSORIUM AND INTELLECTUAL FUNCTIONS

Mental illness commonly involves disturbances in cognitive functioning. A person who is overwhelmed with emotional difficulties (as in depression) or flooded with internal stimuli (as in psychosis) is often unable to focus energy and attention on ordinary intellectual tasks. Such psychiatric disorders as dementia involve, by definition, a loss of intellectual function.

This area of the MSE is the main one in which specific tests can be of use in the clinical interview (see Table 4-3). However, only test particular intellectual functions if the patient's history or behavior in the interview gives you reason to suspect derangement. Further evaluation can be accomplished by observing the patient over time or by obtaining psychological testing.

Consciousness

The presence or absence of a clear sensorium is a crucial factor in diagnosis. Clouded or fluctuating levels of consciousness suggest an organic etiology (drug or metabolic toxicity, organic brain syndromes). Record whether the patient is *hyperalert, alert, drowsy, confused, stuporous,* or *unconscious.* Note whether alertness is steady or varies during the interview.

Orientation

Awareness of time, place, and person are basic cognitive capacities that remain intact even in many severely disturbed patients. Disturbances in orientation are common in delirium, dementia, and drug-induced psychosis, but are less commonly found in patients with acute affective illnesses and schizophrenic disorders. You can test for orientation with a few simple questions:

Time—Time of day (approximate), day of the week, season, year (ask, for example, "What is today's date?")

Place—Building (hospital, office), street, town (ask, for example, "What is the name of this place?")

Person—Identification of self and examiner—doctor, nurse, etc. (ask, for example, "What is your full name? What is my name?")

Concentration

Concentration is the ability to focus and maintain one's attention on a desired set of stimuli. A number of disorders can disturb this capacity, but it is most common in depression, anxiety, and psychosis. Gross disturbances in concentration will affect the patient's ability to pay attention and answer your questions during the interview. If you suspect abnormalities, the following tests are useful:

Serial 7's (or 3's). Ask the patient to subtract 7's (or 3's) in succession, starting from 100. Most patients will be able to perform five or more operations without difficulty, but those who have difficulty concentrating will rapidly lose track of their calculations.

Counting backwards. Particularly if the patient's mathematical ability may be insufficient to perform the task of serial 7's, ask the patient to count backward from 20. Again, those with concentration difficulties are likely to drift away from the task before completing it.

Memory

Memory function is generally divided into three categories: immediate, recent, and remote. Much can be learned about memory as the patient tells his or her story during the interview. Test specific memory functions only when you have reason to suspect memory deficits on the basis of the patient's history and clinical condition.

Table 4-3. Tests of cognitive functioning.

Function	Test
Orientation	
Time	"What is today's date?"
Place	"What is the name of this place?"
Person	"What is your full name?"
Concentration	Serial 7's (or 3's)—ask the patient to subtract 7's (or 3's) in succession, starting from 100. Counting backward from 20.
Memory	
Immediate	Digit span—ask the patient to repeat a series of random numbers, first forward and then backward.
Recent	Ask the patient to remember three unrelated objects and recall them after 15 minutes.
Remote	Ask about names and dates from the patient's earlier life; ask the patient to name the U.S. Presidents beginning with the current one and going backwards.
Fund of knowledge	"Who is the Vice-President of the United States?" "What are the colors of the American flag?" "How far is it from New York to Los Angeles?" "What is a thermometer?"
Abstractions	Proverbs—ask the patient to interpret a proverb (e.g., "A stitch in time saves nine"). Similarities—ask the patient what two things have in common (e.g., table and chair).
Judgment	Ask what the patient would do in a social situation that requires judgment (e.g., on smelling smoke in a crowded theater).

Immediate memory. Use *digit span* to test immediate recall; that is, ask the patient to repeat a series of random numbers (e.g., 2—6—8—9—3—1—5) immediately after you, first forward, and then backward. Normal persons can repeat an average of seven digits forward (± 2) and five digits backward. However, when concentration is impaired (e.g., in depression), the patient may be unable to attend to the task and will *appear* to have a memory deficit when none exists.

Recent memory. Ask patients how they spent the last 24 hours and what they ate for breakfast, lunch, and dinner. Or ask patients to remember three unrelated objects (e.g., lamp, umbrella, telephone) and then recall these objects in 15 minutes.

Remote memory. Ask the patient important names and dates from his or her earlier life (e.g., birth, marriage, school, jobs), or ask about less personal past events (e.g., "Name as many Presidents as you can, starting with the current one and going backward").

If memory impairment is observed, note the patient's reaction to the deficit and any efforts to cope with it. These efforts may include *denial*—acting as if the deficit did not exist; *confabulation*—inventing stories about situations or events that are not remembered; and *circumstantiality*—"beating around the bush" in an effort to mask the memory deficit. Patients who recognize their memory impairment may react to your questions with anxiety, depression, or hostility.

Memory deficits may be confined to particular time spans. In *amnesia*, a specific area of experience becomes inaccessible to conscious recall. *Anterograde amnesia* is memory loss for events that occurred after a significant point in time, while *retrograde amnesia* is memory loss for events that occurred before a significant point in time.

The number of disorders that can impair memory is great, but common causes include:

Organic lesions—Occur as a result of tumors, infarcts, or abuse of alcohol (Korsakoff's syndrome frequently involves short-term memory loss). Both presenile and senile dementia also involve recent memory loss, initially without impairment of remote memory.

Trauma—Post-traumatic amnesia (e.g., after a concussion) is common and is usually predominantly anterograde with a mild retrograde component.

Psychological disorders—Depression, anxiety, and psychosis impair immediate and recent memory, along with concentration, by distracting the patient and making it difficult for him or her to focus on the environment.

Fund of Knowledge

A person's accumulation of knowledge is lifelong and varies with educational and cultural background. However, a person with chronic psychological disturbances may have difficulty in obtaining and processing information for long periods, and will therefore have a poor fund of knowledge. This can usually be judged during the interview. Specific test questions include:

"Who is the President of the United States?"
"Who is the Vice President?"
"What are the colors of the American flag?"
"How far is it from New York to Los Angeles?"
"Name three countries in the Middle East."
"What is a thermometer?"

Abstraction

For adults, normal thought process involves the ability to shift from the specific to the general and to grasp the whole, as well as the particulars, of a given situation. The mind continually categorizes, relying on symbolic thinking to organize details. *Concrete thinking* involves difficulty in shifting from the specific to the abstract. This disorder is prevalent in the various forms of psychosis, particularly in schizophrenia. Concrete thinking can be masked in conversation, so if you suspect psychosis, use the following specific tests to assess the patient's powers of abstraction:

Proverbs. Ask the patient to interpret a proverb, couching it in terms of "How would you explain to someone the meaning of (proverb)?" Use such proverbs as "A stitch in time saves nine," "A rolling stone gathers no moss," and "People who live in glass houses shouldn't throw stones." Obviously, there are no "right answers" in interpreting proverbs. However, patients whose thinking is overly concrete will be unable to infer general meaning from the particulars. For example, a concrete interpretation of the "glass houses" proverb might be "If you throw rocks at others, they'll throw rocks back and break your glass house."

Similarities. Our ability to see relationships among seemingly different things is based on a capacity for abstract thinking. You can test this capacity by asking about similarities—"What do these things have in common?" (for example, apple and orange; table and chair; baseball and tomato). A person whose thinking is very concrete will have difficulty seeing any relationships between these objects.

Judgment

As you listen to the patient's history, you should learn a great deal about his or her ability to make and carry out plans and to discriminate accurately and behave appropriately in social situations. People who have poor impulse control or who have been inadequately socialized will often demonstrate faulty judgment. Drug abuse, organic lesions of the brain, psychosis, depression, and anxiety are among the many causes of impaired judgment.

Formal questions to assess judgment include, "What would you do if you smelled smoke in a crowded theater?" (e.g., run, scream "Fire!", get up and leave, tell the usher). "What would you do if you found a stamped, addressed letter on the ground?" (e.g., mail it, read it).

Insight

Insight refers to patients' awareness and understanding of their illness. Patients vary enormously in how accurately they perceive themselves and their problems.

Some helpful questions in evaluating insight include, "What are your reasons for seeking psychiatric consultation/help/hospitalization?" "Do you feel that you have emotional problems right now?" "Do you feel that you need help in understanding and learning to cope with these problems?"

ATTITUDE TOWARD THE INTERVIEWER

Attitude is the patient's response to you, the interviewer. Psychiatric disorders commonly involve disturbed interpersonal relationships. During a clinical interview, the patient may display such problems by acting them out with you—e.g., by adopting an attitude of hostility or seductiveness that is inappropriate to the interview situation. Patients often adopt surface attitudes in an effort to compensate for deeper problems, e.g., a frightened man may adopt a hostile and aggressive manner in an effort to hide his fear. Attitudes provide valuable clues to how patients defend themselves against unpleasant feelings.

Although it is not sufficient for diagnosis, the patient's attitude can lend support to tentative diagnostic formulations. Paranoid individuals are characteristically suspicious, evasive, and arrogant, while manic patients are frequently impatient and uncooperative. Schizophrenics manifest reserved, remote, and seemingly unfeeling attitudes; depressed people are often apathetic, hopeless, and helpless. Patients with organic brain syndromes (e.g., dementia) classically demonstrate distractibility and apparent indifference to their condition. The following considerations are important in documenting attitude:

- In what ways does the patient engage or distance you?
- Does the patient become more or less comfortable as the interview proceeds?
- Does the patient show an ability to form an alliance and work with you?

REPORTING THE MSE

When you report a mental status examination to others orally or in writing, follow the outline in Table 4-1. Each major category of the MSE (appearance and behavior, speech, emotions, etc.) should be mentioned in its proper order, and when there are no abnormalities you may be brief (e.g., "Speech was clear and normal in rate").

Although you may use many of the terms defined in this chapter, beware of relying heavily on psychiatric jargon, for it does not convey an adequate picture of a person's mental state. Particularly when you document abnormal findings, use specific examples and quotes from the interview to illustrate your points. For example, it is not enough to report "auditory hallucinations"; instead, note that "The patient reported hearing his mother's voice calling his name during the interview."

Report the MSE with enough detail so that a reader or listener who does not know the patient can get a clear understanding of the patient's state of mind at the time of the interview. The two examples presented below are designed to show you how two very different patients might be described.

CASE EXAMPLES

The following examples will give you some perspective on what is involved in recording a mental status examination. It need not be a long and overly detailed endeavor. The MSE report can usually be written in one paragraph, but this will depend on the requirements of the health care facility in which you are working. Be sure to report the findings of the MSE in the order given in this chapter.

Example 1

Mr. A is a well-functioning man who presented to an outpatient clinic with mild anxiety and marital difficulties.

MSE: Mr. A presented as a tall, slender, well-dressed, and meticulously groomed man who looked his stated age of 35. He sat stiffly during the meeting, with a worried facial expression, and made intermittent eye contact with the interviewer. Speech was clear and normal in rate but at times halting, mood was moderately depressed and anxious, and affect varied appropriately with the content of the interview. No abnormalities of thought or perception were noted, and the patient denied any current suicidal or homicidal ideation. Intellectual functioning was grossly intact with apparent above-average intelligence, good judgment, and moderate insight into the nature of his difficulties. Mr. A related to the interviewer in a formal and deferential manner throughout the meeting.

Example 2

Mrs. B is a chronic schizophrenic woman who is being readmitted to a psychiatric hospital for an acute exacerbation of her psychosis and suicidal impulses.

MSE: Mrs. B is an obese, disheveled-looking woman who presented with poor personal hygiene and looked older than her stated age of 46. She sat hunched over in her chair during the interview, with a fixed and bland facial expression, staring at the clock on the wall. She occasionally grimaced and made continuous rapid darting movements with her tongue. Speech was slow and halting, and at times quite loud. She reported "feeling like I'm dead," and her affect was flat and did not vary during the interview. Abnormalities of thought process included occasional episodes of racing thoughts during the interview, loose associations, and tangential replies to questions. The patient also used neologisms infrequently (e.g., "glidders," "crickly"). She insisted that the CIA was trying to poison her, and she reported believing that CIA agents could hear her thoughts. She denied homicidal ideation, but reported urges to harm herself using knives "because I would enjoy seeing the blood run out my veins." She reported seeing men in military uniforms with rifles standing in each corner of the interview room waiting to take her prisoner, but denied any auditory hallucinations. She was oriented to time, place, and person, and her intelligence appeared to be average. There were marked cognitive impairments, notably in concentration (she could only repeat 3 of 7 digits and could not count backwards from 20 beyond 15). Recent memory function was difficult to assess due to her distractibility. Remote memory (date of birth, marital history) was grossly intact. Thinking was markedly concrete on proverb interpretation ("People who have large windows might get them broken with rocks"), judgment was poor, and she had little insight into the nature of her illness. She related to the interviewer in an aloof manner.

REFERENCES

Donnelly J, Rosenbert M, Fleeson W: The evolution of the mental status—past and future. Am J Psychiatry 125:997-1002, 1970.

Nicholi, AM Jr (ed): History and mental status, in The Harvard Guide to Modern Psychiatry. Cambridge, MA, Harvard University Press, 1978, pp 25-40.

A Psychiatric Glossary, 5th ed. Washington, DC, American Psychiatric Association, 1980.

Part II

INTRODUCTION

The third edition of the *Diagnostic and Statistical Manual of Mental Disorders* (DSM-III) lists more than a hundred psychiatric disorders. Obviously, you cannot be introduced to all of them at once, nor would such an introduction be of much use to you as a beginning student. You will get a better understanding of psychiatry if you familiarize yourself with the more common disorders first, and expand your knowledge to more esoteric subjects as your clinical experience deepens.

This section includes the syndromes you are most likely to encounter as you work in outpatient and inpatient psychiatric facilities. They are also the most common psychiatric disorders encountered by practitioners in other areas of medicine.

Chapter 5 focuses on schizophrenia, an illness that accounts for a substantial proportion of chronically disturbed psychiatric patients. Chapter 6 deals with affective disturbances (depression and mania), and Chapter 7 with personality disorders, two categories that encompass much of the psychopathology you will see in your clinical work.

The discussion of personality disorders in Chapter 7 is designed to introduce you to various character styles, as well as to the personality disorders themselves. Since features of human personality such as obsessive-compulsive traits are common to normal people and neurotics, as well as those with personality disorders, an understanding of personality types is relevant to every patient you see, not just those who fit the DSM-III criteria for personality disorders.

A variety of disorders are grouped in Chapter 8. Anxiety disorders are ubiquitous in our society, and both agoraphobia and panic attacks have been the focus of much research and public attention in recent years. Similarly, eating disorders have lately been recognized as being more prevalent in the general population than was previously believed. Somatoform disorders are of concern to every medical practitioner, for these emotional illnesses manifest themselves in physical symptoms for which no organic cause can be found.

Chapter 9 deals with two disorders characterized by global intellectual impairment—dementia and delirium. Dementia, a significant cause of morbidity and mortality in the elderly, is discussed at length. Delirium is discussed only briefly in this chapter, since it commonly stems from underlying somatic illness that is treated by medical and surgical staff.

The literature on each of the disorders in this section is vast. The following chapters are meant to serve as starting points from which you can go on to do further reading.

5

Schizophrenia

MORE THAN A CENTURY AGO, the French psychiatrist Benedict-Augustin Morel watched a 14-year-old boy deteriorate rapidly because of a severe mental illness. The boy had been a good student, but in a matter of months he seemed to have become "demented"—his thoughts were confused and his behavior disorganized. Morel called this devastating illness *demence précoce* (precocious dementia). The term came to be widely used to describe a syndrome we now know as *schizophrenia*.

Schizophrenia has been described as the "cancer" of mental illness—in fact, the two diseases are similar in many ways. We do not know what causes schizophrenia, nor do we know how to prevent it; our efforts at managing the illness once it occurs have met with limited success. Schizophrenia's emotional and financial costs to patients and their families are often astronomical, and the pessimism with which many lay people and mental health professionals approach the schizophrenic patient resembles the aversion often shown to cancer victims.

What is schizophrenia? It is a syndrome that involves a highly altered sense of inner and outer reality to which the afflicted person responds in ways that impair his or her life. This altered sense of reality—the psychotic core of the illness—shows itself in disturbances of perception, thinking, emotion, speech, and physical activity. The term literally means "splitting of the mind," and lay people often misuse the word to describe someone with a "split" or multiple personality. But schizophrenia refers instead to incongruity between different mental functions, e.g., between thought content and feeling, or between feeling and motor activity. The schizophrenic patient may, for example, talk of sad or terrifying events while laughing or showing no emotion whatsoever.

Schizophrenia is a syndrome that probably consists of multiple disorders with varying causes, courses, and treatment outcomes. The diagnostic label covers many different clinical pictures, and symptoms vary so greatly from one individual to another that it is impossible to present a classic picture of the disorder. The diagnosis may, for example, apply equally well to the hypervigilant scientist who suspects others of plotting against him, to the homemaker who believes she is controlled by her dead mother's voice, and to the withdrawn and apathetic teenager who broods incessantly on the reality of existence. Symptoms also vary within the same individual over time, so that a patient who is psychotic and totally unable to function one week may next week be capable of good reality testing and able to perform adequately on the job.

DIAGNOSIS

You must diagnose schizophrenia entirely on the basis of the patient's history and your observations, for we have no independent laboratory tests to verify the presence or absence of the disorder. Since the diagnosis has important implications for prognosis and treatment, psychiatrists have struggled for more than a century to arrive at precise criteria for identifying schizophrenic patients. The latest effort—by the authors of the third edition of the *Diagnostic and Statistical Manual of Mental Disorders* (DSM-III)—is summarized in Table 5-1.

Since these criteria emphasize chronicity, you must get a history of psychotic symptoms over at least six months, or observe the patient for some time, before you can make the diagnosis.

CHARACTERISTIC SYMPTOMS

What are the "characteristic" symptoms that must be present for at least

Table 5-1. Diagnostic criteria for schizophrenia.

Characteristic psychotic symptoms—most importantly, hallucinations or delusions

The presence of these symptoms continuously for more than six months

Loss of functioning in at least two areas of life (e.g., work, school, social relationships, self-care)

Onset before age 45

Chronic course

Symptoms are not due to an affective illness, organic brain syndrome, or mental retardation

---

six months in order to diagnose schizophrenia? The most common ones are described below. Patients may have only one symptom, or they may exhibit many simultaneously. *It is very important that the patient give clear signs of chronically disordered thinking.*

Hallucinations

Auditory hallucinations are most common. They may consist of sounds, identifiable voices, or even continuous dialogues among several voices. These can be particularly dangerous to the patient, or to others, if hallucinated commands are obeyed. Visual, tactile, and olfactory hallucinations occur less often in schizophrenia (they are more commonly associated with organic causes of psychosis).

Also seen in schizophrenia are *coenesthetic hallucinations*—perceptions of altered states in body organs, e.g., "My stomach is rotting" or "My head is growing larger."

Delusions

Falsely held beliefs that cannot be corrected by presenting the patient with the facts are particularly common in schizophrenia. Often these involve erroneous notions about the permeability or transparency of the mind, e.g., that one's thoughts are being controlled by an outside force, that thoughts are being inserted or withdrawn by an outside force, or that thoughts are being broadcast to others. Also common are ideas of reference and delusions of persecution (for discussion of these terms see Chapter 4).

Emotional Disturbance

Blunted or flattened emotional tone is the classic affective symptom of schizophrenia. People who exhibit flat affect can remain so expressionless that they appear to be wearing masks. Other emotional disturbances may accompany this disease, in particular, affect that is inappropriate to thought content (e.g., laughing about a friend's death).

Volitional Disturbance

The patient's will and ability to carry out plans may be paralyzed by negativism, or by an irrational fear of his or her own destructive powers (e.g., a patient may believe that he has the power to single-handedly destroy the universe—and be terrified lest he do so).

Disturbed Speech

Common disturbances of speech include loose associations, incoherence, concreteness, "private" language understood only by the patient, making up new words, and echoing the speech of others.

Disturbed Motor Activity

Activity may be markedly decreased, as in catatonia, or increased, as in excited states. Patients may exhibit automaton-like behavior, bizarre repetitive mannerisms, or echopraxia (mimicking others).

CLINICAL PICTURE

By themselves, these symptoms and diagnostic criteria cannot give you a feel for what people with schizophrenia are like. Although the clinical picture may vary greatly from one patient to another, certain characteristics are common to most people who have the disease.

A person typically develops schizophrenia in adolescence or early adulthood—e.g., a student whose grades begin to decline for no apparent reason and who begins to spend more time lying in bed "daydreaming." Or the patient may be a homemaker who stops spending time with friends, instead spending time apparently lost in thought, and stops paying attention to her appearance. The incipient schizophrenic often begins to communicate in ways that seem odd or nonsensical, e.g., discussing some special personal meaning in a newspaper headline, or using words in eccentric ways. Performance at daily tasks declines as the person withdraws into his or her own world. The patient may initially show considerable anxiety and hypersensitivity to perceptual and interpersonal stimuli, but increasing absorption in an inner world makes it more and more difficult for him or her to pay attention to what is going on in the environment. This *prodromal phase* may last for days or months. However, some people do not develop schizophrenia in this way but suddenly experience a psychotic "break." Thus, the active phase may be the first sign of illness.

Whether or not there is a prodrome to the illness, all schizophrenic patients have what is called an *active phase*, in which their psychosis is most evident and they appear most severely disturbed. It is in this phase that someone is likely to be convinced that he is Jesus Christ, or to believe that the KGB has poisoned his drinking water, or to insist that his intestines are riddled with cancer, despite doctors' assurances to the contrary. In this phase, a patient may believe that her thoughts are controlled by an IBM computer at her husband's office, or that her five-year-old son is trying to murder her, or that she receives messages from her dead mother over a radio station. A patient may hear voices commanding him to collect garbage in his bedroom, or to lead his family in jumping out a fifth-story window. Or he may see snipers shooting at him whenever he attempts to leave his house. Such delusions and hallucinations sound bizarre to us, but they are quite real to schizophrenic patients and may prompt them to act in strange and dangerous ways. To complicate matters, schizophrenic patients may be so withdrawn and guarded that they are unable to describe their psychotic symptoms to you. Or they may describe them without any show of feeling and thus give the false impression that they are not in any real distress.

The active phase of schizophrenia may last indefinitely or only a few weeks. When this phase subsides (with or without treatment), the schizophrenic patient does not return to his or her baseline level of functioning but is left with chronic symptoms that constitute the *residual phase*. In many ways this phase is like the prodromal phase, in that the patient is usually not floridly psychotic or agitated, but is still obviously impaired. If hallucinations or delusions persist in this phase, they are usually less emotionally charged than before. Flattened affect is common, as is poor performance at work, at school, and at household tasks. In fact, impairment of functioning varies, so that some chronic schizophrenics who are in the residual phase of their illness are able to work (albeit with reduced effectiveness), while others are unable to function at all or even to care for themselves.

Some require chronic care in psychiatric hospitals, but most are able to live either on their own or in community-based programs such as halfway houses (see the discussion of Treatment below). Speech and thought commonly remain odd or eccentric, and patients usually continue to behave in peculiar ways (e.g., talking to themselves in public) and remain socially withdrawn.

The most important feature of the residual phase is that the person remains impaired. A return to normal premorbid functioning is the exception rather than the rule. Thus, if you encounter a "schizophrenic" patient who gets back to normal functioning after a psychotic episode, you should question your diagnosis and consider other possibilities (e.g., an affective disorder or drug-induced psychosis).

Once a first psychotic episode occurs, the schizophrenic patient's clinical course is quite variable. A small number of people recover with little or no residual deficit, but the more common course is one of exacerbations and remissions of the illness throughout life. Some patients have increasing residual impairment after each acute exacerbation of their psychosis, while others appear to stabilize at one suboptimal level of functioning.

How do you predict which schizophrenic patients will have a deteriorating course and which will stabilize or get better? To date, we cannot make such predictions with much reliability. Some factors that have been correlated with specific outcomes among schizophrenics are shown in Table 5-2.

A Common and Dangerous Complication

Suicide and *suicide attempts* are common among schizophrenic patients. Suicide is frequently attempted during the onset of a first psychotic episode, when patients feel that something terrible is happening that they do not understand and that is beyond their control. Patients also try to kill themselves during the periods of depression that occur in the course of the illness. Floridly psychotic patients are at particular risk for suicide, since hallucinations or delusions may dictate self-destructive acts and patients may obey these internal commands

Table 5-2. Factors that help predict the clinical course of schizophrenia.

Poor prognosis	Good prognosis
Premorbidly withdrawn and isolative	Good premorbid social functioning
Premorbid personality disorder	No premorbid personality disorder
No identifiable precipitating events	Precipitating events
Insidious onset	Abrupt onset
Early onset (childhood, adolescence)	Mid-life onset
Little confusion in clinical picture	Confusion prominent in clinical picture
No family history of affective illness	Family history of affective illness

quite impulsively. Roughly 20 percent of schizophrenics attempt suicide over the course of their illness, and 2-3 percent of schizophrenics actually kill themselves.

Homicide is much rarer, although catatonic and paranoid patients are more prone to violence than those in other categories.

SUBTYPES OF SCHIZOPHRENIA

It has long been apparent that schizophrenia as a diagnostic umbrella covers a variety of clinical conditions, and psychiatrists have proposed many schemes of subcategories to separate schizophrenics according to symptoms, clinical course, and outcome. The subtypes of schizophrenia listed in DSM-III are of limited value in this respect, and many schizophrenic patients do not fit neatly into any one diagnostic subcategory. Nevertheless, since you will hear these subtypes used in clinical work, they are described briefly below.

Disorganized type includes the primary symptoms of incoherent speech and blunted or inappropriate affect, with extreme social impairment but without well-developed delusional systems. These patients often have a history of poor premorbid functioning, experience an early and insidious onset of the illness, and follow a chronic course without significant remission.

Catatonic type refers to a clinical picture dominated by psychomotor disturbance. This may take the form of catatonic stupor or rigidity, catatonic excitement, catatonic posturing, or negativism (see

Chapter 4). For reasons that are unclear, this type is now relatively rare in Europe and North America.

Paranoid type is quite common and involves the presence of grandiose, jealous, or persecutory delusions or hallucinations with persecutory or grandiose content. Unlike disorganized or catatonic patients, paranoid schizophrenics sometimes show very little impairment in functioning (e.g., a paranoid security expert may function adequately on the job). Gross disorganization of behavior is rare among paranoid schizophrenics—they often speak clearly, and some can behave quite appropriately in social situations that do not arouse their paranoid fears. The onset of this type tends to occur later in life than the other subtypes, and symptoms remain more stable over time.

Undifferentiated type is simply a category for schizophrenic patients whose prominent psychotic symptoms do not fall within any of the main categories listed above.

Subtypes are probably most useful as a kind of shorthand for describing a specific clinical picture of schizophrenia. Do not worry much about classifying a patient by subtype; it is not usually of major importance to the patient's care. What *is* important, however, is that you take utmost care in differentiating schizophrenia from other diagnoses.

DIFFERENTIAL DIAGNOSIS

Accuracy in diagnosing schizophrenia is of critical importance, but it is the ideal rather than the reality in modern psychiatric practice. Many disorders mimic schizophrenia, and schizophrenia varies so greatly in its clinical presentation that it is often mistaken for other syndromes. Because "schizophrenia" implies chronicity and intractability, the diagnostic label can have devastating effects on patients and families when applied incorrectly. On the other hand, correct diagnosis may provide some measure of relief to patients who are struggling to understand their illness and to families attempting to plan for future care and proper treatment.

The process of differential diagnosis is often difficult, because there are several disorders that are commonly confused with schizophrenia and that must be ruled out before the diagnosis can be made with confidence.

Affective Illness

Mania and psychotic depression often present with hallucinations, delusions, and bizarre behavior; they are easily confused with schizophrenia. You should suspect an affective illness:

- When the patient develops prominent affective symptoms of depression or mania *before or along with* the onset of psychosis (schizophrenics often show affective symptoms, but these occur *after* psychosis has developed, often in reaction to it).
- When the patient has a *complete* remission and functions normally between psychotic episodes.
- When the patient has a biological relative who has a history of a remitting psychotic illness, since this is more suggestive of affective illness.

For a detailed discussion of the affective disorders, see Chapter 6.

Schizoaffective Disorder

This diagnosis is made when both chronic psychosis and mood disturbance are prominent and you are unable to distinguish between schizophrenia and affective illness.

Organic Mental Disorders

Organically based psychosis may look exactly like schizophrenia with respect to delusions, hallucinations, incoherence, and bizarre affect and behavior. The cause may be drugs (particularly amphetamines or phencyclidine), metabolic disease, a neurologic condition, or even infection. If disorientation, confusion, and impaired memory are prominent, it is a good rule of thumb to suspect underlying medical illness or drug toxicity. In evaluating acute psychosis, a thorough history, physical examination, and laboratory screening are essential to rule out medical illness (see Chapters 9 and 11).

Personality Disorders

Transient psychotic symptoms may occur in patients with personality disorders—particularly in schizotypal, borderline, and schizoid patients who become psychotic under stress. However, these patients will recompensate completely within hours or days. It is the brevity of the psychosis and the fact that the psychotic symptoms are felt to be "alien" that distinguish such patients from schizophrenics. Paranoid personality disorder involves pervasive suspicion and mistrust that impairs relationships with others, but it does *not* include delusions or other chronic symptoms of psychosis (see Chapter 7).

Paranoid Disorders

Paranoia is the dominant symptom in this condition. Psychosis may take the form of well-systematized delusional beliefs, but disordered thinking is not prominent, as it is in paranoid schizophrenia.

Brief Reactive Psychosis

This condition, which occurs in individuals under severe stress, may look exactly like schizophrenia. It is here that observing the patient over time is crucial, since reactive psychoses clear rapidly (days to weeks) without residual impairment. Reactive psychosis is frequently seen in adolescents.

EPIDEMIOLOGY

Schizophrenia is ubiquitous. It is found in every culture and in every part of the world with roughly the same frequency. It affects men and women equally, and most people develop the illness in their late teens or early twenties. It is estimated that between 100,000 and 150,000 new cases of the disease are diagnosed annually in the United States. Between 500,000 and 1 million cases now exist in this country.

Schizophrenia is more prevalent among lower socioeconomic groups within urban populations—perhaps because of the downward mobility forced on patients by the debilitating effects of the illness, and possibly because the stresses of lower-class life (e.g., poverty, crime) serve as precipitants in those who are susceptible.

WHAT CAUSES SCHIZOPHRENIA?

The cause of schizophrenia, like the cause of cancer, has eluded researchers for years, and few people retain much hope that any single etiologic factor underlies this disorder. Research has been plagued by many difficulties, not the least of which has been the lack of an objective and universally accepted definition of the illness itself. Investigators have looked for a clear relationship between schizophrenia and gross pathologic changes in the brain, early childhood development, metabolic disorders, neurochemical abnormalities, and endocrine dysfunction—thus far, without success.

The Dopamine Hypothesis

To date, the most widely discussed notion of a biologic cause of schizophrenia has been the dopamine hypothesis. It is based on the idea that the mechanism of action of antipsychotic medications can shed light on the pathophysiology of the schizophrenic disorders they treat.

Antipsychotic agents have been shown to block postsynaptic dopamine receptor sites in the brain. This has led investigators to speculate that schizophrenia might involve excessive levels of activity of dopamine as a neurotransmitter. This hypothesis would explain the therapeutic effects of antipsychotic drugs in schizophrenia, but it presents several problems:

- Evidence of increased dopamine activity in the brains of schizophrenics has *not* been found.
- Although the dopamine-blocking effects of these medications appear to coincide with their antipsychotic effects, it has *not* been shown that dopamine blockade is the mechanism by which psychosis is ameliorated.
- These drugs are not specifically antischizophrenic, but have antipsychotic effects in other illnesses, like mania and psychotic depression.

Thus, the dopamine hypothesis remains unproven, and research into the biology of schizophrenia continues.

Heredity versus Environment

To what extent is schizophrenia rooted in human genes? To what extent is it caused by the environment? Recent research has yielded important findings:

Genetics. The case for a genetic basis in schizophrenic disorders has been supported by a variety of studies, including *adoption studies*, which reveal a significant concentration of schizophrenia in the biologic relatives of schizophrenics reared in different environments, and *twin studies*, which show consistently higher concordance for schizophrenia among identical twins (~40 percent) than among fraternal twins (~20 percent). In other words, when one twin is schizophrenic, the other is much more likely to be schizophrenic if the twins have identical genetic make-up.

Such studies lend support to the hypothesis that genetic factors play an important causal role in schizophrenia, but probably a role that varies from patient to patient. It is still unclear whether such genetic predisposition is specific to schizophrenia or occurs broadly within the general population.

Environment. Genetics alone cannot explain why some individuals become schizophrenic while others do not. This is most clearly seen in pairs of monozygotic twins when only one of the twins is schizophrenic.

In looking for environmental causes, researchers have explored the hypothesis that people with one certain personality type (e.g., schizoid personality) are more vulnerable to schizophrenia than others, but in fact many different personality types are found among people who later develop schizophrenia. Investigators looking at family interactions have found evidence that the families of schizophrenics show more communication deviance (i.e., illogical, inconsistent, and/or tangential communications) and lower general competence than families that have no schizophrenia. However, this evidence of preexisting family pathology only establishes a casual (rather than causal) relationship between pathology in family functioning and schizophrenia.

Contrary to earlier hypotheses that certain types of families *cause* schizophrenia, there is increasing evidence that the families of schizophrenics are quite diverse. You must be sensitive to such diversity, helping families to modify behavior patterns that aggravate the schizophrenic's psychotic symptoms, but also helping to alleviate the misplaced burden of guilt many families bear when they feel they are entirely responsible for one member's illness.

Although the appropriate genes may be a necessary precondition for schizophrenia, genetic factors alone do not account for the development of the illness. Thus, the nature-versus-nurture debate is only useful in sorting out the relative contributions of heredity and environment in individual cases. It seems safe to posit an interactive relationship between genes and the environment. It may be that a *vulnerability* to schizophrenia is transmitted genetically but that the development of a schizophrenic phenotype depends on the presence of environmental factors that have yet to be elucidated.

TREATMENT

The treatment of schizophrenia can be an arduous process for patients, families, and clinicians alike. No cure exists for this tenacious disease, so therapeutic efforts are aimed at management of symptoms and at social and psychological rehabilitation. Like cancer, schizophrenia has invited the discovery of "miracle cures," none of which has proved effective. The major treatment modalities we currently use—medications, psychosocial therapies, and hospitalization (see Table 5-3)—are all of limited efficacy and all have the potential to be harmful as well as helpful. Nevertheless, carefully designed treatment programs can help many patients to regain lost functioning and a greater sense of psychological well-being. Long-term support is necessary for most schizophrenic patients to maximize both their ability to function and their quality of life.

Psychosocial Treatments

Hospitalization. Until the middle of this century, the treatment of choice for schizophrenic patients was long-term custodial care. Many patients remained in psychiatric hospitals most of their lives.

Table 5-3. Major modalities used in treating schizophrenia.

Psychosocial treatments
    Hospitalization
    Psychotherapy
    Rehabilitation—social, vocational
    Aftercare—day treatment, halfway houses
    Education about the illness for patients and families

Somatic therapies
    Antipsychotic medications
    Lithium
    ECT
    Antidepressants

Today, long-term inpatient treatment still occurs, but it has been largely eliminated by programs of *deinstitutionalization*. These programs are based on the idea that hospital stays should be short and used for crisis intervention, to stabilize schizophrenic patients so they can return to life in their communities. Obviously, this is less costly than long-term hospitalization.

Advocates of this policy argue that emphasis on returning to the community promotes greater patient autonomy and higher-level functioning than a lengthy stay, during which patients become accustomed to being cared for by others. Advocates of long-term hospitalization argue that lasting psychological change takes time and is more likely to occur in the protective and structured setting of an inpatient unit. At present, deinstitutionalization is the prevailing policy in mental health care; the number of schizophrenic inpatients in the United States has decreased by more than half in the last 20 years.

When should you hospitalize a schizophrenic patient?

At the onset of a first psychotic episode. To facilitate a thorough diagnostic work-up, to keep the patient safe, and to initiate medication and psychotherapy while the patient is under close observation. These treatments can then be continued in an aftercare program when the patient is discharged.

When the patient poses a danger to self or to others. Suicidal and homocidal threats or gestures are especially serious among psychotic patients, who may lack the judgment and impulse control to keep from acting on hallucinated commands or delusional beliefs.

When the patient is unable to care for himself or herself. Patients who cease to be able to protect, clothe, and feed themselves need support until their functioning returns. Some patients have been ill for so long that they have *never* learned to care for themselves. These people can benefit from the intensive social skills programs that are offered in many long-term treatment facilities.

When the patient has lost important social supports. Patients who function well with a network of supportive people and activities (family, friends, therapists, jobs) may decompensate when this network is disrupted. Changes in home life, work, or treatment may precipitate loss of functioning and even psychosis, warranting hospital admission and crisis intervention.

Note that the return of psychotic symptoms is not, in and of itself, an indication for hospitalization of schizophrenic patients. When community support exists and patients are not dangerous to themselves or others, crisis intervention with medication and/or intensified psychological treatment can be attempted on an outpatient basis.

Management of hospitalized patients. During acute episodes of psychosis, patients' behavior may be difficult to manage. Many agitated, suicidal, and violent patients require locked inpatient units. Verbal limits may be sufficient to control behavior, and threatening patients often calm down when confronted with the fact that their behavior is frightening to others. Seclusion rooms (quiet, sparsely furnished areas) are helpful in decreasing the noise and activity around an overstimulated psychotic patient who may be flooded with hallucinations and racing thoughts. When verbal limits, reassurance, and seclusion do not suffice to calm the patient and control dangerous behavior, physical restraint and/or chemical restraint may be necessary (see Chapter 13).

As the acute symptoms subside, the patient can be integrated into the inpatient community. Ideally, the inpatient unit should have structured activities and group meetings in which patients can improve their social skills, modify inappropriate behaviors, and support one another in coping with the stresses of psychiatric illness. This *milieu therapy* provides the backdrop for the action of medications and the individual and family therapies discussed below. A major focus of hospital admission should be careful planning of comprehensive treatment that can continue when the patient leaves the hospital.

The goals of hospitalization usually include resolution of a suicidal or homicidal crisis, improved hygiene and behavior to allow the patient to return to life in the community, improved judgment and reality testing, stable remission of symptoms, the ability to care for oneself (with or without support) outside of the hospital, and the ability to comply with an outpatient treatment program. When these goals are achieved, when the patient has arranged a stable living situation, and when adequate outpatient treatment has been provided for, the patient is usually ready for discharge. Outpatient treatment may include medication, individual and/or group therapy, day treatment, and job rehabilitation.

Repeated hospital admissions are the norm in schizophrenia. Nearly 70 percent of all admissions of schizophrenics are readmissions. Frequently, a life crisis will prompt the patient to become disorganized, discontinue medication and other treatment, and decompensate to the point that hospitalization is required.

Psychotherapy. There is widespread disagreement about the type of psychotherapy that is helpful to schizophrenic patients. *Supportive individual psychotherapy* is nonintensive "here and now" treatment in which the therapist actively assists the patient in understanding and coping with the reality of his or her illness and life circumstances. By contrast, *exploratory psychotherapy* is more intensive and focuses on the therapist-patient relationship as a "laboratory" for patients to gain insight into their psychological make-up and achieve lasting intrapsychic change. Since schizophrenic patients are usually severely handicapped in their ability to be close to others, the first goal of most therapies is to establish a stable, trusting relationship between therapist and patient. Insight-oriented work often emphasizes the importance of helping the schizophrenic to label feelings and connect them to life experiences and to explore feelings that may be so stressful for the patient that he or she lapses into disorganized ways of thinking.

Group therapy has been used with some success in helping patients understand and change their inappropriate ways of dealing with others. As mentioned above, *family therapy* can identify and help to change family patterns of behavior that exacerbate the patient's illness. Family treatment can also be of great help in educating relatives about the illness and what they can expect in dealing with a schizophrenic family member.

The range of approaches to psychotherapy with schizophrenic patients is enormous, and no single approach has been shown to be superior to the others. The diversity of therapies thought to be effective in schizophrenia reflects the tremendous diversity of needs and personalities among schizophrenic patients themselves.

Rehabilitation. Patients uniformly lose functioning in some areas of their lives as a result of schizophrenia, and must overcome intrapsychic and environmental obstacles to leading a productive life in the community again. All too often, the very process of hospitalization prompts patients to allow others to take over their lives for them—one of the unfortunate side effects of chronic institutionalization. Schizophrenics therefore need help in learning or relearning skills for life in the community. Successful rehabilitation can be a tremendous boost to patients' self-esteem as they come to feel more competent at taking care of themselves. Such rehabilitation efforts usually include job training and practice in cooking and other household tasks. Ideally, rehabilitation begins when the patient is in the hospital and continues after discharge.

Aftercare. The extent to which schizophrenic patients can care for themselves on their own, outside a hospital setting, varies enormously. Some are able to live independently, while others need total care on a 24-hour basis. Patients who can live outside a hospital but require supervision in their daily activities (e.g., handling money, buying food) often do well in *halfway houses* or *cooperative apartments*, in which patients are supported by mental health professionals who either live in these facilities or staff them on a regular basis. However, such living arrangements are costly, and many patients are cared for in private homes by family members or friends.

Along with support in a living situation, patients who cannot work full-time or cannot work at all need structured daytime activities. For such people, *day treatment programs* are helpful. These programs are set up so that patients may spend all or part of the day in group activities and meetings designed to increase social and other skills, while providing close supervision of medication regimens for those who have difficulty with compliance. Day treatment programs are usually affiliated with hospitals or community health centers.

Somatic Therapies

Antipsychotic medications. Antipsychotic drugs are the mainstay of somatic treatment in schizophrenia. They have revolutionized the management of the disease, both because of their acute sedative effects and because of their long-term antipsychotic effects. They do not cure the disease, but they have been shown to reduce confusion, anxiety, delusions, hallucinations, social isolation, and other symptoms of schizophrenia. The principles of treatment are discussed in detail in Chapter 15.

Antipsychotic medications are sedating; they may help calm agitated and acutely psychotic patients within hours after treatment is begun. However, the maximum antipsychotic effect of these drugs may not be reached for 6 weeks. Once the acute psychotic symptoms of schizophrenia have been controlled (usually in 4-12 weeks), the dosage can be reduced to a maintenance level of 20-50 percent of the amount needed in the acute crisis. Carefully monitor the tapering of the dosage over several weeks so that it can be increased again at the first sign of a return of symptoms. Patients who cannot comply with an outpatient regimen of oral medication may be maintained on intramuscular injections of fluphenazine decanoate (Prolixin) every 10-14 days. Schizophrenics who are not maintained on antipsychotic medication after an acute psychotic episode have a relapse rate significantly greater than that of those who continue to take their medication once a crisis has passed. Thus, long-term maintenance therapy with antipsychotic medication is indicated for a great many people diagnosed as schizophrenic.

However, patients must not be kept on antipsychotics indefinitely without reevaluation of their need for medication. Patients who have a complete remission that lasts six months or more, and those who are stabilized on low maintenance doses of antipsychotics, deserve a trial off all medications for two reasons:

- To determine whether a first psychotic episode was a reactive psychosis rather than the onset of a schizophrenic disorder (particularly important in young patients, many of whom recompensate quickly after a first psychotic break), and
- To reduce the risk of tardive dyskinesia in patients for whom maintenance medication is no longer essential (see Chapter 15).

Lithium. Lithium therapy has been found to be useful in a minority of patients diagnosed as schizophrenic. It is not clear whether this is because lithium-responsive "schizophrenic" patients have been misdiagnosed and suffer from an affective illness, or because there are some true schizophrenics who happen to respond to lithium. Particularly when the differential diagnosis between schizophrenia and affective illness is difficult to make, a trial of lithium may be both diagnostic and therapeutic. Certainly lithium therapy should be considered whenever affective symptoms are a prominent part of a psychotic illness (see Chapter 15).

Electroconvulsive therapy (ECT). ECT has been found useful in alleviating the symptoms of catatonic stupor and catatonic excitement. However, its efficacy in relieving other symptoms of schizophrenia has not been clearly demonstrated. (see Chapter 15).

Antidepressants. Despite the flat, affectless stereotype, patients with schizophrenic disorders do sometimes become depressed. They are particularly vulnerable to depression after an acute psychotic episode has cleared and they must come to terms with what has happened to them. However, if a schizophrenic patient appears apathetic, inactive, and in low spirits, you must rule out the possibility that he or she has been overtranquilized and is suffering parkinsonian side effects, rather than depression. (This can be done by testing the patient's response to an antiparkinsonian drug or to lowering the dosage of the antipsychotic drug.) For patients who seem genuinely depressed rather than overmedicated, it is often useful to add a tricyclic antidepressant to the medication regimen (see Chapter 15). Observe such patients closely, because tricyclics can precipitate psychosis.

Controversy in the Treatment of Schizophrenia

The introduction of antipsychotic medications has had a powerful effect on the management of schizophrenia. Some psychopharmacologists argue that the only mode of treatment proven effective is drug treatment, and that human intervention in schizophrenia is of little use.

On the other hand, advocates of psychotherapy in schizophrenia argue that drug treatment alone is not sufficient, that the effectiveness of medication depends on the psychosocial context in which it is given, and that medication only reduces psychotic symptoms but does not affect the patient's social or personality development.

In fact, there can be no single correct treatment, since "schizophrenia" almost certainly consists of multiple disorders. The range of treatments and combinations of treatments used effectively reflects the variability inherent in the disease itself. What is useful to some schizophrenic patients may be useless or even harmful to others. *Most effective treatment regimens combine somatic and psychosocial therapies.*

Despite our best therapeutic efforts, schizophrenic patients still occupy nearly half the psychiatric beds in this country. And despite the effectiveness of new antipsychotic medications, the disease continues to leave a significant percentage of patients with real deficits, while the prevalence of schizophrenia in the United States remains unchanged.

REFERENCES

Baldessarini RJ: Schizophrenia. N Engl J Med 297:988-995, 1977.

Cancro R: Advances in the diagnosis and treatment of schizophrenic disorders, in American Handbook of Psychiatry, 2nd rev ed. Edited by Arieti S. New York, Basic Books, 1981, vol. 7, pp 285-296.

Diagnostic and Statistical Manual of Mental Disorders, 3rd ed. Washington, DC, American Psychiatric Association, 1980, pp 181-194.

Green H: I Never Promised You a Rose Garden. New York, New American Library, 1977. (A moving fictionalized account of a young woman's experience of her illness and improvement during intensive psychotherapy.)

Gunderson JG: Drugs and psychosocial treatment of schizophrenia revisited. Psychiatry Digest, December 1977, pp. 25-40.

Gunderson JG: Major clinical controversies, in Psychotherapy of Schizophrenia. Edited by Gunderson JG, Mosher LR. New York, Jason Aronson, 1975, pp 3-22.

Kety, SS: Genetic aspects of schizophrenia. Psychiatr Ann 6:6-15, 1976.

MacKinnon RA, Michels R: The Psychiatric Interview in Clinical Practice. Philadelphia, WB Saunders, 1971, pp 230-258.

Matthysse S, Lipinski J: Biochemical aspects of schizophrenia. Annu Rev Med, 26:551-565, 1975.

Pope HG Jr, Lipinski JF Jr: Diagnosis in schizophrenia and manic-depressive illness. Arch Gen Psychiatry 35:811-828, 1978.

Schader RI, Jackson AH: Approaches to schizophrenia, in Manual of Psychiatric Therapeutics. Edited by Shader, RI, Boston, Little, Brown, 1975, pp 63-100.

6

Affective Disorders

THE AFFECTIVE DISORDERS encompass a spectrum of emotions ranging from deep depression to unbounded elation and mania. An elated or depressed mood dominates the clinical picture, but mood is by no means the only problem for the patient with an affective illness. Physical symptoms, self-destructive behavior, loss of social functioning, and impaired reality testing frequently go hand in hand with depression and mania, posing difficult and sometimes life-threatening problems for patients and their families.

We are all subject to mood changes in our daily lives. Feelings of sadness and disappointment are a normal part of human existence; fortunately, so are feelings of happiness and elation. How, then, do we distinguish "normal" moods from "abnormal" ones? On what basis are mood states labeled abnormal? Here are some questions to use in attempting to identify pathological mood changes:

How intense is the mood, and how long does it last? Pathological mood states are unduly prolonged and severe.

Do physical symptoms accompany the mood change? Impaired body functioning is common, including disturbances of sleep, appetite, sexual activity, and autonomic nervous system functions.

101

Does the mood disrupt normal daily activities?
Impaired performance often occurs in the usual social roles, e.g., home life, work, school, hobbies.

Is the patient's ability to recognize reality impaired? For example, is the mood change accompanied by hallucinations, delusions, or confusion?

Does the mood put the patient or others in danger? The danger may be direct, i.e., suicidal or homicidal intent, or indirect, as a result of impaired judgment.

As in so many other illnesses, the etiologies of affective disorders remain a mystery and are the subject of intense research and heated debate. Diagnosis rests almost entirely on the patient's history, symptoms, and behavior; but, since depression and elation can present themselves in many ways, diagnosis is not always easy. For years, clinicians have debated how best to fit the mood disorders into diagnostic categories, using different etiologic hypotheses and various groupings of symptoms. The most basic and least controversial classification of affective disorders is the bipolar-unipolar dichotomy.

Bipolar affective disorders are conditions in which *both* depression and elation are present at different times in the course of the illness or, more rarely, disorders in which there are only episodes of elation. This category includes *manic-depressive illness* and a milder form of bipolar illness, *cyclothymic disorder.*

Unipolar affective disorders involve episodes of depression, but no episodes of elation. Depression may be chronic or episodic, may occur once or recur again and again. This category includes *major depressive disorder* and the milder and more chronic *dysthymic disorder.*

The distinction between unipolar and bipolar illness has been made not only on the basis of symptoms, but also on the basis of different genetic and familial patterns, different responses to pharmacologic interventions, and different physical and biochemical characteristics.

UNIPOLAR DISORDERS

Depression is the most common of psychiatric illnesses. All of us have friends, acquaintances, or relatives who have at some time been

Table 6-1. Major forms of affective illness.

Type	Key to diagnosis
Bipolar Manic-depressive illness Cyclothymic disorder	History of episodes of elation, with or without a history of depression
Unipolar Major depressive disorder Dysthymic disorder	History of depression without any history of elation

clinically depressed. In fact, at least one in ten adults experiences one or more episodes of depression during his or her lifetime. Some researchers estimate the lifetime risk to be as high as 30 percent.

Some depressed people obtain professional help, but many others do not. Probably only 10 to 25 percent of those with depressive disorders seek treatment. Since many of these seek treatment from internists and general practitioners of medicine, it is critical that practicing physicians and other health professionals recognize the signs and symptoms of these ubiquitous disorders.

The clinical picture of depression varies tremendously. One patient may present with tearfulness and self-reproaches, another with low back pain and chronic fatigue, and a third may be terrified that his spouse is trying to kill him. Yet all three of these patients may have depressive disorders and may even respond to the same treatment modalities. No single symptom is present in all depressive syndromes. Feeling sad or "down in the dumps" is the most common experience of depressed people, but even a depressed mood is not universal. There are patients who report no mood disturbances but have the classic physical signs of depression and respond beautifully to treatment with antidepressant agents.

Symptoms

Given the variety of forms depression assumes, the list of symptoms is long. Some of the most common symptoms of the depressive disorders are listed in Table 6-2 and described below, grouped according to the mental and physical functions they impair. A patient may be troubled by one or by many of these afflictions at any given time.

Affective symptoms

Depressed mood. More than 90 percent of depressed people experience prolonged moods of sadness or discouragement, or a sense of "not caring any more." A depressed mood usually colors the patient's entire mental life; it is pervasive and dominant. A small percentage of depressed people do not experience a depressed mood but manifest other symptoms. One clue to the diagnosis in such cases is that the patient's situation often saddens the interviewer, even though the patient does not report sadness. Depressed children often do not complain of dysphoria but constantly wear sad facial expressions.

Anhedonia. The inability to derive pleasure from previously pleasurable activities is an almost universal symptom of depression. Activities that may cease to be enjoyable include eating, sex, hobbies, sports, social events, and family functions.

Anxiety. Most depressed patients experience anxiety—i.e., inner distress with dread, fear, or anticipation of danger—along with such autonomic nervous system dysfunctions as sweating, palpitations, rapid pulse, or "butterflies in the stomach." Because anxiety and depression often go hand in hand, it may be difficult to distinguish patients who are depressed from those who have primary anxiety disorders.

Vegetative symptoms

Vegetative symptoms are specific physical problems that often accompany a depressed mood. The presence or absence of vegetative symptoms may be crucial in predicting response to somatic therapies for

Table 6-2. The symptoms of depression.

Affective	Motivational
Depressed mood	Loss of interest in usual activities
Anhedonia	Feelings of hopelessness and
Anxiety	helplessness
	Suicidal thoughts or acts
Vegetative	
Sleep disturbance	Cognitive
Appetite disturbance	Sense of guilt, worthlessness, and
Loss of energy	low self-esteem
Decreased libido	Difficulty in concentrating
Psychomotor retardation	Psychosis
Psychomotor agitation	
	Psychosomatic
	Bodily complaints

depression. You should therefore inquire about vegetative symptoms whenever the diagnosis of depression is a possibility.

Sleep disturbance. The majority of depressed patients experience some form of insomnia. This may involve difficulty falling asleep (*early insomnia*); patients with this complaint often report "tossing and turning" while they ruminate on life events. Others complain of waking up during sleep—often from nightmares—and returning to sleep with difficulty (*middle insomnia*). Particularly common is early-morning awakening (*terminal insomnia*); patients wake up at 5:00 or 6:00 a.m. and cannot get back to sleep. Hypnotic medications (e.g., barbiturates, benzodiazepines) are often unsuccessful in prolonging sleep in depressed patients, and antidepressants are generally more effective.

Although insomnia is the norm, some patients (particularly children, young adults, and patients with bipolar illness) experience *hypersomnia*, or sleeping too much.

Appetite disturbance. Many depressed patients experience a loss of appetite (*anorexia*) with or without weight loss. In taking a patient's history, you should always document the amount of any weight loss and the period over which it occurred. Weight loss may be small or quite large, even life-threatening. A minority of patients—particularly young women and people with bipolar illness—will experience overeating (*hyperphagia*) and binge eating (*bulimia*) as a symptom of depression. In such cases, weight gain usually results.

Loss of energy (anergy). Depressed patients commonly experience fatigue and loss of energy in the absence of exertion, and describe this as feeling "run down" or "like all the energy has been drained out of my body." Such patients may believe they suffer from a vitamin deficiency, and some severely depressed patients believe that their decreased energy is caused by cancer or tuberculosis. Some patients experience *diurnal variation* in mood and energy level—i.e., depression is worse in the morning and improves somewhat during the day.

Decreased libido. A loss of sexual interest and energy commonly plagues depressed patients. It may cause an increase in marital tensions and a lowering of the patient's already fragile self-esteem. In men, the most common presenting symptom is impotence. You must inquire specifically about sexual dysfunction when depression is suspected, because many people are too embarrassed to volunteer such information.

Psychomotor retardation. Many depressed patients exhibit an actual retardation of thought, speech, and action. Sparse replies to questions, monotonous and slowed speech, fixed gaze, and slowed body movements are all part of this syndrome, which may be severe enough to resemble catatonia.

Psychomotor agitation. Some depressed patients—particularly elderly patients—experience agitation rather than retardation. This involves an unpleasant restlessness or tension, an inability to relax or to sit still. Such patients appear "fidgety," and unlike elated patients who show purposeful overactivity, agitated patients simply make tension-relieving efforts, such as hand-wringing, pacing, nail-biting, and hair-pulling.

Motivational symptoms

Loss of interest in usual activities. Depressed people not only experience a loss of pleasure, but also a decrease in motivation, often in all areas of life. Work, home life, and other pursuits come to seem dull and uninteresting. Ability to perform one's usual tasks may decline.

Feelings of hopelessness and helplessness. People who are very depressed feel they cannot cope with even the smallest of tasks, including personal hygiene and grooming. Work, school, and household duties can suddenly appear unmanageable to the depressed person. A patient who sees nothing but misfortune in the future may lose all impetus to carry on. Getting out of bed in the morning may take hours.

Suicidal thoughts or acts. Suicide is the most serious complication of depressive disorders and, unfortunately, it is all too common. One percent of all depressed patients kill themselves within 12 months after the onset of a depressive episode. Among patients who suffer from recurrent depressions, 15 percent eventually commit suicide. Depressed patients are at the highest risk for suicide in the 6-to-9-month period *after* they have achieved some symptomatic improvement. Why this seeming paradox? It may be because the patient has regained enough energy and motivation to carry out a suicide plan, but has not regained enough of a positive outlook on life to be able to choose an alternative to self-destruction.

Cognitive symptoms

Sense of guilt, worthlessness, and low self-esteem. Patients who are depressed often berate themselves for perceived shortcomings that they exaggerate but feel are obvious to others. Such patients are unable to realistically evaluate their own performance at daily tasks. Their low self-esteem may vary from mild feelings of inadequacy to severely critical auditory hallucinations as described under "Psychosis" below.

Difficulty in concentrating. Depressed people may be so completely preoccupied with inner thoughts that they have difficulty paying attention to their environment. Patients often complain of "poor memory" or of being unable to keep their minds on such pastimes as reading or watching television. Because demented people also have problems with memory and concentration, it is sometimes difficult to differentiate depression from dementia in the elderly (see Chapter 9).

Psychosis. Depression may be severe enough to include psychotic symptoms, most commonly hallucinations and delusions. The content of these hallucinations and delusions is usually consistent with the depression (*mood congruent*). For example, psychotically depressed patients may suffer from the deluded belief that they are being persecuted because they are sinful or inadequate ("My husband is trying to kill me because I'm a bad wife"); hallucinations frequently take the form of voices that berate patients for their shortcomings.

Somatic symptoms

Bodily complaints. Besides the classic vegetative symptoms of depression, a variety of somatic symptoms are part of the depressive syndrome. In fact, internists and general practitioners are barraged with such complaints; the most frequent are headaches, backaches, muscle cramps, nausea, vomiting, constipation, heartburn, shortness of breath, hyperventilation, and chest pain. Many of these patients undergo various examinations, x-rays, and laboratory tests; some even undergo surgery. Too frequently, the diagnosis of depression is only considered after numerous diagnostic studies have failed to reveal an organic basis for the illness and the doctor concludes that it is "all in the patient's head." Careful inquiry will often uncover other symptoms besides "aches and pains" that point more clearly to the diagnosis of depression.

Classifying Depressive Disorders

The long list above makes it clear that there is tremendous variety in the symptoms of depression. The variations in types of depression become almost infinite when you consider precipitating factors, family histories, and clinical courses. Some people become depressed after obvious traumatic events; others seem to sink into depression for no apparent reason. Some patients have family trees laden with depressed relatives; others have no family history of psychiatric illness. Some patients experience discrete, limited episodes of depressive symptoms; others complain that they have been depressed all their lives.

How can we make sense out of this vast array of clinical presentations? Many classification systems have been proposed, most of them based on unproven theories about the etiology of depression. A newer system, based on symptoms and clinical course, is put forward in the *Diagnostic and Statistical Manual of Mental Disorders*, 3rd edition (DSM-III).

DSM-III defines two basic depressive syndromes: *major depressive episode* and *dysthymic disorder*. In a major depressive episode, symptoms are severe and persistent, and the illness has a discrete, episodic quality. In dysthymic disorder, symptoms fluctuate and are less severe, psychosis is not present, and the illness is long-term. The diagnostic criteria are summarized below.

Major depressive episode
A dysphoric mood that is prolonged and persistent.

At least four of the following symptoms are present nearly every day for at least two weeks:
- Increased or decreased appetite
- Insomnia or hypersomnia
- Psychomotor agitation or retardation
- Loss of interest or pleasure in usual activities
- Decreased sexual drive
- Loss of energy
- Feelings of worthlessness, self-reproach, or guilt
- Impaired ability to think clearly or concentrate
- Suicidal ideation

No psychotic symptoms during periods of normal mood.

Depression is not due to another condition, such as bereavement or an underlying schizophrenic disorder.

Two subtypes of major depressive episode are singled out in DSM-III for special mention:

Depression with psychotic features, which includes gross impairment in reality testing and usually delusions, hallucinations, or depressive stupor (the individual is mute and unresponsive), and

Depression with melancholia, which involves a loss of pleasure in usual activities, and at least three of the following six symptoms: a depressed mood, worsening of depression in the morning, early morning awakening, psychomotor retardation or agitation, anorexia with or without weight loss, and excessive or inappropriate guilt. The emphasis in this subtype is on vegetative signs and diurnal variation in mood—the classic picture of what is often called "involutional melancholia."

Dysthymic disorder (also called "depressive neurosis")

Mild depressive symptoms, present for at least two years, that are not severe or persistent enough to constitute a major depressive episode.

Depression may be episodic or constant, but a period of normal mood lasts no longer than a few months.

Prominent depressed mood or loss of interest in usual activities during depressed periods.

At least three of the following symptoms during periods of depression:

- Insomnia or hypersomnia
- Low energy level
- Feelings of inadequacy or low self-esteem
- Decreased effectiveness at school, work, or home
- Decreased attention or ability to concentrate
- Social withdrawal
- Loss of interest in pleasurable activities
- Irritability or excessive anger
- Inability to respond with pleasure to praise or reward
- Less activity or talkativeness, feeling slowed down or restless
- Pessimistic attitude toward the future, brooding about the past, self-pity
- Tearfulness, crying
- Recurrent thoughts of death or suicide

Psychosis is not present.

Another mental disorder may be present, e.g., a personality disorder or anxiety disorder.

Older systems of classification. The DSM-III diagnostic categories, now widely used, should replace older and less accurate systems. Some more traditional ways of classifying depression will be briefly described here, for they are still used by many clinicians, and you will continue to hear older diagnostic labels used in day-to-day work.

Table 6-3. Comparison of major depressive episode and dysthymic disorder.

Feature	Major depressive episode	Dysthymic disorder
Dysphoric mood	Yes	Yes
Severity of symptoms	Severe	Mild to moderate
Impaired functioning	Common	Less common
Psychosis	May be present	Not present
Persistence of symptoms	Present every day	Usually fluctuating
Duration of symptoms	Every day for two weeks	On and off for two years

Endogenous versus reactive depression

Endogenous depression refers to a syndrome thought to come from *inside* the patient; i.e., it results from internal biological factors and seems to have a life of its own, rather than being dependent on environmental influences. The hallmarks of endogenous depression are prominent physiological disturbances (sleep, appetite, energy); absence of environmental precipitants (deaths, personal losses); and stable premorbid personality patterns without self-pity, hypochondriasis, or self-dramatizing attitudes.

Reactive depression, by contrast, refers to a syndrome triggered by factors in the patient's environment, rather than biological factors. Such depressions are characterized by obvious precipitating events and life stresses, the absence of significant vegetative disturbances, fluctuation of symptoms according to psychological and environmental factors, and unstable, "neurotic" premorbid personality patterns.

The value of the endogenous-reactive dichotomy lies in calling attention to the importance of the vegetative signs of sleep disturbance, weight loss, anergy, and psychomotor retardation or agitation, and in emphasizing the favorable response of these symptoms to antidepressants and electroconvulsive therapy (ECT). However, the problem with this dichotomy is that very few patients fall into one category or the other; most lie somewhere on a continuum between the endogenous and reactive extremes. For example, almost all depressed patients, if pressed, can cite some recent adverse events in their lives that might be termed precipitants. And many patients have both obvious life stresses and clear vegetative signs. To further complicate matters, the presence of precipitating life stresses does not rule out a favorable response to drugs or ECT.

Psychotic versus neurotic depression

Psychotic depression is used quite specifically to denote depression in which the patient has lost the ability to test reality, and this is often manifested by delusions, hallucinations, or profound confusion. Roughly 10 percent of all depressed patients have psychotic symptoms. But the term has also been used more broadly to denote depression with severe impairment in social and personal functioning, inability to perform daily tasks, and withdrawal from others. Psychotic depressions are thought to be biologically based.

In *neurotic depression* reality testing remains intact and, more broadly, day-to-day functioning is not significantly impaired. The term implies social and psychological origins, rather than a biological cause.

This distinction is another dichotomy of limited usefulness. Applied to depression, the term "psychotic" is ambiguous, since it can refer either to specific psychotic symptoms or to the severity of the syndrome. Also, considering the wide spectrum of severity of depressive disorders, it is rather arbitrary to decide that one person has a depression of psychotic severity while another's is simply neurotic.

However, the presence or absence of specific psychotic symptoms is a crucial piece of data in the evaluation of every depressed patient. Besides having implications for long-term treatment (to be discussed later), the presence of psychotic symptoms should alert the clinician to an increased risk of suicide and prompt consideration of a hospital admission.

Agitated versus retarded depression

Agitated depression refers, quite simply, to the clinical picture that includes psychomotor agitation—excessive, unproductive, and tension-relieving activity, like hand-wringing, hair-pulling, nail-biting, and pacing, along with such vocal expressions of psychic pain as sighing or moaning. Agitated depressions are much more common in older patients (peaking in the fifties and sixties), and often include psychotic symptoms. ECT and tricyclic antidepressants are helpful in the treatment of agitated depressions.

Retarded depression refers to a clinical picture that includes psychomotor retardation—slowed, unspontaneous thought and action. The presence of psychomotor retardation predicts a good response to tricyclic antidepressants.

The agitated versus retarded dichotomy is of particularly limited usefulness because many depressed patients show a mixture of agitated and retarded features. Also, many depressed patients have normal rates of psychomotor activity and do not fall into either category.

Differential Diagnosis

In making the diagnosis of major depressive episode or dysthymic disorder, you must rule out conditions that mimic depression and underlying illnesses that manifest themselves secondarily as depression.

Organic causes. These are too numerous to list in their entirety, but the more common ones are:

Drugs—Among the many drugs that can cause depression are reserpine, propranolol, steroids, methyldopa, oral contraceptives, ethanol, marijuana, and hallucinogens. Amphetamine withdrawal can also produce a depressive syndrome, as can withdrawal from benzodiazepines and barbiturates.

Infectious diseases—pneumonia, hepatitis, mononucleosis.

Neoplasms—These often first present as depression, particularly carcinoma of the head of the pancreas.

Endocrine disorders—especially of the thyroid, adrenals, or pituitary.

Central nervous system (CNS) disorders—cerebral vascular insults.

Systemic diseases—including anemias and nutritional deficiencies. The work-up for patients with depression should include the routine screening measures shown in Table 6-4, as well as the additional measures that are done if the patient's history or clinical presentation suggest a particular underlying problem.

Dementia. Because demented patients experience memory loss and difficulty in concentrating, it can be difficult to distinguish between depression and dementia, particularly in the elderly (see Chapter 9).

Psychological reaction to a physical illness. People who suddenly find themselves bedridden or functionally impaired because of a medical condition often react by becoming depressed.

Schizophrenia. Differentiating between psychotic depression

Table 6-4. The medical work-up of the depressed patient.

Routine screening measures
  Medical history—including drug use
  Physical examination
  Complete blood count (CBC)
  Routine blood chemistries (SMA-12)
  Thyroid function tests
  Urinalysis

Additional screening measures
  Neurology consultation
  Chest X-ray
  Electrocardiogram (EKG)
  Computerized tomographic (CT) scan

and schizophrenia may be difficult. *In schizophrenia, depressive symptoms usually follow the onset of psychosis; in psychotic depression, the affective disturbance precedes or coincides with the onset of psychosis.* A history of normal functioning between psychotic episodes suggests affective illness, as does a family history of affective illness. Also, schizophrenic patients may have secondary depressive episodes, particularly on recovering from an acute psychotic break.

   Schizoaffective disorder. This is often called a "wastebasket diagnosis," because the label is given to patients whose symptoms and clinical course make it impossible to differentiate between depression and schizophrenia.

   Bipolar disorders. Those who present initially with depression may later manifest elation or mania as well, taking them out of the unipolar category. At this time, we are unable to predict which people who present as unipolar depressives will go on to reveal a bipolar illness instead.

   Uncomplicated bereavement. A full depressive syndrome is frequently a normal reaction to the death of a loved one. It may include sleep and appetite disturbance. Such a reaction rarely begins more than two or three months following a loss, and it does not result in marked or prolonged functional impairment. Remember that the duration of normal bereavement varies widely among different ethnic groups.

   Personality disorders. Many patients with personality disorders—particularly borderline, histrionic, dependent, and obsessive-compulsive disorders—have depressive symptoms as well. Like the personality disorder itself, the depression is usually chronic, has fluctuating symptoms, and usually meets the criteria for dysthymic disorder.

Chronic alcohol dependence. Alcohol addiction is often associated with depressive symptoms. It is thought that many alcoholics are actually depressed and "self-medicate" underlying depression by drinking, but chronic alcohol abuse can also be the sole cause of depressive symptoms.

Anxiety. Because a large percentage of depressed patients also experience anxiety, the task of distinguishing between anxiety disorders and depressive disorders is not always easy. As more and more studies point out the efficacy of antidepressant medication in treating panic disorders, the overlap between depression and anxiety becomes even greater. Anxious patients usually describe themselves as being primarily anxious, and depressed patients as being primarily depressed. Anxious patients tend to complain more of bodily symptoms than do depressed patients.

Normal mood fluctuations. Obviously, all of us have experienced depressed feelings at some time in our lives. However, normal mood fluctuations are not as prolonged or as severe as those in dysthymic disorder, nor do normal mood changes interfere significantly with day-to-day functioning.

Clinical Course

Major depressive disorder. Symptoms of a major depressive episode usually develop over a period of days to weeks, but they may develop quite suddenly—particularly after a severe life stress. The depressive episode is sometimes preceded by several months of milder symptoms, by anxiety, or by panic attacks.

Most acute depressive episodes are self-limiting and have a good prognosis even without specific therapy, but somatic therapies (antidepressants, ECT) decrease the intensity of the symptoms and hasten recovery. Before the advent of somatic therapies, most acute depressive episodes lasted six to eight months; with these therapies, such episodes now last only several weeks. More than half of those who have a first major depressive episode go on to have one or more recurrences in their lifetime; a minority of patients recover completely after one episode.

Most patients get back to normal—i.e., return to their previous levels of functioning—between depressive episodes, but about 15 to 30 percent of patients with major depressions never return to their premorbid state of mental health; they have residual symptoms and social impairment. Factors that seem to predispose certain depressed patients to a chronic "downhill" course are advanced age, a family history of depression, longstanding personality problems, and lack of social supports.

Patients who have recurrent depressive episodes are more likely to go on to develop a manic or hypomanic episode (i.e., bipolar illness) than those who only experience a single depressive episode.

Dysthymic disorder. Unlike major depressive disorder, dysthymic disorder has no clear onset, but seems to the patient as if it had always been there. A chronic, rather than episodic, course is the rule. Social and occupational impairment may be mild or even moderate, but this is due to the chronicity of the symptoms rather than to their severity. Hospitalization is rarely necessary unless the patient seriously plans or attempts suicide.

Epidemiology

Depressive disorders are ubiquitous. The following figures give a sketch of their distribution in the general population.

Morbid risk. At least 10 percent of adults in the general population have one or more major depressive episodes at some time in their lives. Some estimates place an individual's lifetime risk of developing a major depressive or dysthymic disorder as high as 30 percent.

Age at onset. Dysthymic disorder usually begins early in adult life. Major depressive disorder may begin at any age, and the age at onset is fairly evenly distributed throughout adulthood. Contrary to popular belief, depression is no more common among the elderly than among younger adults.

Sex. Major depressive disorder is roughly twice as common in women as in men, and dysthymic disorder has been estimated to be four to five times more common in women than men. The reasons for this difference are not fully understood.

Socioeconomic status. No strong or constant trend has been demonstrated, but depression appears to be somewhat more common in the higher social strata.

Marital status. There is no appreciable difference among single, married, divorced, and widowed people in the incidence of major depressive disorder. Some reports have shown increased incidence of dysthymic disorder among separated and divorced persons, but this trend is not striking.

Family history. There is a clear tendency for major depressive disorder to run in families. Familial patterns in dysthymic disorder have not been established.

Etiology

No single causal factor has been identified as the basis of depression. Indeed, the depressive syndromes are so varied in their course and symptomatology that discovery of a single cause of all depressive disorders is highly unlikely. Research points to many factors that seem to contribute to the development of depressive illness.

Genetics. Studies of the incidence of depressive illness in twins, families, and the general population strongly suggest a genetic basis for at least some depressive disorders. Evidence includes the fact that relatives of patients with unipolar depressive illness have a higher frequency of depression than the general population. The prevalence of unipolar depression is greatest among first-degree relatives of unipolar depressives. Also, monozygotic twins have a greater concordance rate for depression than do dizygotic twins (i.e., if one twin suffers from depression, it is more likely that the other twin will also suffer from depression if he or she is identical rather than fraternal).

Neurochemical abnormalities. Much attention has been focused on chemicals that transmit nerve impulses from one neuron to another in the brain, particularly norepinephrine and serotonin.

Norepinephrine is found in both the central and peripheral nervous systems and evidence suggests that, in some forms of depression, there is a CNS deficiency of norepinephrine. Abnormally low levels of norepinephrine in the CNS correlate with low levels of its metabolite, 3-methoxy, 4-hydroxyphenylglycol (MHPG), in the urine. And certain tricyclic antidepressants (e.g., imipramine, desipramine) block the reuptake of norepinephrine in presynaptic neurons, increasing the amount of norepinephrine that remains active as a transmitter, and thus remedying the deficiency.

Serotonin is also a CNS neurotransmitter. A lack of serotonin in some depressed patients correlates with low levels of its metabolite, 5-hydroxyindoleacetic acid (5-HIAA) in the cerebrospinal fluid (CSF).

These patients have normal or elevated urinary levels of MHPG, but low levels of 5-HIAA in the CSF. Such patients have been shown to respond clinically to amitriptyline, a tricyclic antidepressant that blocks serotonin re-uptake by presynaptic neurons, and thus increases the amount of serotonin available for neurotransmission.

In summary then, two types of unipolar depression appear to correlate with CNS neurotransmitter deficiency. One is characterized by a norepinephrine deficiency at the synaptic cleft, low urinary levels of MHPG, and a good response to imipramine and desipramine. The other is characterized by a serotonin deficiency at the synaptic cleft, low levels of 5-HIAA in the CSF (but normal or elevated levels of urinary MHPG), and a good response to amitriptyline.

It must be emphasized that many patients who are clinically depressed do not have demonstrable norepinephrine or serotonin deficiencies, nor do they necessarily respond to treatment with antidepressants. Thus, neurotransmitter deficiencies do not sufficiently account for all depressive syndromes.

Other biologic factors. Also investigated for possible roles in the etiology of depression are electrolyte disturbances, electroencephalographic abnormalities, and neuroendocrine abnormalities. Hypothalamic, pituitary, adrenal cortical, thyroid, and gonadal functions have been examined for possible clues. Of particular interest at the time of this writing is the pituitary-adrenal axis and the empirical finding that some depressed patients cannot suppress cortisol production by the adrenal cortex when challenged with a dose of dexamethasone sufficient to suppress cortisol production in normal individuals (see Chapter 15 for a discussion of the dexamethasone suppression test).

Personality and psychodynamic factors. The literature on the psychodynamics of depression is vast. No single personality trait or group of traits has been identified as predisposing one to depression, nor has a single psychological mechanism by which depression comes about been elucidated.

Many psychodynamic theorists note that those prone to depression are characterized by low self-esteem and a high degree of self-criticism. Some conceptualize depression as anger turned inward. Others write about instability and insecurity in early mother-child interactions as laying the groundwork for later sensitivity to separations from loved ones.

In studying the roots of depression, much attention has been focused on the role of interpersonal loss. Freud and his followers examined the similarities (and differences) between normal bereavement and depression, noting that patients commonly seek help for depressive episodes that seem to come on the heels of some setback in personal relationships (e.g., loss of a job, death of a loved one, breakup of a marriage or romance). Researchers have noted an increased incidence of depression among adults who suffered the loss (by death) of a parent in childhood. Such early losses may make individuals particularly sensitive to losses later in life, and thus more vulnerable to depressive illness. But not all those who lose parents in childhood become depressed as adults, and there seem to be many variables that determine one's response to loss. And the variety of psychological factors that contribute to depression is practically infinite.

Treatment

Optimism is usually justified in treating patients with depressive disorders. Currently available therapies have proved effective and afford depressed patients a good prognosis, particularly in cases of acute depressive episodes. A wide range of somatic and psychological treatment modalities is useful in depression. You must be ready to use varying combinations of treatments tailored to each individual patient's needs. Basic approaches to the treatment of depression are outlined below.

Treat emergencies first. *Suicide* constitutes the greatest danger to depressed people, and you must assess the suicide potential of every patient who complains of depressed feelings. Suicidal thoughts and actions may be obvious, or clues to self-destructive intent may be subtle. For example, drug abuse, reckless driving, and other "daring" activities often represent disguised suicide wishes the patient may not recognize (for the assessment of suicide risk, see Chapter 12).

The danger of *homicide* must not be overlooked, since people with depression may try to kill others on the basis of deluded beliefs (e.g., the mother who feels her children would be better off dead).

Acute psychosis must be treated as an emergency, as must severe *starvation* and/or *dehydration* secondary to anorexia. All of the above conditions should prompt you to consider immediate hospitalization to stabilize the patient medically and keep the patient and others physically safe.

Somatic therapies. Medications and ECT are particularly useful in depressive disorders that include psychosis and/or physical

Table 6-5. General indications for hospitalizing a depressed patient.

Significant risk of suicide
Significant risk of homicide
Loss of ability to care for oneself, either because of immobilizing symptoms
or because of psychotic thinking
Acute medical conditions of life-threatening proportion that result from the
depression (e.g., anorexia, dehydration)
Concomitant medical conditions (e.g., severe cardiac disease) that require
special diagnostic and treatment considerations

symptoms (particularly the classic vegetative signs noted above).

Tricyclic antidepressants (TCAs) are the most widely used medications for depression. Their actions seem to be related to their capacity to potentiate the CNS actions of norepinephrine and serotonin. TCAs are used in the treatment of acute depressive episodes, to alleviate more chronic depressive syndromes, and to prevent recurrent depressive episodes. The indications for the use of TCAs are discussed in detail in Chapter 15, along with the principles of prescribing these medications.

Lithium is most widely used as an antimanic drug, but recent studies have shown lithium to be effective in preventing the recurrence of depressive episodes in unipolar depressives. Lithium maintenance is now being used as an alternative to TCA maintenance for the prophylaxis of recurrent depression. However, lithium has not been demonstrated to be useful in treating acute depressive episodes.

The antidepressant action of *monoamine oxidase inhibitors* (MAOIs) is thought to be related to their ability to block the metabolism of norepinephrine and serotonin in the CNS. MAOIs are generally the second-line drugs in treating depression pharmacologically because they are somewhat less effective than TCAs, and adverse reactions are more common with MAOIs than with TCAs. However, MAOIs are useful in treating depression with atypical symptoms, in cases where TCAs are contraindicated or have not proved helpful (see Chapter 15 for more details).

ECT, sometimes referred to as "shock treatment," involves the induction of a seizure by passing a controlled pulse of electrical energy through the brain. The seizure is induced while the patient is partly paralyzed by a muscle relaxant and under general anesthesia. The seizure itself is necessary for the antidepressant effect of ECT, although

ECT's mechanism of action is not known. Courses of treatment vary, but patients often receive between 6 and 20 treatments, given at a rate of 3 or 4 treatments per week. ECT is safe and highly effective. It has the advantage of being *rapidly* effective; response often occurs within days rather than weeks. Thus, ECT is frequently the treatment of choice when depressive symptoms are so severe as to be life-threatening and rapid improvement is essential (see Chapter 15).

Major tranquilizers, also called antipsychotics or neuroleptics, are very useful in depression that is complicated by psychotic symptoms or overwhelming anxiety. They are often used in combination with TCAs or with ECT, since psychotic depression does not generally respond well to antidepressant therapy alone. Symptoms likely to respond to treatment with antipsychotics include delusions, hallucinations, confusion, and overwhelming anxiety.

Sedatives and minor tranquilizers (benzodiazepines, barbiturates, and other sedatives and antianxiety agents) are sometimes used to treat anxiety, restlessness, insomnia, and irritability that are part of depressive syndromes. However, when depression is the basis for these symptoms, they frequently resolve with antidepressant therapy. Like all CNS depressants, these drugs can actually *cause* depression and thereby complicate rather than alleviate the illness.

Note that insomnia associated with a depressive syndrome is best treated by treating the depression itself, not by the chronic use of sedatives or hypnotics.

Psychological therapies. *Individual psychotherapy* based on psychodynamic principles is the most widely used psychosocial treatment for depression. Psychodynamic psychotherapy emphasizes the importance of past experiences and unconscious motivation in determining human behavior.

Short-term therapy (roughly 5 to 20 sessions) is often aimed at support, crisis intervention, and symptom relief for acutely depressed people so that they may cope better with daily activities and in dealing with others. Long-term psychotherapy (several months to several years) allows patients to identify, examine, and resolve intrapsychic conflicts that impair their lives, and to explore ways in which important childhood experiences have served as inadequate models for current relationships. Patients who improve with short-term treatment may or may not need more extended psychotherapy. The decision to continue in long-term treatment is usually based on whether a patient's life is *chronically* hampered by emotional difficulties and the extent to which he or she is motivated to explore these difficulties.

Group psychotherapy can help depressed people improve their social skills and self-esteem. A therapy group provides a mutually supportive environment in which patients can examine their styles of dealing with others and test out new ways of forming relationships.

Cognitive therapy is a specific technique for treating depression and anxiety. It is based on the premise that distorted modes of thinking about oneself and the world in negative and pessimistic terms foster depression and that, by identifying such cognitive distortions and teaching the patient to substitute more realistic and self-enhancing thoughts, painful feelings can be reduced. The therapy is short-term and sessions are more structured than in psychodynamic psychotherapy.

In clinical studies, cognitive therapy has been shown to be of value to many depressed and anxious patients. Clinicians debate whether the therapeutic effects are due to cognitive therapy techniques per se or to the trust and rapport that develop between patient and therapist. Equally controversial is the assumption in cognitive therapy that negative thoughts can actually *cause* painful feelings rather than simply result from them. Cognitive therapy continues to be a subject of active research (see Chapter 15).

Combining different treatment modalities. Used in combination, somatic and psychosocial treatments are generally more effective than either modality alone. Psychotherapy influences social effectiveness and personality functioning, while medications and ECT affect physiologic functions like sleep, appetite, and sexual drive.

Thus, many patients can benefit from both types of treatment. Decisions about treatment must be based on the availability of resources, on the patient's willingness to comply with different regimens, and on the patient's motivation to engage in self-exploratory work.

No one treatment for depression is universally effective, and none has been shown to be the treatment of choice for all types of depression. Ongoing clinical trials are now attempting to evaluate the relative efficacy of different treatments used alone and in various combinations.

BIPOLAR DISORDERS

Bipolar disorders are illnesses that are characterized by two extremes of mood: elation and depression. Stereotypically, the patient with bipolar disorder cycles from wild mania into deep depression and back into mania again. In reality, bipolar illness covers a variety of clinical pictures that will be discussed below.

Depressive episodes in bipolar illness are clinically indistinguishable from those seen in unipolar illness. Thus, the distinctive—and often most dramatic—feature of bipolar illness is elation. Like depression, elation encompasses a broad spectrum of moods, including normal states of euphoria and joy, as well as the pathological elations known as mania and hypomania. *Mania* denotes extreme elation, hyperactivity, agitation, and accelerated speech, often with disordered thinking. *Hypomania* refers to a syndrome similar to, but not as severe as, mania. Many clinicians use "hypomania" to refer to elation without psychosis, and reserve the term "mania" for elation so severe as to include disordered thinking.

The term "elation" warrants an explanatory note. A patient's subjective experience of mania and hypomania can be pleasurable, involving feeling "high," happy, and euphoric, but these mood states are also characterized by extreme irritability, paranoia, and rage. Thus, it would be more accurate to speak of *excited* rather than elated mood states, since the manic patient's subjective experience often varies from extreme euphoria to profound dysphoria.

The major syndromes included under bipolar disorders are *manic-depressive illness* and *cyclothymic disorder*. The two are distinguished on the basis of the intensity and duration of symptoms.

Manic-Depressive Illness

Manic-depressive illness (MDI) generally includes full-blown episodes of mania and depression. Manic episodes may alternate one for one with depressive episodes, or one mood extreme may predominate. While patients who only experience depressive episodes are categorized as having unipolar illness, patients who only experience manic episodes are included in the bipolar category. Such patients are quite rare; the rule in MDI is a history of both depressive and manic episodes.

Symptoms of mania. The symptoms of depressive episodes have already been discussed at length. Since the diagnosis of MDI hinges on the recognition of manic episodes, it is essential that you learn to recognize the symptoms of mania and hypomania. The cardinal symptoms outlined in DSM-III are listed in Table 6-6 and described below.

Mood disturbance. The manic patient commonly experiences

Table 6-6. The symptoms of mania and hypomania.

Mood disturbance (euphoria, irritability)
Hyperactivity (motor restlessness, overinvolvement socially, at work, or
    sexually)
Pressured speech
Flight of ideas
Distractibility
Inflated self-esteem
Decreased need for sleep
Lability of mood
Delusions and hallucinations (in mania)

---

euphoria, and this mood can be quite infectious. In fact, you may find yourself smiling and suppressing the urge to laugh when interviewing a euphoric patient; such a reaction should prompt you to suspect the diagnosis of mania. Those who know the patient well usually recognize that the euphoria is uncharacteristic and excessive. Manic patients have seemingly limitless enthusiasm for interacting with others, and commonly seek people out in an intrusive way (e.g., they may call friends to chat at 4:00 a.m., and be oblivious to others' wish to sleep). As noted above, the predominant mood in some manic patients is *irritability* rather than euphoria. Particularly when their desires are in any way thwarted, manic patients can respond with extreme annoyance, even rage and violence (whence the term "maniac").

Hyperactivity. This includes motor restlessness and overinvolvement in sexual, recreational, occupational, and other activities. Manic patients will plan and enter into a variety of projects, overcommitting themselves and using poor judgment. A patient may, for example, start to repaint his house, begin to write a novel, and rebuild his auto engine—all in one day. Along with poor judgment, manic patients commonly demonstrate expansiveness, grandiosity, and unwarranted optimism—and these characteristics lead to many painful consequences. For example, a patient in the throes of mania can give away an entire fortune, amass huge debts on a buying spree, take off impulsively on a trip around the world, drive recklessly, engage in uncharacteristic sexual behavior, or stand on street corners and engage strangers in conversation.

Pressured speech. Manic patients speak as if they are under pressure to get the words out. They speak loudly and rapidly and are usually difficult to interrupt. Their speech content may be normal, or full of jokes and puns, or full of hostile accusations and angry tirades. Manic patients often have a theatrical style and can be quite entertaining. Associations and word choice may be based on sounds rather than ideas, resulting in *clang associations* (e.g., "talk—tic-toc—what's up doc?").

Flight of ideas. This involves skipping from one idea to another in a continuous flow of accelerated speech. The speaker makes associations that are comprehensible but based on puns, extraneous stimuli, or other chance factors. If it is severe, flight of ideas can make the manic patient's speech impossible to follow.

Distractibility. Manic patients have difficulty in screening out extraneous stimuli. They often react to noises, sights, or smells, shifting their focus of attention rapidly from one irrelevant stimulus to another (hence, the use of seclusion as a means of calming agitated manic patients).

Inflated self-esteem. An unrealistic sense of one's own merits and importance often accompanies an elevated mood. Some patients simply become overconfident and less self-critical; others develop grandiose ideas of delusional proportions. Patients may come to believe, for example, that they have a special relationship with God, that they have a plan to save the universe from destruction, or that they have unparalleled gifts they must share with the world.

Decreased need for sleep. Almost all manic patients experience a decreased need for sleep, feeling full of energy despite little or no rest. Some manic patients actually go without any sleep for days at a time and do not report feeling tired.

Lability of mood. Some manic patients move rapidly from

Table 6-7. The medical work-up of the manic patient.

Medical history—including drug use
Physical examination
Routine laboratory screening
  Complete blood count (CBC)
  Blood chemistries (SMA-12)
  Urinalysis
  Thyroid function tests
Screening of blood and urine for toxic substances

---

euphoria to anger or depression. Mood swings may last for minutes or even several hours at a time, but rarely longer.

Delusions and hallucinations. The content of delusions or hallucinations is usually consonant with an elevated and grandiose mood. For example, a patient may believe that he or she is being persecuted by enemy agents because of possessing special powers. Another patient may believe he or she sees God and speaks directly with Him.

Diagnosis of mania
An **elevated, expansive, or irritable mood.**

At least **three of the following symptoms** persisting for at least one week:
- Increase in activity or physical restlessness
- Increase in talkativeness or pressured speech
- Flight of ideas or racing thoughts
- Inflated self-esteem
- Decreased need for sleep
- Distractibility
- Excessive involvement in activities the person does not realize may have painful consequences (e.g., buying sprees, reckless driving, sexual indiscretions).

No psychosis or bizarre behavior during periods of normal mood.

Symptoms are not due to another condition, such as schizophrenia or a paranoid disorder or to substance abuse.

Differential diagnosis. Many clinical studies have concluded that MDI has been underdiagnosed in the United States in recent years because bipolar disorder is frequently mistaken for other psychiatric illnesses, most notably schizophrenia. Although there are many causes of excited and elated states, only a small number of disorders are commonly confused with manic-depressive illness:

Organic affective syndromes. Organic causes of elation and full-blown mania include the use of such drugs as steroids, alcohol, and amphetamines and specific illnesses like cerebral tumors, multiple sclerosis, and dementia. The work-up of a first acute manic episode should include a thorough physical examination, routine laboratory screening (complete blood count, routine blood chemistries, urinalysis), screening of serum and urine for toxic substances, and a thorough medical and drug history to rule out organic causes of mania.

Schizophrenia. Mania and schizophrenia often look very similar. In some cases it is almost impossible to distinguish between them on the basis of presenting symptoms alone. For example, hallucinations, paranoia, grandiose delusions, loose associations, bizarre behaviors, and irritability are common features of both illnesses. Thus, the clinician must frequently rely on factors other than the patient's mental status to make as accurate a diagnosis as possible. Table 6-8 outlines historical data that favor a diagnosis of MDI and those that favor a diagnosis of schizophrenia.

Schizoaffective disorder. This diagnostic category is used for people who exhibit symptoms of an affective illness (mania and/or depression) but whose chronic impairment of thought and functioning is more consistent with schizophrenia. Many clinicians consider this a "wastebasket" diagnosis, and believe schizoaffective disorder is a variant of MDI or schizophrenia rather than a separate disease entity. The diagnosis is usually made when it is impossible to categorize an illness as MDI or schizophrenia. Lithium and TCAs are often used for schizoaffective patients, but generally with less success than in treating true bipolar or unipolar affective illness. Antipsychotic drugs are also used to treat disordered thinking, and the combination of an antipsy-

Table 6-8. Features which help to differentiate between manic-depressive illness (MDI) and schizophrenia.

Favors MDI	Favors schizophrenia
Previous episode of mania or depression	No previous history of affective disturbance
History of complete recovery between acute episodes of illness	History of residual impairment between acute exacerbations of illness
Good premorbid functioning	Gradual deterioration and poor premorbid functioning
Family history positive for a remitting psychotic illness	Family history negative for remitting psychotic illness
History of favorable treatment response to lithium and/or ECT	Poor response to treatment with lithium and/or ECT

chotic and lithium or a TCA is very common in treating schizoaffective illness.

Cyclothymic disorder. Essentially, this disorder involves periods of depression and hypomania, but with briefer mood swings and less severe symptoms than in MDI. This diagnosis will be discussed at greater length below.

Clinical course. Patients with MDI may initially present with either a manic or a depressive episode. Obviously, a patient who presents with a depressive episode and no history of mania may have either bipolar or unipolar illness. Only time will tell whether that person will go on to have manic episodes or only experience bouts of depression.

In bipolar illness, the first affective disturbance is often manic. Manic episodes generally begin suddenly and escalate rapidly over a few days. Mania may persist for several days or several months, but the episodes are generally briefer and occur more abruptly than major depressive episodes. Particularly if it is not treated early, mania generally goes through stages of severity, beginning with a mild syndrome and progressing to a much more dramatic and disorganized clinical picture. Initially, mood is predominantly euphoric, but the manic patient becomes increasingly irritable and finally panicked and/or enraged. What begins as mildly increased psychomotor activity develops into frenzied and bizarre behavior; initial suspiciousness, grandiosity, and racing thoughts give way to frank delusions, hallucinations, and flight of ideas. This increase in severity is followed by a gradual abatement of symptoms and ultimately a return to normal mood in the majority of manic patients, but the rate at which patients pass through these stages of mania is highly variable.

Almost all patients who have one or more manic episodes will eventually have at least one depressive episode. An episode of either type may be followed immediately by a brief episode of the other kind, but manic and depressive episodes are usually separated by an intervening period of normal mood and functioning. Some patients go for years after an initial affective disturbance without any recurrence; others have clusters of manic and depressive episodes; others have increasingly frequent manic and/or depressive episodes as they grow older.

There is a subgroup of manic-depressive patients (estimates range from 10 to 35 percent) who do not return to normal moods or functioning between episodes, but have a chronic course with significant residual symptomatic and social impairment.

Before lithium, ECT, and antipsychotics were used in the treatment of mania, the average duration of a manic episode was three months; with these modalities, that time has been considerably shortened. Since there is marked variation in both the severity and duration of manic and depressive episodes and the length of intervening periods of normal mood, you should develop a profile of mood cycles for each patient in order to plan for the most effective treatment.

The most common complications in the course of a manic episode are substance abuse and the consequences (personal, financial, etc.) of poor judgment.

Epidemiology. The annual rate of first hospital admission for MDI in men is 8 to 10 per 100,000; in women, it is 15 to 20 per 100,000 population. Between 0.4 and 1.2 percent of the adult population carries the diagnosis. The lifetime risk of developing MDI is roughly 1 to 2 percent.

Age. The first manic episode in bipolar disorder usually occurs before age 30. In fact, a first manic episode in a patient over the age of 50 is so rare that you should strongly suspect an organic cause of mania (e.g., drugs, CNS tumor).

Sex. MDI is roughly as common in men as in women, although studies suggest a slight preponderance of the disease among women (male:female=1.0:1.5). This is in contrast to the unipolar depressive disorders, which are much more common in women than in men.

Socioeconomic status. Although there are no sharp distinctions on the basis of social class, there appears to be a somewhat higher incidence of MDI in the higher social strata.

Marital status. There is no appreciable difference in the incidence of MDI on the basis of marital status.

Family history. The frequency of MDI is markedly higher among the biologic relatives of those who have the disease.

Etiology. The etiology of MDI is not known. As with unipolar depressive disorders, researchers have looked at a wide variety of biological and psychological variables in an effort to find a cause for MDI.

The most substantial information we have to date is about the genetic basis of the illness. Twin studies, family studies, and surveys of the general population support the idea of a genetic predisposition to MDI. Most striking are twin studies that show the concordance rates for MDI to be 68 percent for monozygotic twins and 23 percent for same-sex dizygotic twins.

It is possible that incomplete gene penetrance accounts for the fact that the concordance rate for MDI in monozygotic twins is less than 100 percent. However, it is also possible that other nongenetic factors operate in determining which individuals develop the clinical syndrome of MDI and which do not.

Neurochemical studies of manic-depressive patients have shown decreased levels of urinary MHPG during depressive episodes, but no similar derangement of the levels of biogenic amines during manic episodes. Investigators have speculated that mania results from an increase in dopamine levels in the brain, but this hypothesis has not been proven in research studies. Investigators have also hoped to solve the mystery of MDI by elucidating the mechanism by which lithium exerts its therapeutic effect, but to date we do not know how lithium works.

Treatment

Acute mania. Depending on its severity, an acute manic episode may constitute a psychiatric emergency. You must quickly assess the manic patient for

Self-destructive behaviors. Not only overtly suicidal behaviors, but also acts involving such poor judgment as to be potentially life-threatening (reckless driving, "daredevil" stunts).

Violence. Particularly when paranoia is severe, manic patients can be violent and may even kill others because of a delusional belief that they are acting in self-defense.

Inability to care for himself or herself. In mania, this often takes bizarre forms, e.g., walking naked outdoors in freezing weather, giving away all one's money to strangers, going on wild spending sprees, not sleeping or eating for many days.

Any of the above warrant hospital admission. Hospitalization should also be considered for a first manic episode, to facilitate a complete medical work-up and planning for adequate ongoing treatment.

Treatment of an acute manic episode generally involves both medication and setting limits on manic behavior. Severe mania is often terrifying to the patient—it represents a loss of self-control. Hospital admission to a locked unit can therefore be reassuring, since it conveys the message that others will take control and keep the patient safe.

Similarly, many manic patients initially require locked-door seclusion and physical restraint to keep them from harming themselves or others; this, too, can be reassuring rather than punitive. Physical

Table 6-9. Common therapeutic interventions in manic-depressive illness.

Acute mania
　Setting limits on manic behavior
　　Seclusion
　　Physical restraints
　Antipsychotic medications
　Lithium
　ECT

Acute depression
　Suicide precautions, assistance with self-care
　Antidepressants
　Antipsychotic medications
　ECT

Prevention of further episodes (maintenance)
　Lithium
　Antipsychotic medications
　Antidepressants
　Education about the illness for patients, families
　Psychosocial therapy

restraint should be used only when other measures have proved insufficient to calm the patient. Frequently, unlocked seclusion alone will have a significant calming effect. Manic patients are highly excitable and easily distracted, so the simple act of reducing sensory stimulation in a quiet, secluded room can help to ease severe agitation.

Pharmacologic treatment is aimed at both the rapid amelioration of symptoms and long-term reduction in the frequency, severity, and duration of manic episodes.

Antipsychotics are the mainstay of rapid treatment. They have a marked antianxiety effect and can considerably reduce the manic patient's terror, combativeness, and confusion. Patients generally respond to adequate oral or intramuscular doses of neuroleptics (see Chapter 15) within a few hours to a few days, often eliminating the need for seclusion and restraint. Because lithium takes roughly 10 to 14 days to work, an antipsychotic such as chlorpromazine is often the first-line drug. Lithium is started in addition to the neuroleptic as soon as the necessary preliminary laboratory work has been completed. In many cases, the antipsychotic may be discontinued once the patient has been stabilized on lithium.

ECT has been shown to be a safe and effective treatment for acute mania. It is often used as a second-line measure when antipsychotic treatment is either ineffective or, for some reason, contraindicated in a particular case. ECT and lithium should not be used concurrently (i.e., when ECT is administered, lithium should be temporarily discontinued), since there is evidence that this combination may diminish the therapeutic effects of each modality and increase the risk of neuropsychological side effects.

Lithium produces a response in roughly 70 percent of acutely manic patients in 10 to 14 days. It decreases both the severity and duration of the acute manic episode, and dramatically reduces the rate of relapse. Since mood stabilization is related to the amount of lithium in the bloodstream, serum lithium levels are monitored to titrate the correct dosage of the drug. For a more extensive discussion of indications, contraindications, and guidelines for the use of lithium, see Chapter 15.

Acute depression. There is considerable evidence that lithium is effective in preventing depressive episodes, as well as manic episodes, in MDI, but even in patients maintained on lithium, acute depressive episodes do occur and often require treatment with antidepressants in addition to lithium. The principles of treatment are the same for acute depressive episodes in MDI and in unipolar depression. However, there is a critical distinction between bipolar and unipolar depression in the use of tricyclic antidepressants, because TCAs can precipitate mania in bipolar patients. Thus, the treatment of acute depressive episodes in patients known or suspected to be bipolar must be undertaken with caution, and patients must be carefully monitored for signs of developing mania. If mania develops, TCAs must be discontinued and the mania treated.

Prevention of further episodes (maintenance therapy). *Lithium* is the mainstay of long-term, as well as acute, treatment of MDI. It has been shown to prevent recurrent mania and depression with moderate, if not total, efficacy. Because such underlying conditions as renal disease, cardiac disease, and organic brain syndromes can make lithium administration dangerous, a careful medical screening must be done whenever maintenance therapy is contemplated. In addition, patients' serum lithium levels must be sampled on a regular basis (usually monthly or bimonthly) to ensure adequate dosage, and such metabolic parameters as serum creatinine levels and the white blood cell count must be monitored to prevent toxicity. Thus, lithium can only be used safely in patients who can comply with a precise treatment regimen (see Chapter 15).

In patients who manifest residual thought disorder between episodes of mood disturbance, *neuroleptic drugs* are commonly used on a long-term basis along with lithium.

For some manic-depressive patients in whom recurrent depressive episodes are severe and frequent, maintenance therapy with *tricyclic antidepressants* (with or without lithium) may help to prevent cycles of depression. In such cases, the patient must be carefully monitored lest the antidepressant precipitate a manic episode.

Education. It is important to help patients and their families recognize the signs and symptoms of incipient mania and depression, so that they may seek treatment for acute episodes *early*, and thereby increase the likelihood that a full-scale affective disturbance can be prevented or ameliorated. Patients must have a clear idea of what treatment is available (hospital, emergency room, outpatient clinic) and whom they are to contact when they experience affective disturbances.

There is a good deal of controversy over whether any *psychosocial therapy* is helpful for manic-depressives. Certainly supportive therapy can be useful in helping patients to cope with the devastating social and occupational effects of severe affective illness and in promoting compliance in taking medications. But it has not been demonstrated that insight-oriented, exploratory psychotherapy is useful in treating MDI. Manic-depressive illness can occur in an infinite variety of personality types; some manic-depressives in remission may be psychologically quite healthy and function well, while others may have significant underlying personality disorders. In general, patients who, in remission, manifest personality disturbances that impair their functioning are candidates for psychotherapy, along with routine pharmacologic treatment of MDI.

Cyclothymic Disorder

Clinicians recognize the existence of bipolar affective disturbances that are milder and briefer than those in manic-depressive illness. Cyclothymic disorder describes a syndrome of chronic mood disturbance of at least two years' duration, characterized by numerous periods of depression and hypomania that are less severe and less prolonged than those in MDI. By definition, no psychotic features accompany the affective disturbances in cyclothymic disorder, because the presence of psychosis indicates the full-blown affective syndrome of MDI.

Diagnostic criteria. The diagnostic criteria for cyclothymic disorder outlined in DSM-III are as follows:

• During the past two years, there have been numerous periods during which some symptoms characteristic of both depressive and manic syndromes were present, but not of sufficient severity and duration to meet the criteria for a major depressive or manic episode.

• The depressive periods and hypomanic periods may be separated by periods of normal mood lasting months at a time, they may be intermixed, or they may alternate.

• During depressive periods, there is depressed mood or loss of

Table 6-10. Symptoms of depressive and hypomanic periods in cyclothymic disorder.

Depressive symptoms	Hypomanic symptoms
Insomnia or hypersomnia	Decreased need for sleep
Low energy level or chronic fatigue	More energy than usual
Feelings of inadequacy	Inflated self-esteem
Decreased effectiveness or productivity at school, work, or home	Increased productivity, often associated with unusual and self-imposed working hours
Decreased attention, concentration, or ability to think clearly	Sharpened and unusually creative thinking
Social withdrawal	Uninhibited people-seeking (extreme gregariousness)
Loss of interest in or enjoyment of sex	Hypersexuality without recognition of the possibility of painful consequences
Restriction of involvement in pleasurable activities, guilt over past activities	Excessive involvement in pleasurable activities and lack of concern for painful consequences, e.g., buying sprees, foolish business investments, reckless driving
Feeling slowed down	Physical restlessness
Less talkative than usual	More talkative than usual
Pessimistic attitude toward the future, brooding about past events	Overoptimism or exaggeration of past achievements
Tearfulness or crying	Inappropriate laughing, joking, punning

interest or pleasure in almost all the patient's usual activities and pastimes, along with at least three of the symptoms in Table 6-10.

• During hypomanic periods, there is an elevated, expansive, or irritable mood, along with at least three of the symptoms in Table 6-10.

• There are no psychotic features such as delusions, hallucinations, incoherence, or loosening of associations.

• Symptoms are not due to any other mental disorder, such as partial remission of bipolar disorder. However, cyclothymic disorder may precede bipolar disorder.

Cyclothymic disorder usually begins early in adult life, generally with an insidious onset and a chronic course. The degree to which the illness impairs social and occupational functioning is variable, and may range from mild to severe. The disorder was previously assumed to be rare but, as the syndrome has become more clearly defined in recent years, it has been recognized with increasing frequency, particularly among people seeking outpatient treatment. It appears to be more common among women than among men. It is also more prevalent among those who have biological relatives with major depression and bipolar disorder than it is in the general population.

The most common complication of cyclothymic disorder is substance abuse. As in MDI, cyclothymic patients tend to medicate their depression with stimulants and alcohol, and to abuse stimulants and psychedelics during hypomanic periods.

The differential diagnosis of cyclothymic disorder is essentially the same as that for major depressive and manic episodes. Also, MDI may be superimposed on an underlying, more chronic cyclothymic disorder.

Treatment is similar to that of MDI. Many patients experience a stabilization of their moods when they are maintained on adequate amounts of lithium.

A FINAL NOTE ON MOOD DISORDERS

Affective illness is now the subject of intense research in this country and abroad. Exciting data are emerging that suggest the existence of "affective equivalents"—that is, symptoms that do not look like mood disturbances yet respond to antidepressant medications. Among the symptoms thought to be possible affective equivalents are panic attacks and eating disorders. You will undoubtedly hear more about new categories of affective illness in the coming years.

REFERENCES

Affective disorders, in Diagnostic and Statistical Manual of Mental Disorders, 3rd ed. Washington DC, American Psychiatric Association, 1980, pp 205-224.

Appleton WS, Davis JM: Practical Clinical Psychopharmacology, 2nd ed. Baltimore, Williams and Wilkins, 1980, pp 82-136.

Bibring E: The mechanism of depression, in Affective Disorders. Edited by Greenacre P. New York, International University Press, 1953, pp 154-181.

Carlson, GA, Goodwin FK: The stages of mania: a longitudinal analysis of the manic episode. Arch Gen Psychiatry 28:221-228, 1973.

Childress AR, Burns DD: The basics of cognitive therapy. Psychosomatics 22:1017-1027, 1981.

Freud S: Mourning and Melancholia (1917), in Complete Psychological Works, standard ed, vol 14. Translated and edited by Strachey J. London, Hogarth Press, 1957, pp 237-258.

Isenberg PL, Schatzberg AF: Psychoanalytic contribution to a theory of depression, in Depression: Biology, Psychodynamics, and Treatment. Edited by Cole JO, Schatzberg AF, Frazier SH. New York, Plenum Press, 1978, pp 149-171.

Klerman GL: Affective disorders, in The Harvard Guide to Modern Psychiatry. Edited by Nicholi A Jr. Cambridge, MA, Harvard University Press, 1978, pp 253-282.

Lloyd C: Life events and depressive disorder reviewed, I: Events as predisposing factors. Arch Gen Psychiatry 37:529-535, 1980.

MacVane JR, Lange JD, Brown WA, Zayat M: Psychological functioning of bipolar manic-depressives in remission. Arch Gen Psychiatry 35:1351-1354, 1978.

Pope HG Jr, Hudson JI, Jonas JM, et al. Bulimia treated with imipramine: a placebo-controlled, double-blind study. Am J Psychiatry 140:554-558, 1983.

Pope HG Jr, Lipinski JF Jr: Diagnosis in schizophrenia and manic-depressive illness. Arch Gen Psychiatry 35:811-828, 1978.

Schatzberg AF: Classification of depressive disorders, in Depression: Biology, Psychodynamics, and Treatment. Edited by Cole JO, Schatzberg AF, Frazier SH. New York, Plenum Press, 1978, pp 13-40.

Weiner D: The psychiatric use of electrically induced seizures. Am J Psychiatry 136:1507-1517, 1979.

7

Personality Disorders

THE DIVERSITY AND COMPLEXITY of human personality are highly celebrated in our society. It may seem presumptuous, therefore, to speak of "personality types" or "character styles"—to try to fit ourselves amd our fellow beings into categories according to the way we behave. Yet human beings are generally consistent in their ways of dealing with the world and particularly with other people. Our styles of thinking, experiencing, and behaving usually remain stable as we meet a variety of new challenges in new settings—hence the concept of character.

Character is reflected in our attitudes, our interests, our intellectual inclinations, our job aptitudes, and our social affinities. We all know people who fit certain stereotypes of character styles: the hard-driving unemotional scientist who buries himself in his laboratory work and is oblivious to life around him, or the dazzling actress who is the "life of the party." It would be no suprise to hear that the scientist is fastidious and conservative in dress, or that the actress wears lavish and seductive clothing. Nor would it be surprising that the scientist enjoys complex puzzles and mathematical games, while the actress has little interest in balancing her checkbook. Of course, these are stereotypes; fortunately, most people are flexible enough to have a variety of styles in their repertoire. But most of us have a major personality style that shows itself in many different settings during all sorts of activities—in everything from the hobbies we enjoy to the lovers we choose.

Certainly, the "typing" of personalities does not imply any abnormality. In fact, the traits associated with particular personality types are often highly useful and adaptive, for they allow us to tolerate anxiety, to solve problems, to be creative, and to cope with a variety of life's stresses. For example, medical students would be in trouble if they did not posess some "obsessional" capacities for organizing and concentrating on a variety of tasks. Yet labels like "obsessive-compulsive" and "hysterical" have taken on very pejorative connotations in our daily language, and it is fashionable to use such terms in a sort of diagnostic name-calling.

When do personality *traits* become personality *disorders?* The boundary is not clear but, generally, when character traits are so maladaptive and inflexible that they significantly impair one's work life and social life, or cause major subjective distress, a diagnosis of personality disorder is warranted.

WHAT ARE PERSONALITY DISORDERS?

Personality disorders are common, they are difficult to treat, and the people who have them typically end up being labeled "bad" or "deviant" by others—even by mental health professionals. With that ominous prelude, let us look at some general characteristics of all personality disorders. The following generalizations may not hold true in every case, but they are good rules of thumb to help you put this category of psychopathology into a larger context:

• Personality disorders involve inflexible and maladaptive responses to stress.

• Personality disorders are global—they affect nearly all areas of a person's life, so that he or she is severely handicapped in working and loving. By contrast, neurotics are people whose problems are confined to discrete aspects of their lives, while other aspects remain relatively free of psychological conflict.

• People with personality disorders commonly feel the problem lies not within themselves but in their environment (e.g., "No one understands me!" or "Everyone thwarts my plans!"). Neurotic patients are more likely to locate the source of their problems within them-selves.

• Personality disorders do not, for the most part, involve psychosis. Brief psychotic episodes occur, but florid lapses in reality testing (see Chapter 4) are the exception rather than the rule. Most people with personality disorders are in touch with reality most of the time.

• People with personality disorders are often untroubled by their illness, for they fail to see themselves as others see them. In fact, they may feel themselves to be in the best of emotional health, while others are quite distressed by their behavior. They may be dragged to mental health care facilities by others; the vast majority never seek treatment.

• People with personality disorders have an uncanny ability to get under the skin of others. They are likely, therefore, to be rejected by those close to them. They invariably irritate mental health professionals who try to treat them. Treatment is difficult—failure common.

• The complications associated with personality disorders are many. The most common are depression, suicide, violence and antiso-cial behavior, brief psychotic episodes, and multiple drug abuse.

From this list of features, you may wonder whether the label of "personality disorder" is simply a technical way of saying that someone is obnoxious. Indeed, the diagnostic label is easy to misuse in this way, as an epithet for any patient you do not like. But in fact, individuals with personality disorders have specific and often crippling illnesses, defined not by their unpleasantness but by their social dysfunction and personal inflexibility. They are incapable of responding to life's varied stresses and challenges except in a very rigid manner. They are like musicians who can play only one note.

Causes

Little is known about the causes of specific personality disorders.

Environmental factors have been assumed to play the dominant role in the genesis of these disorders. Psychoanalytic theorists have focused primarily on the significance of childhood experiences within the family. However, few good large-scale studies have corre-lated early deprived or traumatic childhoods with later personality disorders. To date, there are no hard data to answer the perplexing question of why some people who suffer early emotional trauma develop severe character pathology while others, with equally unhappy childhoods, do not.

Genetic factors are under active investigation as possible contributors to the development of personality disorders. There is some evidence for the heritability of certain character traits—particularly for the heritability of introverted personality traits. Work is also being done on the heritability of obsessive-compulsive traits.

Other constitutional factors, such as physical illness, seem to play a role in the development of personality disorders in some people. Neurologic disorders—particularly birth-related insults, postencephalitic states, and temporal lobe epilepsy—have been found to increase both the incidence and severity of personality disorders. In fact, a history of minimal brain dysfunction or the presence of "soft" (nonspecific) signs of neurologic dysfunction in childhood correlate with an increased incidence of personality disorders in adolescence and adulthood.

Course and Prognosis

Personality disorders usually become evident in adolesence, or sometimes earlier. Clinical lore holds that, once you have a personality disorder, you have it for life. However, surprisingly little is known about the course of these illnesses. It may be, for example, that personality disorders seem intractable because such people frequently fail in psychiatric treatment. Also, it may be that personality-disordered patients who "grow up" or "burn out"—or in some way get better—cease to require professional attention, leaving only the truly intractable population in treatment and in correctional facilities. More work needs to be done in charting the course of these illnesses.

Diagnosis

The diagnostic criteria for the personality disorders are described below. Diagnosis is often difficult. The following are points to keep in mind in your assessments:

Be suspicious of reports by family or friends that the patient's personality has changed abruptly. Personality disorders do not begin suddenly. A history of sudden change in character should alert you to the possibility of some other illness, especially a central nervous system lesion, incipient psychosis, or drug or alcohol abuse. Any of these can mimic a personality disorder.

Be curious why someone with a personality disorder comes to you at a particular time. Look for some change in important relationships that upset the former balance and suddenly made the disordered personality obvious to the patient or others.

Pay attention to your feelings about the patient. A person who makes you feel intensely angry, helpless, powerful, or frightened in the first few minutes of the interview may be showing you the nature of his or her personality disorder.

Beware of overdiagnosing personality disorders in people who are ethnically and culturally different from you. Behavior is more likely to look abnormal outside its social context.

Eleven personality disorders are described in the third edition of the *Diagnostic and Statistical Manual of Mental Disorders* (DSM-III). Some of these are new to the third edition. The delineation of the various personality disorders has been a difficult task. First, there is no clear boundary to separate personality disorders from less severe conditions; diagnosis involves a measure of subjectivity. Second, personality is too complex to fit neatly into eleven categories. Many people with personality disorders exhibit features of more than one personality type. Some theorists have suggested that personality disorders are more accurately seen as clusters of pathologic traits that can occur in an almost infinite variety of combinations.

Table 7-1. Categorization of patients with personality disorders.

Patients who appear odd or eccentric and who fear social relationships
    Paranoid personality disorder
    Schizoid personality disorder
    Schizotypal personality disorder

Patients who appear dramatic, emotional, or erratic and who act directly on their environment
    Histrionic personality disorder
    Narcissistic personality disorder
    Antisocial personality disorder
    Borderline personality disorder

Patients who are primarily anxious and careful (rather than fearful) of intimacy
    Avoidant personality disorder
    Dependent personality disorder
    Compulsive personality disorder
    Passive-aggressive personality disorder

As you read through the following descriptions, remember that these are stereotypes—individual patients will have highly individual presentations. DSM-III has sorted the personality disorders into three general groups, as shown in Table 7-1.

PARANOID PERSONALITY DISORDER

Profile

"Paranoid" is a common term in our everyday language, used to describe anyone from a jealous boyfriend to politicians who believe in a heavy build-up of nuclear armaments. *Paranoia* refers to a pervasive and unwarranted suspiciousness and mistrust of others. Suspiciousness may be highly justified and adaptive in war and other stressful situations, but paranoid people cannot abandon their suspicions when presented with convincing contradictory evidence. They remain constantly on guard, because for them there is always a war going on.

Paranoid people are keen observers. They search intently for some confirmation that they are in danger. By disregarding facts that do not confirm their suspicions, they invariably find the plots and threats they so ardently seek. They are hypersensitive, they expect trickery a..d disloyalty from others, and they try to avoid all surprises by anticipating them.

Paranoid people appear tense, guarded, and secretive; they are often litigious and highly moralistic. They are usually humorless and overly serious. They have difficulty expressing warm emotions and tolerating feelings of being dependent on others. They appear cold and may be quite logical. They are often interested in electronics, mechanics, and communication devices. They are also keenly aware of power and rank.

Because paranoid people seize upon irrelevant details to confirm their suspicions, they generally do not see the forest for the trees. They have very poor judgment in matters relating to their fears. They may, under stress, become floridly delusional (e.g., believing themselves wanted by the FBI) or experience ideas of reference. As a rule, however, psychotic episodes are brief and transient. The paranoid individual relies heavily on the defense of *projection* to maintain a psychological equilibrium. Projection simply involves attributing one's motives, feelings, or drives to someone else because one finds them unacceptable in oneself. This all happens unconsciously—i.e., individuals who use projection are unaware that the motives they see in others are really their own. They make their inner world safe by making the outer world dangerous. Not surprisingly, paranoid people often bear a striking resemblance to the "demons" they choose.

In an interview, paranoid people are likely to be very businesslike. They may tell you they see no reason why they were referred to you. They may scan the room anxiously and have great difficulty relaxing. Or their preoccupation with details and constant questions may be the only things that belie their fear and mistrust.

Diagnosis. DSM-III provides a list of items that are characteristic of the paranoid patient's current and long-term functioning (p. 309). These diagnostic criteria are shown in Table 7-2.

Table 7-2. DSM-III criteria for the diagnosis of paranoid personality disorder.

Pervasive, unwarranted suspiciousness and mistrust of people, as indicated by at least three of the following:
   Expectation of trickery or harm
   Hypervigilance, manifested by continual scanning of the environment for
      signs of threat, or taking unneeded precautions
   Guardedness or secretiveness
   Avoidance of accepting blame when warranted
   Questioning the loyalty of others
   Intense, narrowly focused searching for confirmation of bias, with loss of
      appreciation of total context
   Overconcern with hidden motives and special meanings
   Pathological jealousy

Hypersensitivity, as indicated by at least two of the following:
   Tendency to be easily slighted and quick to take offense
   Exaggeration of difficulties (e.g., "making mountains out of molehills")
   Readiness to counterattack when any threat is perceived
   Inability to relax

Restricted affectivity, as indicated by at least two of the following:
   Appearance of being "cold" and unemotional
   Pride taken in always being objective, rational, and unemotional
   Lack of a true sense of humor
   Absence of passive, soft, tender, and sentimental feelings

Not due to another mental disorder such as schizophrenia or a paranoid disorder

---

Causes. The causes of this disorder are unknown. A genetic predisposition to paranoid personality disorder has been considered, but no substantial evidence has emerged to date to support this hypothesis.

Some psychoanalytic theorists suggest that people who were the objects of irrational and overwhelming parental rage may come to adopt their parents' style and project onto others the rage they believed was once directed toward them. Others have characterized the families of paranoids as overly constricted emotionally.

Epidemiology. Little is known about the incidence or prevalence, because many paranoid patients never seek treatment. The disorder is more frequently diagnosed in men than in women. There is no known familial pattern, but the disorder occurs with increased frequency in the biologic relatives of schizophrenics.

Course and prognosis. No good long-term outcome studies have been done on paranoid personality disorder. Some people apparently have the disorder throughout life, while others "grow out of it" as stress diminishes or other circumstances change. Some people diagnosed as having paranoid personality disorder go on to develop schizophrenia.

Differential Diagnosis

There are several conditions from which paranoid personality disorder must be differentiated.

Paranoid disorders. These disorders are characterized by persistent psychotic symptoms (e.g., delusions, hallucinations) that are *not* present in paranoid personality disorder.

Schizophrenia. Like paranoid disorders, schizophrenia is marked by persistent psychosis, which does *not* characterize paranoid personality disorder.

Borderline personality disorder. Although borderline patients may show some paranoid features, they tend to be overinvolved in chaotic relationships with people. Paranoid patients, on the other hand, remain aloof and distant from others.

Antisocial personality disorder. Both antisocial and paranoid personality disorders involve difficulty with intimacy, but paranoids do not have the lifelong history of antisocial behavior that is found in antisocial personality disorder.

Impulse disorders. These may be distinguished from paranoid personality disorder because they are characterized primarily by difficulty with impulse control rather than by suspiciousness.

Treatment

Because paranoid people are so frightened of intimacy and so reluctant to trust, a relationship with a therapist may be both longed for and dreaded. You must be particularly careful to operate in as open and straightforward a manner as possible in dealing with such people. Use humor sparingly and with great care at the start, for patients are prone to feel that others are laughing *at* them rather than with them.

You must be careful to assume a professional manner, *not* one that is overly warm; paranoid patients will be suspicious of and frightened by overtures they do not understand. When paranoid patients develop false beliefs about you (e.g., that you are part of a conspiracy to harm them), their accusations can easily become threats. You must limit any threatening behavior, both for your own and the patient's safety.

Among the most commonly used treatments, individual psychotherapy is probably the treatment of choice, although no good controlled studies on the treatment of paranoid personality disorder have been done. A primary aim of therapy is to help paranoid patients see how they attribute their own unacceptable thoughts and feelings to others, and the ways in which this distorted perspective hampers their lives. Paranoid people have difficulty tolerating confrontation by others in group therapy, or tolerating the directive techniques used in behavior modification.

SCHIZOID PERSONALITY DISORDER

Profile

The term *schizoid* has long been used is psychiatry to describe patients who are socially withdrawn, introverted, eccentric, and uncomfortable with other people. If you consider the schizophrenic disorders as a spectrum (see Chapter 5), then schizoid personality disorder—along with paranoid and schizotypal personality disorder—occupies the healthier end of the schizophrenic spectrum. Schizoid individuals resemble schizophrenics in their odd and withdrawn manner but, while schizophrenics have chronically disordered thinking, schizoids do not.

The avoidance of human contact is a way of life for schizoid patients, and they show little need or longing for emotional ties to others. Instead, they are likely to be quite absorbed in their own private fantasy worlds, in which they carry on relationships with imaginary friends. Their sex life may exist only in this world of make-believe. While they may have violent fantasies, they usually express little emotion to others.

Schizoid individuals actively pursue isolation, and will therefore choose solitary jobs other people find difficult to tolerate. They are likely to work as night watchmen or to bury themselves in the stacks of a library. In fact, schizoid people can be quite absorbed in and successful at such pursuits as mathematics and astronomy, which demand little human contact.

In an interview, you will find the schizoid patient to be uncomfortable with you and eager for the meeting to end. He or she will make infrequent eye contact, show little emotion, and offer little in the way of spontaneous comments—answering your questions but not elaborating on answers at all. Occasionally, you may hear odd word usage, but speech and thought content do not generally appear abnormal.

Why does the schizoid person flee from other people? Although he or she is seemingly indifferent to others, the schizoid person usually feels quite vulnerable and finds human interaction confusing, frightening, and painful. The isolation is thus sought in self-defense. One schizoid patient described her situation as that of a tiny, naked baby locked inside a steel drawer (Guntrip, 1973, p. 152).

Diagnosis. The diagnostic criteria given in DSM-III for schizoid personality disorder (p. 311) are shown in Table 7-3.

Table 7-3. DSM-III criteria for the diagnosis of schizoid personality disorder.

Emotional coldness and aloofness and the absence of warm, tender feelings for others

Indifference to praise or criticism or to the feelings of others

Close friendships with no more than one or two persons, including family members

No eccentricities of speech, behavior, or thought that are characteristic of schizotypal personality disorder

Not due to a psychotic disorder such as schizophrenia or paranoid disorder

If under 18, the patient does not meet the criteria for schizoid disorder of childhood or adolescence

---

Causes. No one knows why some individuals become schizoid and others do not. In psychotherapy, schizoid patients commonly report bleak childhoods devoid of emotional warmth, but no prospective studies have been done to see which factors in childhood can be correlated with schizoid personality traits in adult life. There is also considerable speculation, but no clear evidence, of possible genetic factors in the genesis of schizoid personality disorder.

Epidemiology. The incidence, prevalence, and sex ratio of schizoid personality disorder are not known. Many schizoid people never seek treatment.

Course and prognosis. Schizoid personality disorder generally begins in childhood and may last throughout life. Neither the frequency of remission nor the frequency with which schizoid people go on to develop schizophrenia is known.

Differential Diagnosis

Schizoid personality disorder must be differentiated from the following:

Schizophrenia. The presence of a thought disorder at some time during the course of schizophrenia differentiates it from schizoid personality disorder. Also, schizoids usually function better than schizophrenics in work situations.

Schizotypal personality disorder. The schizotypal and schizoid disorders both involve an odd and eccentric manner, but schizotypal personality disorder is closer to schizophrenia in the following respects: poor work history, oddities of perception and communication, and a high frequency of schizophrenic relatives.

Avoidant personality disorder. Individuals with avoidant personalities are similar to schizoid people in that they avoid most human interaction. Unlike schizoid individuals, they profess to long for relationships with others and hang back from them because of extreme sensitivity to rejection.

Paranoid personality disorder. This disorder involves a greater ability to engage others socially. Paranoid people are more verbally aggressive than schizoid people, and less absorbed in fantasy.

Treatment

Individual psychotherapy with schizoid patients is difficult, but by no means impossible. Such patients engage in any human interaction reluctantly, and a therapeutic relationship is no exception. However, as schizoid people begin to trust the therapist, they begin to share their fantasy lives, as well as their intense fears about becoming close to the therapist.

The value of group psychotherapy in treating schizoid people has not been established, but some schizoids manage to become involved in and use groups to experiment with interpersonal closeness.

Since schizoids do not have disordered thinking, antipsychotic medication is not likely to benefit them.

SCHIZOTYPAL PERSONALITY DISORDER

Profile

Schizotypal personality disorder is a new diagnostic category, used to describe a condition that is like schizoid personality disorder but characterized by additional symptoms; it is believed to be genetically linked to schizophrenia. Although it is not always easy to differentiate schizotypal from schizoid individuals, schizotypals are likely to look more obviously strange and eccentric, even to those who meet them in passing.

Patients with schizotypal personality disorder suffer from clear disturbances of thinking and communication. Although they may never have a frank psychotic episode with hallucinations or bizarre delusions, they show milder forms of thought disorder, such as derealization, ideas of reference, and perceptual illusions (see Chapter 4). They are extremely sensitive to others, and so retreat into a world of imaginary relationships and vivid fears and fantasies.

In an interview, you will find schizotypal patients to be withdrawn and to have a great difficulty with face-to-face interaction. They show little feeling, and their affects are at times grossly inappropriate to the subject being discussed. Speech is usually peculiar, in that they use words in odd ways and express ideas unclearly; you may often need to ask for clarification. Although schizotypal patients will be guarded about their inner worlds, they may admit to unfounded beliefs, e.g., that they have special powers, or that they are the focus of special attention.

Diagnosis. DSM-III lists the following characteristics of schizotypal personality disorder (p. 313). At least four must be present for diagnosis:

- Magical thinking, e.g., superstitiousness, clairvoyance, telepathy, sixth sense, "others can feel my feelings" (in children and adolescents, bizarre fantasies or preoccupations).
- Ideas of reference.
- Social isolation, e.g., no close friends or confidants, social contacts limited to essential everyday tasks.
- Recurrent illusions, sensing the presence of a force or person not actually present (e.g., "I felt as if my dead mother were in the room with me"), depersonalization, or derealization not associated with panic attacks.
- Odd speech (without loosening of associations or incoherence), e.g., speech that is digressive, vague, overelaborate, circumstantial, metaphorical.
- Inadequate rapport in face-to-face interaction due to constricted or inappropriate affect, e.g., aloof, cold.
- Suspiciousness or paranoid ideation.
- Undue social anxiety or hypersensitivity to real or imagined criticism.

Causes. This diagnostic category was created in DSM-III for persons who are believed to share a genotype with schizophrenics. This disorder is more common among the biologic relatives of schizophrenics than among the general population, but no studies have clearly demonstrated particular causal factors.

Epidemiology. Because schizotypal personality disorder is a classification new to DSM-III, no epidemiologic information is available on patients who fit into this specific category.

Course and prognosis. The course of patients with schizotypal personality disorder is marked by chronic impairment of role performance and social isolation.

Differential Diagnosis

The validity of this new diagnostic category has yet to be confirmed in clinical studies. The three major disorders from which schizotypal personality must be distinguished are schizoid personality disorder, schizophrenia, and borderline personality disorder.

Schizoids do not show the oddities of speech, perception, and behavior seen among schizotypals. Schizotypals are not frankly psychotic, unlike schizophrenics who have gross psychotic disturbances at some point in their illness. Although many of the cognitive and perceptual oddities of schizotypal personality disorder are also found in borderline personality disorder, borderlines are more likely than schizotypals to have intense, stormy interpersonal relationships.

Treatment

As with schizoid patients, schizotypals are absorbed in fantasy and private belief systems that they may share, with great difficulty, in psychotherapy. Therapy is aimed at establishing a relationship and weathering the difficulties these patients encounter in dealing with another human being. Exploratory psychotherapy is often resisted; supportive treatment is less threatening to many of these patients.

Antipsychotic medication may be of help to diminish disordered thinking in schizotypal personality disorder, but it is not clear that the side effects of these medications outweigh their therapeutic effects in schizotypal patients.

HISTRIONIC PERSONALITY DISORDER

Histrionic personality disorder is really a descendent of *hysteria*, a term used in clinical settings all the time. It is one of the oldest psychiatric diagnoses in Western civilization, and has acquired a bewildering variety of uses over the years.

The four most common uses of the term "hysteria" describe (a) a specific personality style, (b) a conversion reaction (e.g., hysterical paralysis), (c) a neurotic illness characterized by phobias and anxiety, and (d) certain pathological character traits. It has also been used in our culture as a term of disapproval, particularly toward women. We will focus here on hysteria as a normal personality style, and then look at histrionic personality disorder as a pathological exaggeration of that style.

Hysterical people are typically warm and imaginative, with well-developed intuition. They tend to look at the world in global, impressionistic terms rather than focusing on details—i.e., they are "headline readers." They gravitate toward activities that do not require intense concentration on facts but allow for the use of intuitive faculties. Thus, hysterics are less likely to be technicians and scholars than they are to be actors or artists. Hysterics tend to see those things in life that are vivid, colorful, and immediately striking; they often overlook more subtle or more neutral details. They are emotive, and often act as the life of the party in groups. Stereotypically, hysterics are seductive and somewhat superficial in their relationships, getting carried away by exaggerated emotionality that is not founded on deep convictions.

Hysterics characteristically rely on the defense of *repression* to maintain their psychological equilibrium. Repression is akin to forgetting, in that it involves banishing unacceptable ideas, feelings, or impulses from one's conscious awareness in order to decrease anxiety. Thus, the hysteric might simply repress the fact of an upcoming examination and forget to arrive on time. This tendency to "forget" unpleasant facts often makes the hysterical individual appear to be more scatterbrained and less intelligent than he or she really is.

Now let us go on to look at histrionic personality disorder, in which hysterical traits are highly inflexible and maladaptive.

Profile

Although people with histrionic personality disorder may be colorful and outgoing, they are also highly excitable and have great difficulty maintaining deep and lasting attachments to others. They tend to use displays of emotion to control other people—to get attention, to avoid unwanted responsibilities, and to coerce others into taking responsibility for their welfare. Typically, these people can induce guilt in others by throwing temper tantrums or bursting into tears, and their control by these means can be quite powerful. Their affections and loyalties are extremely fickle, and this frustrates those who try to get close to them. While these people are often quite seductive, their purpose in attracting partners is not always sexual—e.g., they may seduce lovers who will then satisfy their wishes to be taken care of and nurtured.

Diagnosis. The diagnostic criteria given in DSM-III for histrionic personality disorder (p. 315) are shown in Table 7-4.

Causes. The etiology of histrionic personality disorder has not been demonstrated in any prospective studies.

Epidemiology. Little information is available on the prevalence of this disorder, because people with this condition previously were included in the larger and more ambiguous category of hysterical personality. The disorder is diagnosed much more frequently in women than in men, but this may reflect sex-role bias on the part of diagnosticians.

Course and prognosis. Little is known about the outlook for this disorder, but it is thought to improve with advancing age.

Table 7-4. DSM-III criteria for the diagnosis of histrionic personality
disorder.

Behavior that is overly dramatic, reactive, and intensely expressed, as
indicated by at least three of the following:
    Self-dramatization, e.g., exaggerated expression of emotions
    Incessant drawing of attention to oneself
    Craving for activity and excitement
    Overreaction to minor events
    Irrational, angry outbursts or tantrums

Characteristic disturbances in interpersonal relationships, as indicated by at
least two of the following:
    Perceived by others as shallow and lacking genuineness, even if
        superficially warm and charming
    Egocentric, self-indulgent, and inconsiderate of others
    Vain and demanding
    Dependent, helpless, constantly seeking reassurance
    Prone to manipulative suicidal threats, gestures, or attempts

---

Differential Diagnosis

Histrionic personality disorder and borderline personality disorder are
quite similar. However, borderline patients generally feel chronically
empty, lack a sense of identity, experience brief psychotic episodes, and
engage in overtly self-destructive acts. Histrionic patients do not exhibit
these features with any regularity.

    Along with histrionic personality disorder, people may suffer from
a *somatization disorder* (akin to the old category of conversion hysteria)—see Chapter 8.

Treatment

Psychodynamic, insight-oriented psychotherapy is the treatment of
choice for histrionic personality disorder. Both individual and group
therapy have been found useful. The therapist must work on helping
histrionic patients to clarify their genuine feelings, since the experience
of deeply felt emotion is foreign to them. The therapist must help
patients learn to take responsibility for the consequences of their
actions, and to use their rational cognitive abilities rather than remaining "helpless" and "scatterbrained."

NARCISSISTIC PERSONALITY DISORDER

Narcissus, legend tells us, was a beautiful Grecian youth who fell madly in love with his own reflection when he happened upon a pool one day. Realizing that he could never possess what he so ardently desired, he killed himself.

Narcissism has come to represent many things in our culture, including self-centeredness and the ethos of the "me generation." In one sense, narcissism simply refers to self-love, and loving self-regard is both desirable and healthy. Only when self-absorption impairs one's ability to form lasting attachments to others do we term it pathological. Ironically, the crippling self-doubt and insecurity involved in pathological narcissism are a far cry from simple self-regard.

Profile

People with narcissistic personality disorder have severe problems maintaining a realistic concept of their own worth. They generally set goals and make demands of themselves that are utterly unrealistic, and then feel inadequate and helpless when they fail to meet these standards. They constantly crave love, attention, and admiration from other people as a means of bolstering their faltering self-esteem. Their demands for such love and praise can be insatiable, and they are likely to fly into a rage when these demands are not met. They are exquisitely sensitive to perceived slights from others, and approach people expecting to be disappointed. Thus, the narcissist struggles to keep a tenuous balance between the intense need to be admired by an important person and rage at that person's disappointing qualities. This struggle makes intimacy difficult and threatening. The narcissist often idealizes other people, only to come to devalue and despise them when they reveal themselves to be in some way imperfect.

Narcissistic people are preoccupied with fantasies of unlimited success, and tend to overestimate their abilities and their own specialness. This inflated self-importance often coexists with an unrealistic sense of worthlessness. Fantasies of achievement may take the place of actual work, but some people with this disorder are highly successful, pursuing fame and power with a relentless driven quality, never feeling satisfied with their achievements.

People with narcissistic personality disorder have difficulty recognizing how other people feel. They usually expect special favors from others without feeling any need to reciprocate; in this respect, they have a characteristic sense of *entitlement*. Narcissists are more concerned with how they look to others than with genuine feeling. They often use other people for their own ends.

All of this, it must be remembered, is in the service of protecting the narcissistic person's very fragile self-esteem. Narcissists feel devalued easily, and they may react to perceived slights not only with inappropriate rage, but also with emotional withdrawal, depression, and even suicide. The "insults" that trigger such rage and depression are often as minor as a misunderstood remark or a canceled appointment.

Diagnosis. DSM-III presents diagnostic criteria for narcissistic personality disorder (p. 317) that are shown in Table 7-5.

Causes. No specific genetic or environmental factors have been clearly demonstrated to cause narcissistic personality disorder. Many psychoanalytic theorists believe the disorder stems from early childhood experiences in which parents did not encourage or appreciate the

Table 7-5. DSM-III criteria for the diagnosis of narcissistic personality disorder.

Grandiose sense of self-importance or uniqueness, e.g., exaggeration of achievements and talents, focus on the special nature of one's problems

Preoccupation with fantasies of unlimited success, power, brilliance, beauty, or ideal love

Exhibitionism and the requirement of constant attention and admiration

Cool indifference or marked feelings of rage, inferiority, shame, humiliation, or emptiness in response to criticism, indifference of others, or defeat

At least two of the following characteristic disturbances in interpersonal relationships:
Entitlement: expectation of special favors without assuming reciprocal responsibilities, e.g., surprise and anger that people will not do what is wanted
Interpersonal exploitativeness: taking advantage of others to indulge one's own desires or for self-aggrandizement; disregard for the personal integrity and rights of others
Relationships that characteristically alternate between the extremes of overidealization and devaluation
Lack of empathy: inability to recognize how others feel, e.g., inability to appreciate the distress of someone who is seriously ill

---

child's efforts at self-assertion, and did not help the child take pride in accomplishments. The child is left emotionally hungry and unable to maintain a stable sense of self-worth without constant support from important people (see Chapter 2).

Epidemiology. No good data on the prevalence of narcissistic personality disorder are available. Reports in the literature indicate that the diagnosis is made more frequently in men than in women, but it is not yet clear whether men are actually more susceptible to the disorder.

Course and prognosis. No good data are available on the outlook for this disorder.

Differential Diagnosis

Some theorists have questioned the validity of narcissistic personality disorder as a separate diagnostic category because many patients with other disorders have prominent features of pathological narcissism. In particular, it may be difficult to differentiate narcissistic personality disorder from the following:

Histrionic personality disorder. Although both disorders involve seductiveness and self-dramatization, the person with a histrionic personality disorder is generally more playful and warm, while the narcissist is likely to be haughty, cold, and more obviously exploitative in dealings with others.

Borderline personality disorder. As a rule, borderline patients show poorer impulse control and are more socially and occupationally dysfunctional than narcissistic patients. Borderline patients often appear to be very emotionally needy, while narcissistic patients appear to be more self-sufficient.

Antisocial personality disorder. People with antisocial personality disorder are more impulsive than narcissists and show a constant calculated disregard for social standards. Narcissistic patients either do not recognize their violations of social norms or else view themselves as deserving to be above society's rules.

Compulsive personality disorder. Both compulsive people and narcissistic people set high standards and pursue perfection with a driven quality. However, the narcissist is haughty and claims perfection to maintain an idealized self-image; the compulsive strives for perfection in order to feel capable and in control.

Treatment

Individual and group psychotherapy are the treatments of choice, but treatment is fraught with difficulties. Narcissistic patients will often idealize you at the outset of treatment and then find it difficult to tolerate later recognition that you are not all-giving, all-knowing, and all-caring. This disappointment may cause disruptions in treatment; you and the patient must weather the storms of rage and periods of haughty devaluing that ensue.

In group therapy, the patient may act out this scenario with group members or the group leader. The aim of therapy is to provide a consistent, caring relationship in which narcissistic patients can develop more realistic concepts of themselves and of other people as neither perfect nor worthless.

ANTISOCIAL PERSONALITY DISORDER

Profile

"Antisocial personality disorder" may sound quite judgmental and pejorative, but it is in fact an accurate label for this illness. The most salient diagnostic feature is a long history of antisocial behavior in which the rights of others are repeatedly violated. This is *not* simply the medical term for criminality, but describes a longstanding illness that impairs most important areas of the patient's life. In clinical settings, you may also hear the more informal term *sociopath* used to refer to people with antisocial personality disorder.

People with this disorder are not usually patients—i.e., they do not commonly appear in mental health care settings—but are more likely to end up in courts, prisons, and welfare offices. When they do appear in psychiatric clinics, it is often either because they were brought there unwillingly or because they are trying to avoid the legal consequences of some recent act.

By definition, the people with this disorder begin their antisocial behavior before age 15. In childhood, they typically lie, steal, fight, and have pervasive difficulties with authority. In adolescence, sexual behavior begins early and may be unusually aggressive, and there is generally excessive drinking and drug use. By the time they reach adulthood, these people are usually unable to hold a responsible job or maintain family ties; most of them habitually break the law. Alcoholism, vagrancy, and social isolation are common, and a substantial number commit suicide. What is often striking and exasperating about socio-paths is their apparent lack of anxiety or depression in situations where one might expect such emotions.

People with antisocial personality disorder often turn on their charm at will in order to subtly manipulate others. You may find yourself baffled in an interview with somebody who has an antisocial personality disorder, for they can present a charming and strikingly "normal" facade. In fact, if an interview discloses nothing that seems abnormal, think first about the possibility that your patient has no disorder, but then consider whether you may have been "conned" by a sociopath.

Obviously the diagnosis of this disorder depends not on the mental status examination but on the patient's history. You are more likely to get reliable historical data from the family or from law enforcement officials than from the patient. Despite a healthy facade, the sociopath may show you some signs of stress in the interview—complaining of tension, of vague somatic symptoms, of feeling depressed, or of feeling (often correctly) that others are hostile toward him or her.

Diagnosis. The diagnostic criteria for antisocial personality disorder given in DSM-III (pp. 320-321) are shown in Table 7-6.

Causes. Both environmental and genetic factors seem to play a role in the genesis of antisocial personality disorder. The main environ-mental factor seems to be the sustained deprivation in early childhood of any consistent emotional ties with a significant person. The classic example of such deprivation is parents who are inconsistently available to the child and who are impulsive and erratic in their behavior. It is therefore no surprise to find that antisocial personality disorder is frequently found in the parents (particularly among the fathers) of those who have the disorder.

The evidence for genetic factors in antisocial personality disorder comes from studies which show that having a sociopathic or an alcoholic father is a powerful predictor of developing a sociopathic personality, *even* among children who were adopted at birth and not raised by their biologic parents.

There also appears to be a modest correlation between (a) hyperac-tive behavior and having "soft" (nonspecific) neurologic abnormalities in childhood and (b) later development of antisocial personality disor-der.

Table 7-6. DSM-III criteria for the diagnosis of antisocial personality disorder.

Current age at least 18

Onset before age 15, as indicated by a history of three or more of the following before that age:

Truancy (at least five days per year for at least two years, not including the last year of school)

Expulsion or suspension from school for misbehavior

Delinquency (arrested or referred to juvenile court because of behavior)

Running away from home overnight at least twice while living in parental or parental surrogate home

Persistent lying

Repeated sexual intercourse in a casual relationship

Repeated drunkenness or substance abuse

Thefts

Vandalism

School grades markedly below expectations in relation to estimated or known IQ (may have resulted in repeating a year of school)

Chronic violations of rules at home and/or at school (other than truancy)

Initiation of fights

At least four of the following manifestations of the disorder since age 18:

Inability to sustain consistent work behavior, as indicated by too frequent job changes, significant unemployment, serious absenteeism from work, or walking off the job without another job in sight (similar behavior in an academic setting may substitute for this criterion for those who have not had an opportunity to demonstrate occupational adjustment)

Lack of ability to function as a responsible parent, as evidenced by child's malnutrition, child's illness resulting from lack of minimal hygiene standards, failure to obtain medical care for a seriously ill child, child's dependence on neighbors or nonresident relatives for food or shelter, failure to arrange for a caretaker for a child under six when parent is away from home, or repeated squandering of money required for household necessities

Failure to accept social norms with respect to lawful behavior, as indicated by repeated thefts, illegal occupation (pimping, prostitution, fencing, selling drugs), multiple arrests, or a felony conviction

Inability to maintain enduring attachment to a sexual partner as indicated by two or more divorces and/or separations (whether legally married or not), desertion of spouse, promiscuity (ten or more sexual partners within one year)

Irritability and aggressiveness, as indicated by repeated physical fights or

---

assault (not required by one's job or to defend someone or oneself), including spouse or child beating

Failure to honor financial obligations, as indicated by repeated defaulting on debts, failure to provide child support, failure to support other dependents on a regular basis

Failure to plan ahead, or impulsivity, as indicated by traveling from place to place without a prearranged job or clear goal for the period of travel or clear idea about when the travel would terminate, or lack of a fixed address for a month or more

Disregard for the truth, as indicated by repeated lying, use of aliases, "conning" others for personal profit

Recklessness, as indicated by driving while intoxicated or recurrent speeding

A pattern of continuous antisocial behavior in which the rights of others are violated, with no intervening period of at least five years without antisocial behavior between age 15 and the present time (except when the individual was bedridden or confined in a hospital or penal institution)

Antisocial behavior is not due to severe mental retardation, schizophrenia, or manic episodes

---

Contrary to what you might expect intuitively, antisocial personality disorder is *not* correlated with such factors as living in a high-crime area, keeping bad company, or being a member of a deviant subgroup in society.

Epidemiology. The prevalence of antisocial personality disorder is estimated to be roughly 3 percent for American males and less than 1 percent for American females.

The disorder is more common among lower socioeconomic groups, probably because (a) most people with antisocial personality disorder have very poor work records and, therefore, impaired earning capacity, and (b) since the fathers of those who have the disorder frequently had it themselves, many of these people grew up in impoverished homes. However, the disorder is found in all social classes, including the most privileged.

The prevalence of the disorder among prison populations is very high—perhaps as high as 75 percent.

Course and prognosis. The disorder begins in childhood, and antisocial behavior reaches its peak in adolescence and young adulthood. Two changes seem to occur later in life. First, for some people, the disorder seems to remit. Among those who have the disorder, roughly 2 percent improve (i.e., stop their antisocial behavior) each year once they get beyond age 21. Second, many of those patients who stop their antisocial behavior in their adult years develop hypochondriacal concerns and depression.

Differential Diagnosis

There are several conditions from which antisocial personality disorder must be differentiated.

Criminality. As noted above, antisocial personality disorder is not simply another term for criminality. It is a disorder that impairs all aspects of the individual's life—social functioning, work capacity, and the ability to achieve and maintain intimate relationships. Many people with this disorder manage to keep their actions within the limits of the law but nevertheless violate social norms and harm others by their behavior. Conversely, some people who commit crimes may act with loyalty and a sense of responsibility toward others in their lives (e.g., spouses, parents) and could not be accurately labeled sociopaths.

Borderline personality disorder. Both borderline and antisocial personality disorders may involve impulsive and destructive behavior, directed at the self as well as others. However, borderlines are more likely than sociopaths to behave self-destructively. Also, although sociopaths often act aggressively toward others without anger or guilt, borderlines usually become hostile only when feeling deprived by people who are important to them, and they commonly feel guilty about their anger. Borderline personality disorder is more frequently diagnosed in women, while antisocial personality disorder is more frequently diagnosed in men.

Manic episode. Mania may involve antisocial behavior, but such behavior is clearly episodic rather than chronic and longstanding, and it accompanies a highly altered mood.

Substance abuse disorder. Drug and alcohol abuse can certainly result in global impairment of functioning and chronic antisocial behavior (stealing, lying, etc.) as the individual struggles to maintain and conceal an addiction. In these cases, antisocial behavior stops when the drug abuse stops. Often, however, substance abuse is simply secondary to an underlying antisocial personality disorder, and both diagnoses may be warranted in such cases.

Treatment

Sociopaths look unreachable and untreatable in an outpatient setting. They appear to lack anxiety, to lack any motivation for change, and to learn nothing from experience. However, these are only the characteristics of a sociopath who is in flight. When people with an antisocial personality disorder are immobilized—i.e., when they are held in a treatment or prison facility and can no longer act to avoid unpleasant feelings—a very different picture emerges. Sociopaths begin to experience considerable anxiety and become convinced that this anxiety will be intolerable to others. The fear of getting close to others becomes much more apparent, as does the sociopath's sensitivity to criticism and rejection.

Thus, actual control over the behavior of sociopaths is the cornerstone of treatment. They must be prevented from running away, or from hurting themselves or others when feelings seem intolerable. This control is usually impossible to achieve on an outpatient basis, and can only be achieved in prison or on a locked inpatient unit. The goal of treatment is to show these patients that they and others can tolerate their anxiety. Sociopaths often need much more support than is possible in individual therapy. Peer support groups of all kinds are probably the most effective treatment, since the sociopath can use such groups to identify with others who struggle with similar problems.

You may be tempted to try to rescue charming sociopaths, and to shield them from the consequences of their own behavior (e.g., legal proceedings, prison sentences). This is antitherapeutic. People with antisocial personality disorder cannot be treated without the clear understanding that they are responsible for whatever they do.

BORDERLINE PERSONALITY DISORDER

For years, psychiatric thinkers taught that an individual could be either psychotic or neurotic, not both. Yet therapists reported many cases in which people became transiently psychotic under stress, recompensated quickly, and in most situations remained completely in touch with reality. Some thought these people had a mild form of schizophrenia; others called them severely neurotic. Out of this confusion, contemporary theorists developed the concept of the borderline personality— *borderline* referring to the line between psychosis and neurosis.

Profile

Many borderline patients do indeed move in and out of psychosis. When they lose touch with reality it may take the form of frank hallucinations and delusions, but more often the psychosis involves dissociative states, derealization, and depersonalization (see Chapter 4). These episodes are usually brief—lasting several minutes to several days—and occur in response to stress (e.g., a break-up with a lover).

But reactive psychosis is by no means the only prominent feature of the borderline syndrome. Intense and persistent anger is one of the hallmarks of this disorder. Borderline patients are characteristically rageful and demanding, going to great lengths to get others to feel responsible for their woes and their welfare. Borderline patients form chaotic relationships with others because they struggle with intense dependence upon and intense hostility toward those to whom they become attached. Borderlines are adept at manipulating others to do their bidding. But their use of emotional blackmail (e.g., suicide threats) and angry outbursts ultimately drive away the people who are important to them.

The borderline patient is easily overwhelmed by anger and frustration, and generally acts impulsively when feelings become intolerable. This usually involves repeated self-destructive acts (e.g., wrist slashing, overdoses, car crashes) and may also include drug abuse, sexual promiscuity, and abrupt changes in job and living situations.

Borderline patients usually possess a facade of sociability and adaptiveness that makes them quite engaging in superficial contact. Thus, many borderlines are very good at interviews but function erratically and below their apparent capabilities in work situations.

People with borderline personality disorder chronically experience feelings of emptiness and uncertainty about who they are. This disturbed sense of identity can be seen in a variety of areas—gender identity, personal goals, the difference between their own and others' feelings, their self-image, and their body image. When borderlines complain, "I don't know who I am," they generally reflect a profound sense of internal chaos and confusion. This is particularly acute when there is no one around from whom the borderline can take his or her cues; therefore, the borderline has difficulty being alone and will seek out companionship, at times frantically, in order to avoid it.

Diagnosis. DSM-III gives the diagnostic criteria for borderline personality disorder (pp. 322-323) shown in Table 7-7. In addition to the

Table 7-7. DSM-III criteria for the diagnosis of borderline personality disorder.

At least five of the following:

    Impulsivity or unpredictability in at least two areas that are potentially self-damaging, e.g., spending, sex, gambling, substance use, shoplifting, overeating, physically self-damaging acts

    A pattern of unstable and intense interpersonal relationships, e.g., marked shifts of attitude, idealization, devaluation, manipulation

    Inappropriate, intense anger or lack of control of anger, e.g., frequent displays of temper, constant anger

    Identity disturbance manifested by uncertainty about several issues relating to identity, such as self-image, gender identity, long-term goals or career choice, friendship patterns, values, and loyalties, e.g., "I feel like I am my sister when I am good"

    Affective instability: marked shifts from normal mood to depression, irritability, or anxiety, usually lasting a few hours and only rarely more than a few days, with a return to normal mood

    Intolerance of being alone, e.g., frantic efforts to avoid being alone, depressed when alone

    Physically self-damaging acts, e.g., suicidal gestures, self-mutilation, recurrent accidents or physical fights

    Chronic feelings of emptiness or boredom

If under 18, does not meet the criteria for identity disorder

criteria listed in the table, some clinicians insist that true borderline personality disorder must involve psychotic experiences that are brief, reversible, and stress related.

Causes. Most of the major work on the etiology of borderline personality disorder has come from psychoanalytic theorists. They focus on early childhood, particularly between the ages of six months and two years, when the child learns to separate from the mother and gains a sense of himself or herself as a separate being. Many psychoanalysts postulate that disturbances in the mother-child relationship during this separation-individuation phase of development can leave children with a poorly developed sense of self and render them extremely vulnerable to separations from important others. One theorist (Kernberg) has hypothesized that borderline patients may have an inborn deficit in their ability to tolerate anxiety.

Empirical studies are now under way to try to validate the theories mentioned above, and to explore possible biologic factors in the etiology of borderline personality disorder.

Epidemiology. Little is known about the prevalence of this disorder, since diagnostic criteria have only been established in the past decade and are still the subject of some debate. In recent years, roughly 10 to 20 percent of hospital admissions have been of patients with this diagnosis. Women are diagnosed as borderline more than twice as often as men, but it may be that clinicians underdiagnose the disorder in men and overdiagnose it in women.

Course and prognosis. There is considerable disagreement about what happens to borderline patients over time. While the disorder begins in childhood or adolescence and continues well into adult life, it may be that the disorder remits somewhat after age 40, since the diagnosis is made in people over 40 much less frequently. Whether borderline patients "burn out," become more stable in their functioning, or simply stop seeking help as they get older is unclear. Further research needs to be done in this area.

Differential Diagnosis

Other personality disorders. Borderline patients often have features consistent with other personality disorders—particularly histrionic, narcissistic, schizoid, schizotypal, and antisocial personality disorders. If a patient meets the criteria for more than one personality disorder, more than one diagnosis is warranted.

Affective disorders. Because the patient with borderline personality disorder has intense and highly changeable emotional storms, it is easy to confuse symptoms of the disorder with mood swings due to an underlying affective illness. Recent studies suggest that up to 50 percent of patients with borderline personality disorder have a concurrent affective disorder; in such cases *both* disorders should be diagnosed and treated.

Treatment

While psychotherapy is the treatment of choice for borderline patients, treatment is extremely difficult for patient and therapist. Borderlines often cannot tolerate the intense feelings they develop for the therapist, and their responses range from abruptly breaking off treatment to intense verbal abuse to severe self-destructive acts. Patients frequently threaten and attempt suicide, using this and other maneuvers to try to elicit signs of the therapist's love and concern. This behavior is designed in part to manipulate others, but it is nonetheless dangerous. Suicide is common. You may become overwhelmed by your own emotional responses to borderlines. Intense anger is common, as is an unrealistic sense of responsibility for the patient's safety.

Two differing views of psychotherapy with borderline patients predominate. Some clinicians advocate intensive individual psychotherapy (two or more sessions per week) aimed at in-depth exploration of how patients relate to others in their lives and, most important, how they relate to the therapist. Another view is that such intensive work prompts the borderline patient to become irreversibly clinging and dependent on the therapist, that treatment should instead be limited to weekly sessions that focus on "here-and-now" issues of improving job performance, stabilizing the patient's living situation, etc. Group therapy is often advocated as an adjunct to both intensive and supportive individual therapy, since groups can often confront borderlines with their manipulative behavior quite effectively. Treating borderline patients in groups is very difficult because of their wish to have an exclusive relationship with the therapist.

Medication has proved to be of little use in borderline personality disorder. Psychotic episodes are too brief to require antipsychotic medication, and mood swings are too rapid and dependent on life events to be stabilized by antidepressants or lithium. However, patients who have an affective disorder in addition to borderline personality disorder often benefit from medication.

Whatever treatment regimen is decided upon, it is crucial that the *therapist* have support. This should always include the option to hospitalize the patient when self-destructive activities or psychosis make it impossible to continue treatment on an outpatient basis. Supervision, peer group support, and consultation with other clinicians can also help the therapist to maintain some perspective on the treatment during particularly difficult periods.

AVOIDANT PERSONALITY DISORDER

Profile

The hallmark of the avoidant personality disorder is extreme sensitivity to rejection. Avoidant individuals stay away from relationships—not because they want to, but because they are so afraid of rejection. Only when guaranteed uncritical acceptance can they feel safe enough to get attached to other people.

Avoidant people generally lack self-confidence, which they attempt to bolster by seeking out unusually supportive companions. They are often afraid to speak up, and feel uncomfortable in the limelight and in positions of authority.

In the interview, people with avoidant personality disorder will be anxious about what you think of them. They may seem fragile and waiflike. If you attempt to clarify something they have said, they are likely to interpret your comments as critical even when you did not mean them to be.

Diagnosis. The diagnostic criteria for avoidant personality disorder given in DSM-III (p. 324) are shown in Table 7-8.

Causes. The causes are unknown. Childhood experiences and inborn temperament may exert some influence in the genesis of this disorder.

Epidemiology. Since the diagnosis is new to DSM-III, there is no information on prevalence, sex ratio, or familial patterns of the disorder.

Course and prognosis. These are also unknown.

Table 7-8. DSM-III criteria for the diagnosis of avoidant personality disorder.

Hypersensitivity to rejection, e.g., apprehensively alert to signs of social derogation; interprets innocuous events as ridicule

Unwillingness to enter into relationships unless given unusually strong guarantees of uncritical acceptance

Social withdrawal, e.g., distances self from close personal attachments, engages in peripheral social and vocational roles

Desire for affection and acceptance

Low self-esteem, e.g., devalues self-achievements and is overly dismayed by personal shortcomings

If under 18, does not meet the criteria for avoidant disorder of childhood or adolescence

Differential Diagnosis

Avoidant personality disorder was not included in diagnostic manuals prior to DSM-III. There is considerable disagreement about whether the avoidant personality constitutes a true personality disorder or merely represents a trait common to a variety of personality types.

The individual with an avoidant personality disorder longs for and responds to genuine attention and support from others; the person with a *schizoid personality disorder* expresses no desire for social relations.

Unlike people with dependent, borderline, and histrionic personality disorders, avoidant people suffer quietly and are not demanding of others' attention.

Treatment

Psychotherapy is the treatment of choice. In individual therapy, a strong alliance is difficult to form because it is so easy for the avoidant individual to feel rejected. However, once formed, this alliance can help the avoidant patient learn to weather the storms inherent in human interaction.

Group therapy can demonstrate to avoidant individuals the difficulties their hypersensitivity poses for other people. But avoidant individuals are likely to be very reluctant to take the risk involved in entering into group therapy in the first place.

Some clinicians feel that an important distinction between avoidant and schizoid personality disorders is that the avoidant individual is more inclined than the schizoid to seek and profit from psychotherapy.

DEPENDENT PERSONALITY DISORDER

Profile

Dependent personality disorder is another new diagnostic category in DSM-III. Clinicians disagree about whether extreme dependence is a trait common to many types of personality disorder or whether it is truly a unique disorder in its own right.

People with dependent personality disorder structure their lives so that other people will take responsibility for their welfare. They feel unable to function on their own, and so seek out lovers, bosses, and friends who will allow them to be passive and who will tell them how to live their lives. They avoid making decisions whenever they can get others to do it for them—e.g., whom to see socially, where to work, and even what to wear.

The person with this disorder will put up with a great deal from others in order to preserve a dependent relationship and avoid having to function autonomously—for example, the wife who puts up with verbal and physical abuse from her husband because she feels incapable of functioning without him. Dependent people lack self-confidence and are preoccupied with fears of being abandoned.

Diagnosis. The diagnostic criteria for dependent personality disorder given in DSM-III (p. 326) are as follows:

• Passively allows others to assume responsibility for major areas of life because of inability to function independently (e.g., lets spouse decide what kind of job he or she should have).

• Subordinates own needs to those of persons on whom he or she depends in order to avoid any possibility of having to rely on self, e.g., tolerates abusive spouse.

• Lacks self-confidence, e.g., sees self as helpless, stupid.

Causes. Most theorists who write about the roots of extreme passivity and dependence emphasize early childhood experiences. One hypothesis is that parents can foster dependent personality traits by giving their children the implicit or explicit message that independent behavior is bad and will lead to abandonment.

Evidence has begun to emerge that suggests that dominant and submissive personality traits may be genetically transmitted. Researchers have found a higher rate of concordance for these traits among identical twins than among fraternal twins. However, submissiveness and dependence are not the same thing, and it is not clear whether these two traits usually coexist in the same person.

Epidemiology. The diagnosis is more often assigned to women than to men, and more often to people who are the youngest children within their family constellations.

Course and prognosis. Functioning depends on the patient's maintenance of dependent relationships. When these are disrupted in some way (e.g., the death of a spouse), a person who previously functioned well may seriously decompensate and seek psychiatric help.

Differential Diagnosis

Dependent traits are common in other personality disorders, particularly in borderline, histrionic, avoidant, passive-aggressive, and schizoid personality disorders. Some diagnosticians believe that masochism—i.e., the pleasure obtained from pain, failure, and disability—is the more central trait in dependent personality disorder than dependence per se. This calls into question whether dependent personality disorder is a valid diagnostic category.

Agoraphobia (Chapter 8) may be mistaken for dependent personality disorder, but the agoraphobic individual is much more *active* in demanding that others take responsibility for his or her life (e.g., the agoraphobic husband who insists that his wife drive him everywhere). Dependent individuals "can't" do things because of a sense of inadequacy and incompetence, while agoraphobics "can't" do things because of overwhelming fear and anxiety.

Treatment

Psychotherapy can be very helpful for people with dependent personality disorder. In the relationship with the therapist, patients can begin to examine the effects of their passivity, and to recognize their own competence and self-worth. In the beginning, it is important that the therapist respect the patient's need for dependent relationships (even abusive ones) and not push the patient to give them up until he or she is ready.

COMPULSIVE PERSONALITY DISORDER

The "obsessive-compulsive" is an infamous character familiar to every hard-working student. We often use this label to lampoon ourselves or others for being too careful, too preoccupied with detail, and too diligent or perfectionistic. The terms *obsessive* and *compulsive* are used in psychiatry in three major ways: (a) to describe a classic preoccupation with unwanted thoughts or behaviors (obsessive-compulsive neurosis), (b) to describe a general personality style, and (c) to describe a specific personality disorder.

Obsessive-compulsive neurosis. *Obsessions* are persistent unwanted ideas or images that seem as if they come from outside the mind and force themselves on the victim's thoughts against his or her will. One might, for example, be obsessed with the thought that one has accidentally hurt someone, or be terrified of being contaminated by touching a door knob. People who suffer from this disorder may be hopelessly preoccupied with obsessions despite realizing that these preoccupations are absurd and irrational. They usually feel powerless to keep obsessive thoughts out of their awareness, and become anxious when they attempt to do so.

Compulsions are the behavioral equivalents of obsessions—repetitive urges to perform acts that are contrary to one's ordinary wishes or standards. Common compulsive acts include hand-washing, counting (e.g., money), and checking (e.g., to be certain the stove has been turned off). The action usually seems senseless; performing the act is not pleasurable, but it does relieve tension. When the problem is severe, people may need to spend most of their waking moments carrying out compulsive acts (e.g., cleaning) to avoid massive anxiety.

According to psychodynamic theory, obsessive thoughts and compulsive acts serve as benign substitutes for more threatening *unconscious* ideas or impulses (e.g., the wish to kill one's parent). True obsessions and compulsions (i.e., discrete and isolated symptoms) are relatively rare—estimated at 0.05 percent of the general population.

Obsessive-compulsive style. Much more common than true obsessions or compulsions is the obsessive-compulsive personality style, which may be both normal and highly adaptive. Like hysterical traits, obsessive-compulsive traits can be very useful—e.g., when studying for an anatomy exam, or organizing a business venture, or even planning a wild party.

Obsessive-compulsive people have the ability to focus their attention and screen out distractions. Thus, they can be skilled at highly detailed work; many obsessive-compulsives are technicians, physicians, and scientists. Obsessive-compulsives are perfectionists and they are list-makers. They are usually intensely and continuously active at some kind of work. Their deliberateness makes them less open than others to spontaneous experiences. Obsessive-compulsives rarely get hunches, and often immerse themselves so completely in small details that they cannot step back and see the "big picture."

In contrast to hysterics, obsessive-compulsives are characteristically serious. They generally apply great pressure to themselves to live up to high standards of performance and morality, for they live according to the dictates of a very demanding conscience. "I should..." is their motto. They are their own harshest taskmasters and never feel that they are free. In fact, many obsessive-compulsives are uncomfortable in situations where they are truly free, e.g., on vacation.

Decisions are the bane of the obsessive-compulsive's existence, and he or she will try to find a rule or moral dictum to avoid having to exercise free choice. Obsessive-compulsives have difficulty when faced with decisions in which no duty is involved and they must act wholly according to their own desires, because they are generally unaware of their desires.

Profile of Compulsive Personality Disorder

As with other personality types, the line between what constitutes *style* and what qualifies as a *disorder* is not at all clear in the case of the obsessive-compulsive. This is a judgment call, based on the extent to which personality traits are inflexible and impair one's ability to love and to work.

Individuals with compulsive personality disorder are very limited in their ability to express warm and tender feelings toward others. Feelings provoke anxiety, and compulsives focus on facts instead of feelings to overcome anxiety. They are preoccupied with the "right" way of doing things, and often alienate others by their insistence on having their own way. They can be moralistic to the point of absurd rigidity and extreme insensitivity to the needs of others.

Lists and routines dominate their lives. They may focus on their bowel habits, for example, to the point that any irregularity leaves them unable to function at their usual daily activities. Decision making will often be reduced to a "science." When this is not possible, compulsives may be paralyzed by indecision and the fear of making a mistake.

Other compulsive traits include parsimony, extreme cleanliness, and orderliness. At the healthier end of the spectrum, the individual with a compulsive personality disorder may have a stable marriage and hold a responsible job, but is constantly tense and driven, unable to have fun.

When you interview people with compulsive personality disorder, you will most likely find them neatly and conventionally dressed. They may sit stiffly, and will be serious in demeanor. They are likely to drone on and on in a monotonous tone of voice as they give detailed and often circumstantial answers to questions. In fact, when you ask how they feel about something, they will usually give an answer consisting of facts and circumstances instead of emotions. They will be slow to "warm up" to you, and preoccupied with ideas about what you expect of them in the interview.

Diagnosis. According to DSM-III (pp. 327-328), at least four of the following must be present for a diagnosis of compulsive personality disorder:

• Restricted ability to express warm and tender emotions, e.g., the individual is unduly conventional, serious and formal, and stingy.

• Perfectionism that interferes with the ability to grasp the "big picture," e.g., preoccupation with trivial details, rules, order, organization, schedules, and lists.

• Insistence that others submit to his or her way of doing things, and lack of awareness of the feelings elicited by this behavior, e.g., a husband stubbornly insists his wife complete errands for him regardless of her plans.

• Excessive devotion to work and productivity, to the exclusion of pleasure and the value of interpersonal relationships.

• Indecisiveness: decision-making is either avoided, postponed, or protracted, perhaps because of an inordinate fear of making a mistake, e.g., the individual cannot get assignments done on time because of ruminating about priorities.

Causes. Classic psychoanalytic thinking emphasizes the importance of the anal phase of development (age two to four years) in the genesis of compulsive personality disorder. Toilet training is the standard metaphor for this stage: children want to gratify their urges wherever and whenever they occur, but these urges conflict with the desires of parents and society. The tension, then, is between the assertion of autonomy and the development of self-control.

Many therapists write about the role of rigid, controlling parents in fostering compulsive personality disorder in their overdisciplined offspring. However, these ideas have yet to be validated in long-term prospective studies.

Compulsive personality disorder is more prevalent among family members of identified compulsive patients than in the general population, and newer studies suggest that genetic as well as environmental factors play a role in determining which people develop this condition.

Epidemiology. Prevalence is unknown, because much depends on where the diagnostician draws the line between the personality style and the disorder. It is more common in men than in women.

Course and Prognosis. The course of the disorder varies tremendously. Compulsives are quite vulnerable to unexpected life changes, and are prone to bouts of depression. However, some compulsive people appear to "loosen up" with age and exhibit fewer symptoms of the disorder as they grow older. Still others develop frankly compulsive behaviors, and a small number appear to adopt compulsive symptoms as a prelude to a schizophrenic break. Unfortunately, many severely compulsive people continue to lead an emotionally barren existence throughout life.

Differential Diagnosis

People with obsessive-compulsive neurosis report being plagued by obsessive thoughts, or of feeling unable to resist performing compulsive acts, and these symptoms are disturbing to those who have them. By contrast, compulsive personality disorder is not characterized by ego-dystonic obsessions or compulsions.

People who fulfill the criteria for compulsive personality disorder may also show features of other personality disorders—particularly schizoid and paranoid personality disorders.

Treatment

Psychotherapy is the treatment of choice; medication has not proved effective in this disorder.

Compulsive people differ from many others with personality disorders in that they see themselves as troubled and seek help on their own. Therapy is a long and slow process, because the compulsive sees therapy, like every other relationship, as a struggle for control. The therapist must carefully sidestep potential battles and point out the patient's extreme sensitivity to issues of power and authority. The focus must be clearly maintained on the patient's feelings, because the compulsive tends to use his or her intellect to defend against feelings that are less controllable than ideas and therefore more threatening.

Group psychotherapy has also proved effective, either alone or in combination with individual therapy. Group members can have a powerful influence on the compulsive patient, by pointing out the maladaptive ways of dealing with others revealed in the group. They can also reward the compulsive with praise when positive changes are made.

Behavior therapy, while useful for specific compulsive behaviors, has not been shown to be effective for more global compulsive personality traits.

PASSIVE-AGGRESSIVE PERSONALITY DISORDER

Passive aggression is a powerful means of controlling other people. Hunger strikes, sit-ins, and work slow-downs are common examples of how doing nothing can be a highly effective means of gaining attention or power. Where more openly aggressive behavior is impossible, passive resistance may be the only reasonable course of action. Gandhi made masterful use of this technique on a national scale in India. However, as a global and pervasive style of dealing with life, passive-aggressive behavior is usually self-defeating and self-destructive.

Profile

Individuals with passive-aggressive personality disorder spend their lives saying "yes" and behaving as if they had said "no." They fail to live up to demands made on them by their jobs and by people who are important to them. They do not fail directly or deliberately but "by accident"—e.g., by forgetting, procrastinating, or misplacing things. Typically, passive-aggressive individuals are largely unaware of their obstructiveness and feel that they are doing their best. They feel that no one appreciates how hard they try and how many difficulties the world puts in their way. They do not get angry at others directly, nor are they direct about their own needs and desires. People usually experience the passive-aggressive person's behavior as punitive; initial guilty acquiescence gives way to anger and even abandonment. Thus passive-aggressive people are not only underachievers who infuriate their bosses, but they are also tyrants who hold captive those friends and lovers who remain close to them.

Diagnosis. The diagnostic criteria for passive-aggressive personality disorder given in DSM-III (p. 329) are shown in Table 7-9.

Causes. There have been no prospective studies of the causes of passive-aggressive personality disorder. Certainly, early childhood experiences seem to be of primary importance in the genesis of the disorder, particularly in conveying the message to the developing child that the direct expression of aggression is in some way taboo.

Epidemiology. The prevalence, sex ratio, and familial patterns of this disorder have not been well studied.

Course and prognosis. People with this disorder are prone to depression and to alcohol and drug abuse.

Differential Diagnosis

Borderline and histrionic patients may use a great many passive-aggressive maneuvers, but they are more flamboyant and more openly aggressive than people with passive-aggressive personality disorder.

Because passive-aggressive behaviors are used defensively in a wide range of disorders, many clinicians question the validity of passive-aggressive personality disorder as a separate diagnostic category.

Treatment

Psychotherapy is the treatment of choice for passive-aggressive personality disorder. Patients invariably attempt to put the therapist in the same bind that they put others in their lives: if the therapist gratifies the patient's covert demands for assistance, the patient will make further

Table 7-9. DSM-III criteria for the diagnosis of passive-aggressive personality disorder.

Resistance to demands for adequate performance in both occupational and social functioning

Resistance expressed indirectly through at least two of the following: procrastination, dawdling, stubbornness, intentional inefficiency, and "forgetfulness"

As a consequence of the above, pervasive and long-standing social and occupational ineffectiveness (including roles of housewife or student), e.g., intentional inefficiency that has prevented job promotion

Persistence of the behavior pattern even under circumstances in which more self-assertive and effective behavior is possible

Does not meet the criteria for any other personality disorder and, if under age 18, does not meet the criteria for oppositional disorder

---

and more unreasonable demands. However, the patient will take a refusal to honor these requests as rejection. The therapist must constantly try to sidestep this dilemma by bringing the patient's covert aggression out into the open. This means confronting veiled threats and manipulative efforts, and asking what the patient hopes to gain by such tactics.

SOME FINAL THOUGHTS ON TREATMENT

People with personality disorders are notoriously difficult to treat. Their pathological ways of dealing with the world are deeply ingrained, yet they act as if the problem lies with the world and not with them. They are often angry, demanding, and abusive toward therapists and have an extraordinary capacity to home in on the weaknesses and vulnerabilities of those who try to help them. They will attempt to form the same type of pathological relationship with you that they form with others in their lives. They are generally reluctant to see their behavior as a problem and are likely to blame you when their wishes are not fulfilled in therapy.

You may become so angry at such patients that you will unwittingly retaliate when they are abusive. You may, for example, withdraw your emotional investment from your work with them in subtle ways, prompting patients to feel increasingly worthless. You must pay close attention to the hostile feelings that invariably arise toward the patient with a personality disorder; by being aware of these feelings and tolerating them, you can avoid acting on them.

The following ground rules may be helpful to you in dealing with a personality-disordered patient, whether you are doing a single interview or embarking on long-term therapy:

• Focus on the patient's behavior, *not* on his or her explanations of that behavior.

• Do not listen to repetitious complaints. When patients recount the supposed injustices the world has dealt them, direct the focus to their own role in these events.

• Maintain the stance that you and your patients are collaborating—i.e., that you are doing something *with* them rather than *for* them or *to* them.

• Pay close attention to your own fantasies of "rescuing" the patient. You are bound to be disappointed.

• Set limits on any behavior that threatens your safety, the patient's safety, or the future of the treatment. This may range from ending your meeting early, to putting the patient in the hospital against his or her will. When patients try to push you into the role of savior, friend, or co-conspirator, show them what they are doing.

• Scoldings and guilt trips are of no use to your patients. You must simply hold them responsible for their behavior, rather than making any moves to shield them from its consequences.

• Provide *yourself* with support. Seek supervision from a more senior person, or "let off steam" with a peer. Use *all* the help available to you to weather the difficult times that are unavoidable in treating people with personality disorders.

REFERENCES

Akhtar S, Thompson JA: Overview: narcissistic personality disorder. Am J Psychiatry 139:12-20, 1982.

Chodoff P, Lyons H: Hysteria, the hysterical personality, and "hysterical" conversion. Am J Psychiatry 114:734-740, 1958.

Diagnostic and Statistical Manual of Mental Disorders, 3rd ed. Washington, DC, American Psychiatric Association, 1980, pp 305-330.

Frances A: The DSM-III personality disorders section: a commentary. Am J Psychiatry 137:1050-1054, 1980.

Frosch JP (ed): Current Perspectives on Personality Disorders. Washington, DC, American Psychiatric Press, 1983.

Gunderson JG: Diagnoses of personality disorders. Presented at the annual meeting of the American Psychiatric Association, May 1982, Toronto, Canada.

Gunderson JG, Singer MT: Defining borderline patients: an overview. Am J Psychiatry 132:1-10, 1975.

Guntrip H: The schizoid problem, in Psychoanalytic Theory, Therapy, and the Self. New York, Basic Books, 1973, pp 145-173.

Kernberg O: Borderline personality organization. J Am Psychoanal Assoc 15:641-685, 1967.

Shapiro D: Neurotic Styles. New York, Basic Books, 1965. (An excellent and highly readable discussion of personality styles.)

Stanton AH: Personality disorders, in The Harvard Guide to Modern Psychiatry. Edited by Nicholi AM Jr. Cambridge, MA, Harvard University Press, 1978, pp 283-295.

Vaillant GE: Sociopathy as a human process: a viewpoint. Arch Gen Psychiatry 32:178-183, 1975.

Vaillant GE, Perry JC: Personality disorders, in A Comprehensive Textbook of Psychiatry, 3rd ed. Edited by Kaplan HI, Freedman AM, Sadock BJ. Baltimore, Williams and Wilkins, 1980, vol. 2, pp 1562-1590.

8

Anxiety, Phobias, Somatoform Disorders, Dissociative Disorders, and Eating Disorders

ANXIETY

WHAT IS ANXIETY? Each of us has experienced it, and ours has been called "the age of anxiety." Yet precise definition of the term is difficult, for it has been applied to a wide range of emotional responses.

Fear is a normal reaction to a consciously recognized external source of danger. It is appropriate to the source of danger, both in its intensity and in its duration, and it dissipates when action is taken that leads to escape or avoidance. Fear involves both subjective feelings of apprehension and objective physiological changes that usually include tachycardia, rapid respiration, tremor of skeletal muscles, and redistribution of blood from the skin and viscera to the large muscle groups. These changes prepare the body for the violent muscular activity (fight or flight) that may be necessary in responding to a threat.

Anxiety, by contrast, involves tension, apprehension, or even terror about danger, the source of which is largely unknown or unrecognized. Like fear, anxiety is accompanied by increased activity of the sympathetic nervous system, with such physical signs as sweating, tachycardia, tremor, hyperventilation, and gastrointestinal distress. But, unlike fear, anxiety stems from sources that are not obvious to the one who suffers, or that seem minor compared with his or her intense emotional reaction. Anxiety is common, and in many instances consists of an overreaction to mildly stressful events (e.g., excessive concern over a relatively unimportant examination). We regard anxiety as pathological when it interferes with daily functioning, the achievement of desired goals, or reasonable emotional comfort.

Situational anxiety occurs in response to a specific stress and ends shortly after the stress is removed. *Free-floating anxiety*, by contrast, involves apprehension that is not clearly linked to a specific situation.

What Causes Anxiety Disorders?

Anxiety disorders do not have a single cause—there are both psychological and somatic factors that foster the development of anxiety.

Psychological factors. Psychoanalytic theorists postulate that anxiety stems from intrapsychic conflict. When a young child's wishes come into conflict with parental expectations and the realities of the world, the child may imagine being punished for these wishes (e.g., a youngster who harbors murderous wishes toward his little brother may fear that he will be severely punished for these feelings). These conflicts may be within a young child's awareness, but they are repressed as children grow up. In adulthood, circumstances may reactivate an unconscious conflict and foster anxiety. Typical childhood fears that may be repressed and lead to anxiety disorders in adult life are:

• Loss of, or separation from, a parent or other caretaker on whom one depends.

• Loss of love through anger or disapproval of an important person.

• Damage to or loss of the genitals (also called *castration anxiety*).

• Loss of self-esteem when one fails to live up to one's moral standards adopted from early caretakers.

Thus, for example, a woman may become terrified when her husband leaves on a business trip, not on the basis of any actual danger to herself or her husband, but because the separation revives her early fears of separation from parents.

Biologic factors. Genetic predisposition to anxiety disorders is now the subject of intense research. Specific syndromes like panic attacks (discussed below) have been shown to be familial diseases, and researchers are currently looking for possible biological markers of panic and other anxiety disorders.

Underlying somatic illnesses. Many organic disorders are accompanied by symptoms of anxiety. Some of the most common of these are listed in Table 8-1.

Among people who come to health care facilities complaining of anxiety, medical illness is found in only a minority of cases. Nevertheless, the possibility of underlying somatic disease must not be overlooked when you evaluate anxious patients, and everyone who is being evaluated for anxiety for the first time should have a thorough medical evaluation as well as a psychiatric one.

Generalized Anxiety Disorder

The system of classification outlined in DSM-III divides the anxiety disorders according to whether the symptoms are nonspecific (generalized anxiety disorder) or specific (phobic disorders, panic disorders).

Generalized anxiety disorder, also called "anxiety neurosis," is characterized by persistent anxiety for at least one month without specific phobias or panic attacks. The symptoms of anxiety vary greatly from person to person, but usually include the following manifestations:

Motor tension—trembling, muscle aches and tension, easy fatigability, inability to relax, and restlessness;

Autonomic hyperactivity—sweating, palpitations, rapid respirations, rapid pulse, dry mouth, clammy hands, dizziness, paresthe-

Table 8-1. Somatic illnesses that are commonly accompanied by anxiety.

Cardiovascular	Neurologic
Angina pectoris	Partial complex seizures
Cardiac arrhythmias	
Mitral valve prolapse	Toxic metabolic
Hyperkinetic heart syndrome	Medication side effects
Recurrent pulmonary emboli	Substance abuse
	Withdrawal states
Endocrine	
Hyperthyroidism	
Pheochromocytoma	
Hypoglycemia	
Hypoparathyroidism	
Cushing's syndrome	

sias (tingling in hands or feet), nausea, stomach pain, frequent urination, diarrhea, hot or cold spells, flushing, pallor;

Apprehensiveness—continual worry and anticipation that
something bad will happen to oneself or another; and

Vigilance—hyperattentiveness, impatience, irritability, distractibility, difficulty concentrating, insomnia, and fatigue on awakening.

Generalized anxiety often accompanies other psychiatric disorders,
particularly depressive syndromes, schizophrenia, and various personality disorders. The diagnosis of generalized anxiety disorder is not made
when another mental disorder or an underlying organic disorder is
responsible for the patient's distress.

Patients commonly attempt to medicate their anxiety by abusing
such drugs as alcohol, barbiturates, and antianxiety agents. In such
cases, substance abuse often stops when the anxiety disorder is treated.
The extent to which anxiety interferes with work and social life varies
greatly among patients with this disorder, but impairment is usually
mild.

Treatment may employ a variety of modalities. *Antianxiety
medications* (e.g., benzodiazepines) are used to relieve symptoms and
improve functioning. However, these are prone to abuse, and dependence on them is a common problem among anxious patients. Thus,
you must closely monitor their use and limit their administration to
short periods of time. *Psychotherapy* is often effective in helping
patients to understand and master the underlying conflicts that prompt
anxiety; a therapeutic relationship provides much-needed emotional
support to anxious patients. *Behavior therapy* can teach patients techniques of relaxation that they can use in anxiety-provoking situations to
overcome fears and decrease symptoms (see Chapter 14).

PHOBIAS

A phobia is a persistent and irrational fear of a specific object, activity, or
situation that results in a compelling desire to avoid what is feared. Even
though the afflicted person recognizes the fear as excessive or unrealistic
given the actual dangerousness of the object, activity, or situation, he or
she nevertheless goes to some lengths to avoid it. If this avoidant
behavior has no major effect on the person's life, the phobic behavior
does not constitute a disorder (e.g., being afraid of spiders). However,

Table 8-2. Major categories of phobias.

Social phobias
  Fear of embarrassment or humiliation in public situations

Simple phobias
  Fear of specific objects or situations (other than being alone, being away
    from home, or embarrassment in public)

Agoraphobia
  Fear of being alone or in public places from which escape might be diffi-
    cult or help unavailable in case of sudden incapacitation

---

when the phobia impairs one's ability to function at normal daily tasks, the diagnosis of a phobic disorder is warranted.

Phobias are generally divided into three major categories, as shown in Table 8-2. *Agoraphobia* involves a fear of being alone or in public places from which escape might be difficult (e.g., crowds or closed spaces) and where help might not be readily obtainable. *Social phobias* involve a fear of embarrassment or humiliation in situations in which one must interact with other people (e.g., fear of speaking in public, using public lavatories, or eating in public). *Simple phobias* involve fear of specific objects or situations other than being alone, being away from home, or embarrassment in public (e.g., fear of snakes, fear of heights). For most patients with phobias, anxiety occurs not only when they are faced with the dreaded stimulus, but even when they anticipate encountering it (anticipatory anxiety).

Psychoanalytic theory holds that phobias begin as perceived dangers from within—that one's own fears of forbidden sexual or aggressive impulses become transposed onto some external object (e.g, snakes). Internal dangers cannot be avoided but a danger in the external world can be; thus, by using the defense mechanism of *displacement*, the phobic patient achieves a partial solution to the problem.

Behavioral treatment of simple and social phobias is often quite successful in alleviating the symptom and restoring the patient's lost ability to function at daily tasks. *Systematic desensitization* is a widely used behavioral technique that involves the creation of a hierarchy of anxiety-producing stimuli (e.g., thinking about a snake, then looking at pictures of snakes, and finally watching a live snake). The therapist then uses this hierarchy of stimuli to desensitize the patient, presenting them to the patient gradually until they no longer produce anxiety (see

Chapter 14). Psychotherapy that focuses on the childhood origins and symbolic meanings of the patient's fears has also been found to be helpful in some cases. Benzodiazepines and other antianxiety drugs can alleviate anticipatory anxiety, but are generally not suitable for long-term treatment. Some clinicians have found the phobic anxiety itself responsive to treatment with imipramine or phenelzine (see Chapter 15). At present, behavior therapy is the mainstay of treatment for simple and social phobias.

Since agoraphobia is usually associated with panic attacks, the treatment of agoraphobia will be discussed in the next section.

PANIC DISORDER

Panic disorder is a dramatic syndrome characterized by discrete spontaneous panic attacks—crescendos of fear and apprehension—associated with multiple physical symptoms. Attacks resemble the body's normal physiologic response to a life-threatening situation or extreme physical exertion but, in panic disorder, attacks come on suddenly and unpredictably without provocation.

Panic attacks are characterized by feelings of fear, extreme tension, and a sense of impending doom. Various physical symptoms accompany these feelings, most commonly:
- Shortness of breath
- Palpitations
- Chest pain or discomfort
- Choking or smothering sensations
- Dizziness, vertigo, or unsteady feelings
- Feelings of unreality
- Paresthesias (tingling in hands or feet)
- Hot and cold flashes
- Sweating
- Faintness
- Trembling or shaking
- Fear of going crazy, dying, or doing something uncontrolled during an attack
- Nausea, vomiting, diarrhea

Attacks commonly last for several minutes or, more rarely, for an hour or more. They recur with varying frequency. Psychotic disorders, medical illnesses (listed above), and substance abuse and withdrawal can all produce symptoms of panic and must be ruled out before you make this diagnosis.

Conversely, because the symptoms of panic attacks mimic many organic disorders, patients often consult internists for these symptoms and may have extensive medical work-ups and numerous consultations before the idea of a panic disorder is considered. The disorder is common; it occurs in an estimated 1 to 2 percent of the general population, although it frequently goes unrecognized. It is diagnosed more often among women than men, and typically begins in late adolescence or early adulthood. Panic disorder tends to run in families, and an accumulating body of evidence suggests both that biochemical factors play a crucial role in the etiology of this condition and that there may be a genetic vulnerability to it.

Panic disorder may be limited to one brief period of illness lasting several weeks or months, it may recur several times, or it may become chronic. Patients usually develop nervousness and apprehension between attacks; when this is severe, agoraphobia ensues.

Agoraphobia with panic attacks. Agoraphobia and panic attacks are so frequently encountered together that you are unlikely to encounter them separately in your clinical work.

How do the two go together? Many clinicians postulate that panic attacks come first, and that the fear of being alone and in public places where help is unavailable develops in response to these terrifying episodes of panic. Patients who experience recurrent symptoms of panic become preoccupied with a fear of developing subsequent attacks, and develop an increasing number of phobias about the settings in which they have experienced attacks in the past (e.g., in the supermarket, while driving a car). The number of situations they avoid increases until they are considered truly agoraphobic—afraid of being on their own in public places or of staying alone at home. Between panic attacks, they develop chronic anticipatory anxiety about having another attack.

They often do not seek psychiatric help until they have had symptoms for many years, and by that time they may have agoraphobia with multiple particular phobias, and chronic anticipatory anxiety in addition to the panic attacks themselves. Sadly, some patients with this syndrome become shut-ins, unable to leave the house or stay alone for even short periods of time.

Treatment must be aimed at each of the three aspects of this syndrome: panic attacks, anticipatory anxiety, and agoraphobia. It begins with a careful history, physical examination, and laboratory studies to rule out underlying organic illnesses. Panic attacks can be blocked effectively by maintaining patients on a tricyclic antidepressant (e.g., imipramine) or a monoamine oxidase (MAO) inhibitor. Anticipatory anxiety and free-floating anxiety can be treated with selective intermittent use of a benzodiazepine (e.g., diazepam). Recently, some clinicians have advocated the use of the benzodiazepine alprazolam (Xanax) alone, since it is thought to have properties that both reduce anticipatory anxiety and block panic attacks.

Agoraphobia may be treated with behavior therapy designed to expose patients gradually to feared experiences, so that they can slowly master their fear of recurrent attacks in specific situations (e.g., in supermarkets, at parties). Dynamically oriented psychotherapy may be necessary when anxiety is due to conflicts or to reactions to the environment that must be explored before symptoms will resolve.

POSTTRAUMATIC STRESS DISORDER

This disorder occurs among people who have survived traumatic events that are outside the realm of normal human experience—e.g., rape or assault, physical injury, military combat, bombings, torture, and floods or earthquakes. The afflicted person reexperiences the traumatic event through painful, intrusive recollections or nightmares. Episodes may last from several minutes to several days. During an episode, the person may behave as if he or she were reliving the event.

This disorder also involves a kind of "psychic numbing" or decreased responsiveness to the environment, which may be experienced as decreased ability to receive pleasure from life's activities, or diminished capacity to feel interest in and tenderness toward other people. Anxiety and depression commonly occur with this disorder.

People who experienced traumatic events with others may also feel guilty about having survived when others did not (e.g., concentration camp survivors). Some people are only minimally impaired by this disorder, but others are severely incapacitated by phobic avoidance of all situations that might remind them of the traumatic event and trigger further episodes. This disorder has received increasing attention in recent years because of its prevalence among those returning from the Vietnam War.

Psychotherapy, antianxiety agents, and antidepressants have all been used in the treatment of this disorder. Group psychotherapy with survivors of the same traumatic situation has been found useful, particularly for war veterans.

SOMATOFORM DISORDERS

Somatoform disorders are, quite literally, psychiatric disorders that assume the form of somatic illness. As any internist will tell you, these disorders are very common in general medical practice. Patients afflicted with them are often called "doctor-shoppers" or "hypochondriacs." They go from one medical facility to another, seeking help for an illness for which physicians can find no organic basis. It is a frustrating situation for patients, their families, and their physicians. They are told that there is nothing wrong, or that it is "all in their heads," yet they remain convinced that their pain and physical symptoms are real.

In fact, their symptoms and concerns *are* real—as if there were visible physical lesions to account for them. And patients with these disorders do not experience their symptoms as being within their control—i.e., they do not feel that they have voluntarily produced these problems. Yet the symptoms are linked to psychological factors that these patients are generally reluctant to explore, and so they persist in searching for an organic cause.

The somatoform disorders fall into the four major categories

Table 8-3. Major categories of somatoform disorders.

Somatization disorder
  Multiple recurrent somatic complaints of several years' duration which are not due to any physical disorder

Conversion disorder
  Sudden, dramatic loss of physical functioning that has no known pathophysiological cause and appears to be a manifestation of a psychological need or conflict

Psychogenic pain disorder
  Pain in the absence of adequate physical findings or pathophysiologic explanations, and in association with psychological factors that seem to play an etiological role

Hypochondriasis
  Unfounded fears of having serious illness

---

outlined below. All are characterized by physical symptoms that cannot be accounted for by any demonstrable physical findings or known physiological mechanisms.

Somatization Disorder

This disorder, also called *Briquet's syndrome* or *Briquet's hysteria*, is characterized by multiple somatic complaints that are recurrent and of several years' duration, for which medical attention has been sought but for which no physical cause can be found. Complaints are often general, vague, and dramatically presented. Any or all body systems may be involved, but the most common complaints are neurological (e.g., pseudoseizures), gastrointestinal, gynecologic, sexual, and cardiopulmonary. Chronic pain is generally present (e.g., back pain, joint pain), and abdominal pain is probably the most frequent specific complaint encountered among people with this disorder.

Somatization disorder begins before age 30 and has a chronic course, usually involving consultation by many physicians and frequently complicated by multiple hospital admissions and unnecessary surgical procedures. Abuse of both prescribed and nonprescribed substances is common. Anxiety and depression often accompany this disorder. When afflicted individuals seek psychiatric help, it is often for symptoms of depression, or after suicide threats or gestures. The disorder is much more commonly diagnosed among women than men, with estimates that one percent of women in the general population suffer from it.

Before you make this diagnosis, you must rule out organic illnesses (e.g., multiple sclerosis, systemic lupus erythematosus) that can present with vague and diffuse symptomatology. Also, some schizophrenic patients suffer from somatic delusions as part of their illness (e.g., "my insides are rotting"); it is important to differentiate such psychotic patients from people with somatization disorder, who are, by definition, not psychotic and do not benefit from treatment with antipsychotic medication.

Conversion Disorder

Also called *conversion hysteria*, this is the "classic" disorder that fascinated Freud and other pioneers in the field of psychoanalytic psychiatry. It typically involves the sudden and dramatic onset of blindness, paralysis, seizures, or other symptoms that seem to suggest neurological disease but that have no known pathophysiological cause. It is different from somatization disorder in that it generally involves a single symptom during any one episode, and this symptom results in the loss or alteration of a particular physical function.

In addition to the symptoms mentioned above, typical conversion symptoms include loss of speech, involuntary movements, inability to walk, loss of coordination, tunnel vision, and anesthesia or paresthesia of a body part. Although symptoms appear to be neurological, careful examination and tests reveal discrepancies between the loss of function and known anatomical distribution of motor and sensory nerves. For example, anesthesia of a hand typically occurs over a "glove" distribution, rather than along lines of anatomical sensory innervation.

Conversion symptoms are not under the patient's voluntary control, yet they appear to be the expression of a psychological conflict or need. These symptoms are thought to provide patients with two sorts of gains. The *primary gain* from the symptom is thought to be relief from an emotional conflict and the reduction of anxiety. The symptom actually represents the conflict and achieves a partial solution to it. In such cases, there is usually a temporal relationship between an event that provokes conflict and the onset of the symptom (e.g., conflict about expressing overwhelming rage at a spouse, which results in loss of speech).

The *secondary gain*, common to all somatoform disorders, is that, by assuming a sick role, the disabled patient can avoid unwanted responsibilities and get support from others that would not otherwise be forthcoming. Because the conversion symptom diminishes anxiety and intrapsychic conflict, patients may be blind or paralyzed and yet seem relatively unconcerned about their severe physical disability—a phenomenon called *la belle indifference.*

Conversion disorder usually begins in adolescence or young adulthood. Episodes of conversion begin suddenly during times of severe stress and resolve abruptly. Functioning may be greatly impaired, and the patient may develop physical complications (e.g., limb contractures) due to prolonged loss of function. Unnecessary medical procedures can also produce serious complications. Although it was more common several decades ago, the disorder is now relatively rare in clinical practice in industrialized nations.

Psychogenic Pain Disorder

Psychogenic pain disorder involves the predominant complaint of pain in the absence of any physical findings or pathophysiologic explanation. It differs from somatization disorder in that pain, rather than a variety of symptoms, is the primary presenting complaint. Pain generally does not follow the anatomical distribution of motor and sensory nerves, and laboratory studies reveal no underlying lesions. There is usually a relationship between the exacerbation of psychological conflict or need and the onset of or increase in pain. Secondary gain is generally an important motivating force in the illness (e.g., the man whose chronic back pain worsens every time his wife plans an outing with friends). However, the patient does not experience the pain as being within his or her voluntary control.

The disorder typically begins in adolescence or early adulthood, but it can occur at any age and may remit spontaneously or become chronic. It is more common in women, but the reasons for this are not clear. As you might expect, frequent medical consultations, unnecessary surgery, and abuse of analgesics are common complications of this disorder.

Hypochondriasis

Unlike the other somatoform disorders, hypochondriasis involves unfounded *fears* of having serious illness. It is based on a preoccupation with body functions and the unrealistic interpretation of physical signs or sensations as abnormal, e.g., an occasional cough may be interpreted as a sign of lung cancer. Although these concerns are not frankly delusional, patients cannot shake their fears of physical illness despite repeated reassurance from physicians and persistently negative physical and laboratory findings.

Hypochondriasis is equally common in men and women. It begins most frequently among men in their thirties and among women in their forties. It is quite common in general medical practice, and its chronic course invites extensive work-ups and unnecessary surgery. Although some patients can continue to function with only mild impairment at home and at work, others become invalids. One danger in this disorder is that real organic pathology may go unnoticed because of repeated '"false alarms."

Treatment of Somatoform Disorders

The treatment of somatoform disorders is difficult. Patients usually refuse to accept the possibility that the roots of their problems are psychological. Insight-oriented psychotherapy can help some patients explore and resolve conflicts that foster physical symptoms; with conflict resolution, symptoms often disappear spontaneously. However, many of these patients are particularly resistant to exploratory psychotherapy. Biofeedback and other behavior modification techniques can help patients to relax and control pain and anxiety.

Antianxiety medications are helpful for some patients on a short-term basis, but the potential for abuse and dependence on such drugs limits their value in the treatment of these disorders. Antidepressant medication has been found to be helpful for patients who have prominent symptoms of depression along with somatic complaints.

One great service a therapist can provide patients with somatoform disorders is to coordinate their medical care, so that "doctor-shopping" ends and unnecessary surgical procedures are avoided. This requires a good working relationship between the psychiatrist and other physicians responsible for the patient's medical care.

DISSOCIATIVE DISORDERS

Dissociative disorders are relatively rare phenomena in psychiatric practice. Their discussion here will therefore be brief. They are, however, quite dramatic and have received much publicity in literature, in films, and on television. The four major disorders are described below.

Psychogenic Amnesia

This disorder is a sudden inability to recall important personal information (e.g., name, occupation, family). This may be amnesia for the patient's entire life up until the moment of onset, or it may be amnesia for a circumscribed period of time (e.g., for the events surrounding a car crash). Amnesia may be selective; that is, some events during a specified period of time are forgotten, while others are still subject to recall.

Unlike amnesia that is due to organic mental disorders, psychogenic amnesia usually has an abrupt onset following a traumatic or

Table 8-4. Major categories of dissociative disorders.

Psychogenic amnesia
   Sudden inability to recall important personal information

Psychogenic fugue
   Amnesia combined with sudden travel away from home, usually in
     flight from an intolerable situation

Multiple personality
   The existence of two or more distinct personalities within an individual,
     each of which is dominant at a particular time

Depersonalization disorder
   Feelings of self-estrangement or unreality that impair social or occupa-
     tional functioning

---

unusually stressful experience. It generally resolves abruptly as well, and recurrences are rare.

Psychogenic Fugue

In this disorder, amnesia is combined with physical flight, usually from an intolerable situation. The individual assumes a new identity and is unable to recall his or her previous one. This is generally a short-lived phenomenon, involving a minimal amount of travel, but it may be quite prolonged and may result in the assumption of a whole new life in another locale (e.g., a man may leave his family, move to another city, get a new job, and make a new set of friends).

    Recovery is usually as abrupt as the onset, and recurrences are rare.

Multiple Personality

Multiple personality involves the existence within the individual of two or more distinct personalities, each with its own unique set of memories, attributes, and social relationships. Each is dominant at different times, and the transition from one personality to another is often abrupt.

    The personalities are usually distinct, and represent different unintegrated aspects of the person's identity. For example, a patient may have one shy and inhibited personality, another that is gregarious and promiscuous, and a third that is hostile and suspicious. The personalities may call themselves by different names. Each one may be unaware of the existence of the other personalities, and aware only of lost periods of time when the other personalities are dominant.

This disorder is exceedingly rare, and its course is generally more chronic than those of the other dissociative disorders mentioned. Intensive psychotherapy is usually the treatment of choice, with the goal of helping the patient to integrate the different personalities into one coherent self.

Interesting case studies of multiple personality in the popular literature include *The Three Faces of Eve* and *Sybil*.

Depersonalization Disorder

This disorder involves the occurrence of one or more episodes of depersonalization, manifested by feelings of self-estrangement or unreality. Patients often report feeling as if they were watching a play rather than participating in real life, or as if they were watching themselves from a distance.

Such episodes are extremely common in normal persons, especially young adults during times of stress. They only constitute a disorder when they impair social or occupational functioning. The disorder is often chronic, commonly waxing and waning as the patient's degree of anxiety or depression increases or decreases.

EATING DISORDERS

Eating disorders have become the focus of much interest among mental health professionals in recent years. An increasing number of people (predominantly women) report gross disturbances in their eating behavior. The two most prevalent syndromes are *anorexia nervosa* and *bulimia*. Although these eating disorders are described as primary—i.e., as not resulting from some medical illness—a great many patients with anorexia and bulimia also suffer from other diagnosable mental disorders. In fact, eating disorders occur in people who span the entire range of psychopathology, from psychosis to anxiety disorders and neurosis. In particular, many people with severe disturbances in their eating behavior suffer from personality disorders.

Thus, when you see patients who report eating problems such as binge eating and vomiting, or who engage in self-starvation, you should look carefully for underlying psychosis, affective disturbances, and personality disorders before assuming that the eating disorder is an isolated problem.

Anorexia Nervosa

Anorexia nervosa is a syndrome of self-starvation in which the patient willfully restricts food intake and overexercises in an effort to ease the intense fear of becoming obese. Anorectics report feeling fat when they are at normal body weight and even when they are emaciated, because weight loss does not decrease their fear of obesity. They suffer from a distorted perception of their bodies, and have difficulty identifying bodily sensations, including the feeling of hunger. However, anorexia nervosa is not primarily a disturbance in appetite. Rather, it is related to disturbances in the sense of self, identity, and autonomy. The anorectic struggles desperately to control appetite and weight, often to combat an underlying and global sense of helplessness.

Anorectics are almost exclusively female (95 percent)—most commonly adolescent girls and young adults. The syndrome often begins unnoticed by others, as the anorectic goes on a diet "to slim down." But as weight loss progresses and food intake decreases, family and friends gradually become alarmed, while the anorectic remains adamant in her desire to lose weight because she is fat. Many anorectic teenagers give histories of being overly compliant "model children," who become angry and negativistic as the syndrome develops and they begin to struggle with their families over eating practices. Besides using diet and exercise to accomplish their starvation, anorectics also use self-induced vomiting, laxatives, and diuretics. Weight loss, by definition, proceeds to at least 25 percent of the anorectic's original body weight (or projected normal body weight in growing teenagers), and may go well beyond this mark to total emaciation.

Anorectics typically deny that they have a problem, and do not want treatment. Anorectic adolescents often manifest delayed sexual development, and adults show little interest in sex. (Amenorrhea is often one of the earliest results of the anorectic's stringent dieting.) Many theorists postulate a fear of sexuality as contributing to the anorectic's drive to become emaciated.

Fortunately, most anorectics experience a single episode of the eating disorder and then recover completely without recurrence. However, some people have recurrent periods of anorexia, and a sizable proportion take an unremitting course, with progressive starvation. Factors associated with a good prognosis include onset of the problem before age 15 and weight gain within two years after treatment is begun.

If weight loss becomes profound, physical signs ensue, including hypothermia, pedal edema, slowed heart rate, hypotension, and lanugo (fine, soft body hair). Medical complications include severe electrolyte disturbances, coma, and death. *Anorexia nervosa is a potentially lethal disease*—mortality ranges from 15 to 21 percent. Hospitalization and forced feeding are often necessary to prevent starvation, and procedures such as feeding by means of a nasogastric or gastrostomy tube come to be the focus of the severely anorectic patient's angry struggles to maintain rigid control over her body.

Treatment of anorexia nervosa is extremely difficult. The first goal must be improvement of the patient's nutritional status, both to stabilize the patient's medical condition and to reverse the psychological disturbances (such as difficulty in assimilating new information) that specifically result from starvation. Only when the worst malnutrition is reversed can you get an accurate picture of the patient's baseline psychological condition (e.g., the presence of a thought disorder or severe personality disturbance). Underlying illness must be treated with psychotherapy and, where indicated, medication.

Clinicians have reported some success in treating anorexia nervosa with a combination of behavior therapy aimed at maintaining weight at an adequate level and insight-oriented psychotherapy aimed at elucidating and correcting patients' inner confusion and misconceptions

Table 8-5. Major categories of eating disorders.

Anorexia nervosa
> Intense fear of becoming obese and a disturbance of body image that leads to willful restriction of food intake, significant weight loss, and refusal to maintain a minimal normal body weight

Bulimia
> Recurrent episodes of binge eating accompanied by a fear of not being able to stop eating, and followed by depressed mood and self-deprecating thoughts

Bulimarexia
> Features of both bulimia and anorexia nervosa—particularly binge eating and refusal to maintain a minimal normal body weight

about their own feelings and needs, their self-worth, and their ability to control their lives. An important adjunct to this treatment is family therapy aimed at decreasing the family's characteristic overinvolvement with the patient, and helping the family to allow the patient more autonomy.

Bulimia

Bulimia is a disorder characterized by recurrent episodes of binge eating that are frequently associated with self-induced vomiting or laxative abuse. Binge eating involves rapidly consuming large amounts of food in a short period of time. In contrast to patients with anorexia nervosa, bulimics are generally aware that their eating patterns are abnormal, and they fear not being able to stop eating voluntarily. Bulimics often become depressed after binges, and frequently berate themselves for their behavior.

Binges commonly consist of high-calorie foods, many of which are sweet and can be eaten quickly. Eating is usually done secretively, and the binge eater often stops only when abdominal pain becomes severe, sleep intervenes, or social circumstances make it impossible to continue gorging. Bulimics frequently vomit after binges to relieve abdominal pain, reduce guilt, and control their weight. Their weight may fluctuate widely, because of alternating periods of binge eating and fasting, or it may remain stable. When it is severe, bingeing may disrupt bulimics' social and occupational lives, since they may spend hours secretly procuring food, gorging themselves, and rushing to a bathroom to induce vomiting after each binge.

Bulimia typically begins in adolescence or early adulthood. It is much more common in women than in men. It generally follows a chronic course, occurring intermittently over many years, and episodes of binge eating are often precipitated by life stresses. The etiology of bulimia is not known but, in many cases, the eating disorder is related to more global psychopathology (e.g., an underlying personality disorder).

A variety of treatment modalities have been used with bulimic patients, including behavior modification techniques, insight-oriented psychotherapy, and cognitive therapy—all with limited success (see Chapter 14). Recently, research has focused on a possible link between bulimia and affective disorder, and new studies suggest a role for antidepressant medication in the treatment of bulimic patients.

Bulimarexia

This term is used to describe patients who exhibit features of both bulimia and anorexia nervosa—i.e., binge eating, vomiting, and self-starvation with severe weight loss. The overlap between the two syndromes is significant; it is estimated that between 40 and 50 percent of patients with primary anorexia nervosa exhibit bulimic behavior.

REFERENCES

Bruch H: Anorexia nervosa: therapy and theory. Am J Psychiatry 139:1531-1538, 1982.

Bruch H: Eating Disorders: Obesity, Anorexia Nervosa, and the Person Within. New York, Basic Books, 1973.

Diagnostic and Statistical Manual of Mental Disorders, 3rd ed. Washington, DC, American Psychiatric Association, 1980, pp 225-252.

Dietch JT: Diagnosis of organic anxiety disorders. Psychosomatics 22:661-669, 1981.

Garfinkel PE, Moldofsky H, Garner DM: The heterogeneity of anorexia nervosa: bulimia as a distinct subgroup. Arch Gen Psychiatry 37:1036-1040, 1980.

Pope HG, Hudson JI, Jonas JM, Yurgelun-Todd M: Bulimia treated with imipramine: a placebo-controlled, double-blind study. Am J Psychiatry, 140:554-558, 1983.

Schreiber F: Sybil. New York, Warner Books, 1974. (An account of the psychotherapy of a woman with multiple personalities.)

Shader RI, Goodman M, Gever J: Panic disorders: current perspectives. J Clin Psychopharmacology 2 (6 Suppl): 2S-10S, 1982.

Shader RI, Greenblatt DJ, Ciraulo DA: Benzodiazepine treatment of specific anxiety states. Psychiatr Annals 11:16-20, 1981.

Sheehan DV: Current concepts in psychiatry: panic attacks and phobias. N Engl J Med 307:156-158, 1982.

Thigpen CH, Cleckley HN: The Three Faces of Eve. New York, Popular Library, 1974. (A highly readable case study of a woman with multiple personalities.)

9

Dementia and Delirium

DEMENTIA AND DELIRIUM are conditions characterized by *global* intellectual impairment. Patients with these disorders commonly suffer from deficits in memory, in abstract thinking, in the ability to learn new tasks and solve problems, and in orientation to time, place, and person. These syndromes generally result from diffuse disease of the brain and consequent loss of function of large numbers of neurons.

Delirium is commonly referred to as an *acute organic brain syndrome*. It is characterized by a clouded state of consciousness, often with a rapid onset, a fluctuating course, and short duration. In addition to diffuse intellectual deficits, the delirious patient is likely to suffer from hallucinations, delusions, and increased motor activity (see Table 9-1).

Dementia, by contrast, is often called a *chronic organic brain syndrome*. Consciousness is not usually clouded in dementia until the end stages of the dementing process. The onset of dementia is usually insidious, the course is one of slow but persistent deterioration, and the demented patient is much less likely than the delirious patient to manifest hallucinations or other signs of disordered thinking. The demented patient is not generally agitated or hyperactive; rather, motor activity is usually normal or slow.

Table 9-1. Comparison of dementia and delirium.

Dementia	Delirium
"Chronic organic brain syndrome"	"Acute organic brain syndrome"
Consciousness unimpaired (until late in the course of disease)	Consciousness clouded
Normal level of arousal	Agitation or stupor
Develops insidiously over months or years	Develops rapidly
Often chronic, progressive	Often reversible
Common in nursing homes, psychiatric hospitals	Common on medical wards in general hospitals

Both dementia and delirium are included under the general diagnostic category of *organic brain syndromes*. But the term is not particularly useful, for it is nonspecific and conveys little information about the conditions it is meant to describe. It is also somewhat misleading, in that it implies that we can neatly separate disorders that have "organic" causes from other psychiatric illnesses that are functional in origin. It makes more sense to refer to dementia and delirium, as well as other "organic" syndromes (such as those caused by drugs and alcohol), by their specific names.

Dementia and delirium are *not* diseases—they are conditions that can result from a large number of underlying organic processes affecting brain tissue, and a vast array of underlying somatic illnesses can give rise to them. Stereotypically, delirium is reversible, while dementia is irreversible. However, there are remediable causes of both dementia and delirium, and you must diligently search for such treatable illnesses whenever a patient presents to you with global cognitive deterioration.

You need not memorize all the possible organic etiologies of dementia and delirium, but it *is* important that you:

• Learn to recognize the signs of dementia and delirium, so that you will not overlook these syndromes.

• Be aware of possible underlying causes that are treatable.

• Understand the need for careful examination and laboratory work-up of every patient who presents with altered cognitive functioning.

• Understand the course and treatment of those common syndromes that are not reversible.

DEMENTIA

Dementia is defined as a deterioration in intellectual abilities that is of sufficient severity to interfere with social or occupational functioning. The deficit involves many aspects of cognition—particularly memory and judgment. Higher cortical functions such as language, abstract reasoning, and the ability to follow directions are also commonly impaired. Although dementia is most common in the elderly, it is *not* synonymous with old age, nor is it a normal part of the aging process; rather, it implies diffuse disease of the brain that has impaired the functioning of larger numbers of cerebral cortical neurons. The *Diagnostic and Statistical Manual* (DSM-III) criteria for the diagnosis of dementia (pp. 111-112) are shown in Table 9-2.

Table 9-2. DSM-III diagnostic criteria for dementia.

A loss of intellectual abilities of sufficient severity to interfere with social or occupational functioning

Memory impairment

At least one of the following:
  Impairment of abstract thinking, as manifested by concrete interpretation of proverbs, inability to find similarities and differences between related words, difficulty in defining words and concepts, and other similar tasks
  Impaired judgment
  Other disturbances of higher cortical function, such as aphasia (disorder of language due to brain dysfunction), apraxia (inability to carry out motor activities despite intact comprehension and motor function), agnosia (failure to recognize or identify objects despite intact sensory function), "constructional difficulty" (e.g., inability to copy three-dimensional figures, assemble blocks, or arrange sticks in specific designs)
  Personality change, i.e., alteration or accentuation of premorbid traits

State of consciousness not clouded (i.e., does not meet the criteria for delirium or intoxication, although these may be superimposed)

Either (a) evidence from the history, physical examination, or laboratory tests of a specific organic factor that is judged to be etiologically related to the disturbance or, in the absence of such evidence, (b) an organic factor necessary for the development of the syndrome can be presumed if conditions other than organic mental disorders have been reasonably excluded and if the behavioral change represents cognitive impairment in a variety of areas

---

Clinical Picture

As noted above, dementia normally has an insidious onset, evolving over many months or even many years. It often begins with vague, nonspecific physical complaints, increased moodiness or irritability, and subtle withdrawal of interest from life. Patients often seem to be "not themselves," and their personalities appear to lose their sparkle. The early symptoms are so subtle that families often cannot identify any specific disorder, and instead are likely to be hurt by the seemingly willful moodiness and emotional withdrawal of their loved one. Patients begin to have trouble with any activity that requires new or original thought or learning. Dementia may thus be apparent earlier in those who are involved in more intense creative and intellectual endeavors.

Early memory loss may go unnoticed by the patient and the family. For example, patients may begin to forget dates or telephone numbers, but may compensate for this quite well by writing things down. They may forget instructions or directions, and may need to ask that these be repeated several times before they can commit the information to memory. Some patients notice such deficits in memory themselves, while others remain oblivious to them even when they become obvious to family and friends. Demented people may even fabricate false details (*confabulation*) to fill in gaps in their memory. As the dementia progresses, patients become increasingly distractible. They may, for example, begin tasks but forget to return to them after an interruption. Patients who live alone may forget to turn off the stove and thereby put themselves in danger.

Demented patients eventually begin to lose more skills, and their deficits become more obvious. They commonly become lost on their way to familiar places, and it is then that their condition may begin to seem more serious to those around them. Language initially remains unimpaired but, as other intellectual functions deteriorate, language usually begins to become more stereotyped and to convey less and less information. Patients may perseverate in speech (i.e., repeat the same word or phrase over and over again), or may continue to perform work, such as arranging chairs, long after the task has been completed. Although they normally become more quiet and socially withdrawn, some demented people become more active in socially inappropriate ways, such as going on spending sprees or becoming physically assaultive.

When dementia becomes severe, patients are unable to perform such simple tasks as feeding themselves, despite the fact that motor functions remain intact. They forget the names of friends, are unable to recognize even close relatives, and finally forget their own name and date of birth (although this information is usually the very last to be forgotten). They increasingly neglect their personal hygiene and begin to disregard normal rules of social conduct. More infantile behaviors, such as incontinence and extreme emotional lability (fits of laughing and crying) may appear. Finally, many patients become totally mute and unresponsive to the environment. At this stage, death often occurs within a few months, but patients with end-stage dementia may linger on in this stage for several years.

Although dementia occurs most frequently in the elderly, the age at which it develops and the course it takes depends on the underlying cause. Patients may remain unaware of and unconcerned by their growing deficits, or they may recognize them and react with anxiety, depression, or paranoia. When personality changes occur, they are usually exaggerations of preexisting character traits (e.g., a man who has always been somewhat suspicious by nature may become floridly paranoid as dementia progresses). Demented patients sometimes develop hallucinations, delusions, hypochondriacal concerns, and even suicidal ideation as a result of such personality change and deterioration. All the symptoms of dementia can be exacerbated by stress, such as a move to unfamiliar surroundings, hospitalization, loss of a loved one, or concurrent medical illness. Dementia is not a lethal condition in and of itself, but the inability to care for oneself predisposes patients to malnutrition, decubitus ulcers, and aspiration pneumonia (which is the most common cause of death).

Irreversible Causes

Senile and presenile dementia (Alzheimer's disease). This disease, the most common form of dementia, accounts for roughly half of all cases. It is of unknown etiology and is associated with diffuse atrophy of the cerebral cortex. Clinicians have traditionally made a distinction between senile and presenile dementia, based on whether the disease began before or after age 60, but there is in fact little clinical or pathological basis for such a distinction. The illness is very similar, whether it begins at age 45 or at age 95. The term *Alzheimer's disease* was once synonymous with presenile dementia, but you will now hear it used to describe *idiopathic primary dementia* without reference to age of onset.

Alzheimer's disease usually begins after age 60, but it is seen as early as age 40. Estimates of the prevalence of Alzheimer's disease among those over age 65 range from 5 to 12 percent, and it is a leading (although often unreported) cause of death among the aged.

Its symptoms begin very gradually and progressively worsen, often over several years. At present, the disease process is irreversible. Afflicted individuals may live as long as 10 years after the onset of the disease, but they eventually require total care and succumb to secondary illnesses, e.g., aspiration pneumonia.

Physical findings are generally absent in Alzheimer's disease, or are present only in the end stages of the illness, when there may be hyperactive deep tendon reflexes, positive Babinski signs, and snout, suck, and rooting reflexes (signs of frontal lobe release). Patients with Alzheimer's disease often have normal computed tomography (CT) scans, although they typically show some atrophy of the cerebral cortex and dilatation of the cerebral ventricles, particularly if the disease is far advanced. Electroencephalogram (EEG) abnormalities are present in about 80 percent of patients (usually diffuse slowing and decreased alpha rhythm), but these changes are not diagnostic. Thus, there are no diagnostic laboratory studies; the clinical diagnosis of Alzheimer's disease is made only when the history, physical examination, and laboratory work-up have ruled out other causes of dementia.

At autopsy, patients with Alzheimer's disease have characteristic brain pathology that includes:

- Senile plaques—microscopic lesions of the cerebral cortex, consisting of neurons tangled around an amyloid core.
- Neurofibrillary tangles, helical filaments tangled within neurons throughout the cortex.
- Granulovacular degeneration of nerve cell bodies.

Such changes occur in normal aging brains, but much less extensively than they do in the brains of patients with dementia.

Despite recent intensive research into the causes and treatment of this devastating and common illness, its etiology remains a mystery. Several hypotheses about the cause of Alzheimer's disease have received a great deal of public attention. In particular, the theory that Alzheimer's disease is caused by abnormally high levels of aluminum in the central nervous system (CNS) has not been substantiated by empirical research, nor has the notion of a viral etiology. Much attention has recently been focused on the hypothesis that patients with Alzheimer's disease have abnormal (decreased) cholinergic activity in the CNS, but at present this too remains unproven.

Pick's disease is similar to Alzheimer's in its clinical manifestations and pathology, but involvement spares the parietal lobes. Since this incurable familial disorder is rare and almost impossible to differentiate clinically from Alzheimer's, it need not be discussed in detail.

Cerebrovascular dementia. "Hardening of the arteries" was once thought to be responsible for most cases of dementia. Alzheimer's disease has since been recognized as the major dementing illness in the elderly, but cerebrovascular disease is thought to account for a significant number of cases as well (perhaps 15 to 25 percent).

Atherosclerosis, in and of itself, does not seem to result in dementia; rather, it predisposes patients to cerebral damage from emboli, thrombi, and hemorrhage. In fact, it appears that multiple small infarctions of brain tissue produce dementia, and the condition often has a fluctuating, "stuttering" course with stepwise deterioration in functioning. Patients with this disease commonly have high blood pressure or diabetes. Some give a history of several strokes in the past, but many have had "silent" infarcts and have no awareness of discrete episodes of neurologic illness. There are usually focal neurological signs (e.g., weakness of one limb). In some cases, cerebrovascular disease and Alzheimer's coexist, and both contribute to the picture of dementia.

Although atherosclerosis in major arteries (e.g., stenosis of the internal carotid artery) may be surgically correctable, much atherosclerosis occurs diffusely among smaller intracranial vessels and is therefore not amenable to any specific intervention. Hypertension can be controlled in most cases, and early treatment of asymptomatic patients can help to prevent or arrest the development of multi-infarct dementia. Patients who have had or are at risk for strokes may benefit from the administration of anticoagulants or aspirin, which may prevent thrombus formation.

Treatable Causes

Tumors. Most intracranial neoplasms cause focal neurological signs (e.g., weakness on one side of the body), and are therefore not likely to be confused with Alzheimer's disease. However, depending on their anatomical location, tumors may initially present with psychiatric symptoms and no other obvious disturbances, and so may be mistaken for signs of "senility." The most common forms of intracranial tumors are gliomas (which constitute 30-50 percent of all brain tumors), meningiomas (20 percent), and secondary metastases (20 percent), most often from lung or breast carcinomas or malignant melanomas. Tumors of the frontal lobe, thalamus, and corpus callosum, as well as olfactory groove meningiomas, are particularly likely to present with psychiatric symptoms but no neurologic findings. Thus, it is generally recommended that every patient with dementia (indeed, every patient who has undergone a major personality change) have a CT scan to rule out a tumor. Obviously, how treatable neoplasms are depends largely on the location of the tumor and whether it is malignant or benign, but in some cases intellectual impairment can be completely reversed by successful surgical intervention.

Brain trauma. Trauma to any part of the nervous system usually results in maximal impairment immediately after the event. Victims of brain injury continue to recover lost function for up to a year. Such obvious cases of trauma are not generally mistaken for Alzheimer's disease or other forms of primary dementia. However, *chronic subdural hematoma* is easy to confuse with Alzheimer's, and the consequences of failing to recognize this life-threatening problem may be disastrous.

Subdural hematoma denotes a collection of blood that is extracerebral but within the cranium. It often results from head trauma but, particularly in elderly patients, the trauma may be minor or not recalled at all. When blood collects slowly and puts gradually increasing pressure on the brain, the patient may become demented over days or even weeks without focal neurological signs or impaired consciousness. A CT scan will generally reveal these mass lesions (which are often bilateral). Surgical evacuation of the hematoma may be life-saving, and will frequently reverse the intellectual impairment.

Normal-pressure hydrocephalus (NPH). A small subgroup of people who present with dementia have been found to have hydrocephalus (excessive accumulation of cerebrospinal fluid dilating the ventricles of the brain) with normal CSF pressure. The flow of CSF from the ventricles to its usual site of absorption in the subarachnoid space surrounding the cerebral cortex is somehow obstructed, so fluid collects within the ventricles and causes the characteristic syndrome of *dementia, gait apraxia,* and *urinary incontinence.* (Gait apraxia is a particular type of abnormality of locomotion in which the patient has normal strength and coordination, but literally loses the intellectual ability to organize the act of walking, and therefore has difficulty in lifting each foot in succession.)

Although some people with NPH have a history of meningitis, subarachnoid hemorrhage, or trauma that might account for the obstruction of the normal flow of CSF, in many cases there is no apparent cause for this abnormality. The syndrome develops gradually, often over 6 to 12 months. A CT scan reveals dilated ventricles, out of proportion to the degree of atrophy of brain tissue.

Treatment is surgical: a shunt allows CSF to flow from the cerebral ventricles to another body cavity, such as the peritoneal cavity. In cases that are accurately diagnosed, this procedure can result in dramatic improvement in symptoms. (The degree of gait disturbance that results from drawing off CSF by lumbar puncture may predict improvement.) However, in some cases no improvement ensues—perhaps because of misdiagnosis—and the shunt procedure has many complications. Although NPH occurs infrequently, it must be considered in the differential diagnosis of dementia because it is potentially treatable.

Dementia Secondary to Systemic Illness

As noted above, a great many systemic illnesses—including metabolic disturbances, infections, and exposure to toxins—can present with gradual intellectual deterioration. These conditions run the gamut from porphyria to pellagra, from lead poisoning to tuberculous meningitis. It is therefore critical to do a careful screen for these disorders so that you will not overlook treatable causes of dementia. These illnesses are well described in general medical texts. Table 9-3 lists some of the most common diseases that may present with dementia.

Pseudodementia

Despite the implication of its name, this condition is a true dementia, but it is due to a functional psychiatric disorder—depression. When dementia is seen in elderly people, it is assumed to be due to Alzheimer's disease. In fact, many older people who present with a deterioration in personality, retardation of thought and action, apathy, disorientation, sleep disturbance, and global loss of intellectual functions are not demented, but depressed.

It may be impossible to differentiate depression from dementia on the basis of clinical findings, but if you take a careful history from

Table 9-3. Some diseases that may present with dementia.

Metabolic disorders
  Hepatic encephalopathy (liver failure)
  Wilson's disease
  Uremia (kidney failure)
  Hypoxia (congestive heart failure, anemia)

Deficiency diseases
  Wernicke-Korsakoff syndrome (thiamine)
  Pernicious anemia (vitamin B_{12}, folate)
  Pellagra (niacin)

Endocrine disorders
  Thyroid disease (hypothyroidism, thyroid storm)
  Hypercalcemia (parathyroid disorders)
  Cushing's disease
  Pancreatic disease (diabetic ketoacidosis, hypoglycemia)

Toxins (exogenous)
  Drugs of abuse: amphetamines, cocaine, alcohol, LSD
  Prescription drugs: bromides, steroids, reserpine, methyldopa, L-dopa, pro-
    pranolol, scopolamine, atropine
  Industrial toxins: lead, mercury, manganese, carbon monoxide, organic
    solvents

Infections
  Chronic meningitis (tuberculosis, cryptococcosis)
  Viral meningitis
  Syphilis (tertiary lues)
  Creutzfeld-Jakob disease (slow virus)

Neurologic diseases (often accompanied by movement disorders)
  Huntington's chorea
  Parkinson's disease
  Spino-cerebellar degeneration

Neoplasms

family or close friends, you are likely to find that patients with pseudodementia have not deteriorated over many months or years, but have been "demented" for only a few weeks. Moreover, you are likely to see that this deterioration is associated with feelings of sadness. Be particularly alert to pseudodementia in anyone with a family history of depression or manic-depressive illness.

The differential diagnosis is extremely difficult, because demented patients who recognize their growing deficits may react with depression, and depressed patients may also have mild dementia. The important point is that, whenever you suspect a depressive component to the illness, it is worth giving "demented" patients a trial of antidepressant therapy or electroconvulsive therapy (ECT), for they may respond. In fact, some people who appear floridly demented recover all their baseline mental abilities when the underlying depression is treated. If pseudodementia goes undetected, it may be fatal, because the patient may lapse into total self-neglect, or attempt suicide.

Interview and Evaluation

Demented patients are often brought to physicians by family members when they can no longer tolerate such symptoms as increased emotional outbursts, socially embarrassing or dangerous behavior, and suspiciousness. Demented people are less likely than delirious patients to be psychotic or to appear medically ill. They are often quite alert, neatly dressed, and socially appropriate when they meet you. Evidence of dementia in the course of conversation may be difficult to find, and may only take the form of an apparent hesitancy in answering questions. Patients may cover their memory deficits by dismissing a question as unimportant (e.g., "I don't need to know the date any more, doctor, since I retired") or by giving a tangential answer.

Only by performing a careful mental status examination will you pick up early signs of dementia. Patients will have difficulty with tests of recent memory, and so be unable to remember three unrelated objects (e.g., apple, tree, chair) several minutes after they are given the task. Their interpretations of proverbs will be concrete if their abstract thinking is impaired, and they will have difficulty naming objects, doing simple calculations, following directions, or copying geometric patterns.

If dementia is more advanced, signs of memory impairment, distractibility, and other cognitive difficulties will be readily apparent in conversation before you get to the mental status examination.

A word of caution in interviewing demented patients: It is important to be particularly gentle in testing cognitive functioning. A patient who is suddenly forced to confront his or her intellectual deficits during the interview may become acutely embarrassed, anxious, depressed, or agitated. Such "catastrophic reactions," as they are called, can sometimes be avoided if you proceed slowly, respectfully, and with tact in conducting a mental status examination.

Taking a history. As you do a general psychiatric evaluation, keep the following in mind:

Document the course of the illness. When did problems first begin? What were the earliest changes noted? What intellectual functions seem to have deteriorated? Was deterioration rapid or slow, stepwise or gradual? Has the patient become unable to care for himself or herself, and in what ways?

Note any accompanying psychiatric symptoms. Have there been mood changes (depression, sadness, elation)? Has the patient shown signs of disordered thinking (e.g., hallucinations, paranoia)?

Note accompanying physical symptoms. Have there been vegetative signs (sleep disturbance, weight loss) or other signs of systemic illness (e.g., fever)? Has the patient suffered from headaches, seizures, or paralysis? Has he or she begun to make any involuntary movements?

Take a medical history. Note major medical or neurological illnesses. Be sure to document any history of psychiatric illness as well (e.g., affective illness, psychotic episodes).

Note all medications, drug use, and possible exposure to toxins at home or work (and their relationship to the onset of symptoms). Do not forget over-the-counter preparations.

Obtain a careful family history. Has anyone else in the family been demented or suffered from other neurologic disease? Is there a family history of depression or mania?

Pay attention to the patient's social supports. How much can the patient do for himself or herself? How much assistance is required? Who is available to assist? Have the patient's support systems been stressed beyond their limits, or can the patient continue to receive adequate care at home if the condition is not reversible?

The mental status examination. Take particular care in doing a mental status examination (MSE) on a person who presents with suspected dementia, for it is essential that you document the nature and extent of the existing cognitive deficits. The MSE is discussed at length in Chapter 4.

In examining demented patients, be sure to proceed gingerly, to minimize the patient's anxiety as you ask about intellectual impairment. Focus on cognitive functions, particularly the following:

- Orientation

- Memory—immediate, recent, and remote (be careful to test concentration as well, and note attention span)
- Fund of information
- Calculations
- Abstraction
- Judgment
- Language—spontaneous speech, naming objects, reading and writing.

Physical examination. A thorough physical examination should be performed on every patient who presents with intellectual deterioration. Look for signs of systemic illness, and pay particular attention in the neurologic examination to:

- Focal neurologic signs (weakness, sensory loss)
- Papilledema
- Frontal lobe release signs (snout, suck, palmomental, and rooting reflexes)
- Hyperreflexia, Babinski signs

Laboratory studies. Basic laboratory studies should include:

- Urinalysis
- Chest x-ray
- Blood studies—complete blood count (CBC) with differential metabolic screening battery (e.g., electrolytes, glucose, blood urea nitrogen (BUN), creatinine, liver function tests, serum calcium), serological test for syphilis, thyroid function tests, serum B12 and folate
- CT scan
- Electrocardiogram (EKG)

Other studies that may be indicated, on the basis of the patient's history and physical examination, include:

- Lumbar puncture
- Toxic screen
- Arterial blood gases
- EEG

Treatment of Dementia

Treatment is likely to be most successful when there is an underlying remediable cause. Whether treatment will result in reversal of the cognitive deficits depends on the underlying illness and how far it has progressed before the initiation of therapy.

In more than three-quarters of all cases of dementia, no treatable cause exists, and therapy is designed to provide symptom relief and support. Such therapy can be remarkably effective in helping patients and their families to deal with the stresses of dementing illness. Individual psychotherapy and family therapy can help clarify many of the problems the illness presents, and help patients and families find ways of dealing with this chronic debilitating illness. Intervention in the patient's environment may be necessary, e.g., arranging home care by professionals, or care in a nursing home.

Drug treatment has been helpful in treating specific symptoms in many cases of progressive dementia. Depressive symptoms often respond to treatment with antidepressants (e.g., a tricyclic such as desipramine). Anxiety, insomnia, and agitation are commonly alleviated by minor tranquilizers (particularly the benzodiazepines), although these drugs may cause paradoxical agitation in some patients. In cases of severe agitation and psychosis, antipsychotics (e.g., haloperidol) are often effective. Drug treatment in elderly patients must be undertaken with caution, for they generally require smaller doses than younger adults, and are more prone to such side effects as postural hypotension. However, medication need not be avoided, for it can provide them with considerable relief from the psychiatric symptoms that accompany the dementing process.

You may do the initial evaluation on an outpatient basis, but hospitalization often allows for a more thorough work-up and enables you to monitor the patient more carefully if a trial of medication is indicated. The decision to hospitalize a patient who presents with dementia will depend on the severity of the condition, the social supports available to the patient, and whether serious systemic illness is suspected.

A Word About Aging

The notion that "senility," or dementia, is an inevitable part of the aging process pervades our youth-oriented culture. In reality, among more than 25 million Americans over the age of 65, only 1 to 2 million suffer from significant intellectual impairment. The overwhelming majority of the elderly care for themselves and live outside of institutions.

The majority of older people maintain their intellectual competence as they age, although the speed with which they perform mental functions (e.g., recalling names or dates) declines somewhat. While mild or "benign" impairment in memory is common among the elderly, this is easily compensated for by keeping notes and establishing routines. The notion that dementia is synonymous with old age is a myth. Dementia is a pathological state, *not* a part of the normal human life cycle.

DELIRIUM

Delirium is a syndrome in which consciousness is clouded, the attention span is shortened, sensory misperception is common, and thinking is often disordered. Like dementia, delirium involves global cognitive deficits but, in addition, there is a change in the patient's level of arousal and marked disorientation. Delirious patients often present to emergency rooms or on hospital wards with extreme agitation and disordered thinking, while demented people more often come to medical attention in less dramatic ways and hide their deficits rather well in the early stages of the condition.

Delirium develops over hours or days, rather than over months or years. The delirious patient may initially show only mild symptoms of sleeplessness, anxiety, depression, irritability, forgetfulness, nightmares, or incoherent speech. More severe delirious states often include florid hallucinations, rapid or slowed thoughts, severe agitation or stupor, extreme distractibility, and fits of uncontrollable crying or laughter. The DSM-III criteria for the diagnosis of delirium (p. 107) are shown in Table 9-4.

Underlying medical illness is almost always identifiable in cases of delirium. Illnesses that can produce delirium include virtually all of those listed as causes of dementia. Such acute medical conditions as infection, anemia, hypertensive encephalopathy, cerebral edema, and dehydration and fluid and electrolyte imbalance commonly cause delirium. A long list of medications and street drugs (see Appendix B) can cause this condition—not only through intoxication but also during withdrawal. Alcohol withdrawal resulting in delirium tremens (DTs) is discussed in Chapter 11.

Delirium often occurs in hospitalized patients, particularly among patients in intensive care units. Almost all patients undergoing open-heart surgery with cardiac bypass become at least temporarily delirious sometime after they awaken from anesthesia. Renal dialysis patients

Table 9-4. DSM-III diagnostic criteria for delirium.

Clouding of consciousness (reduced clarity of awareness of the environment), with reduced capacity to shift, focus, and sustain attention to environmental stimuli

At least two of the following:
Perceptual disturbance: misinterpretations, illusions, or hallucinations
Speech that is at times incoherent
Disturbance of sleep-wakefulness cycle, with insomnia or daytime drowsi-
ness
Increased or decreased psychomotor activity

Disorientation and memory impairment (if testable)

Clinical features that develop over a short period of time (usually hours to
days) and tend to fluctuate over the course of a day

Evidence, from the history, physical examination, or laboratory tests, of a
specific organic factor judged to be etiologically related to the disturbance

---

frequently become transiently delirious because of toxic metabolic
products or electrolyte imbalance. Refer to a general medical text for a
more detailed discussion of the various medical conditions that can
cause delirium.

The elderly are more prone to develop delirium than younger
patients. Nearly one-third of those over 65 who are hospitalized for any
reason become delirious at some point during their stay. You are likely
to encounter this on general medical units, where older people often
experience transient confusion at night ("sundowning").

The treatment of delirium usually involves discovering the underlying cause and remedying it. A thorough history is essential to your
evaluation, and often must be obtained from those who accompany the
patient. Careful physical and mental status examinations are also part of
the work-up. You may learn a great deal about the patient's condition
by simply observing at the bedside. If the cause of the condition is not
obvious, laboratory studies (as noted for dementia above) are indicated
and should include a toxic screen. Not all delirium is reversible, but a
great many cases resolve completely when the acute medical condition
is effectively treated.

A word of caution: Delirium may look like an acute episode
of a functional psychosis (e.g., a schizophrenic or a manic episode).

Anyone who presents with an acute psychotic episode and no prior history of psychotic illness must have a thorough medical work-up. Otherwise, you may miss life-threatening and potentially treatable medical conditions that masquerade as psychiatric disorders.

REFERENCES

Adams RD, Fischer CM, Hakin S, et al: Symptomatic occult hydrocephalus with "normal" cerebrospinal fluid pressure. N Engl J Med 273:117-126, 1965.

Caine ED: Pseudodementia: current concepts and future directions. Arch Gen Psychiatry 38: 1359-1364, 1981.

Diagnostic and Statistical Manual of Mental Disorders, 3rd ed. Washington, DC, American Psychiatric Association, 1980.

Hoffman RS: Diagnostic errors in the evaluation of behavioral disorders. JAMA 248:964-967, 1982. (An enlightening survey of patients on medical and surgical wards who develop behavioral disturbances. Many of these are of organic etiology, but are misdiagnosed as primary psychiatric disorders.)

Kaufman DM: Clinical Neurology for Psychiatrists. New York, Grune and Stratton, 1981, pp 89-111. (A clear and highly readable textbook of neurologic disorders, including a discussion of the neurologic aspects of dementia.)

Lipowski ZJ: Organic brain syndromes: overview and classification, in Psychiatric Aspects of Neurologic Disease. Edited by Benson DF, Blumer D. New York, Grune and Stratton, 1975.

Schneck MK, Reisberg B, Ferris SH: An overview of current concepts of Alzheimer's disease. Am J Psychiatry 139:165-173, 1982.

Wells CE: Chronic brain disease: an overview. Am J Psychiatry, 135:1-12, 1978.

Part III

INTRODUCTION

The chapters included in this section cover subjects that every health care professional must understand. They are clinical problems that cross all diagnostic boundaries and often present as manifestations of other medical and psychiatric conditions.

Chapter 10 deals with sexual dysfunctions and deviations—concerns that are often overlooked in diagnostic evaluations. Drug and alcohol abuse are discussed in Chapter 11. Problems of substance abuse have reached epidemic proportions in our society, but they, too, are missed in many medical and psychiatric work-ups. Both of these chapters therefore emphasize diagnosis, with specific techniques for eliciting a history of problems with drugs or sexual functioning.

Suicide and violence are two of the most anxiety-provoking problems you will encounter in your clinical work. Chapters 12 and 13 focus on suicidal and violent patients respectively, highlighting ways in which you can assess patients' potential for carrying out threats of harming themselves or others, and strategies for managing emergency situations.

10

Human Sexuality:
Function and Dysfunction

IN OUR SOCIETY, physicians are the professionals most often consulted about sexual problems. Ironically, although they are assumed by many to be "experts" in this field, they are frequently less knowledgeable about and less comfortable with various aspects of sexual behavior than some nonprofessionals. As a physician-in-training, you must gain some understanding of the broad range of human sexual behaviors, as well as an understanding of your own attitudes toward sex. Such awareness is essential to good clinical work in any specialty of medicine.

TAKING A SEXUAL HISTORY

To learn about the sexual aspects of your patients' lives, you must be comfortable in eliciting such information.

General medical work-ups and psychiatric histories should routinely include questions that will allow you to establish the patient's general attitude toward sex, his or her sexual functioning, and its bearing on important relationships. Sexual functioning should be explored in depth whenever the patient's complaints suggest possible sexual difficulties or concerns. Such common complaints as fatigue,

219

headaches, dysmenorrhea, and depression should also alert you to the possibility of underlying sexual dissatisfaction.

When is it best to broach the subject during an interview? Obviously, if the patient's chief complaint is of a sexual nature, begin with a sexual history immediately. When this is not the case, it is usually best to wait until you and the patient have established some degree of rapport in the interview. A relaxed, matter-of-fact display of interest is most helpful. Ask questions as straightforwardly as possible.

The natural openings for discussion of sexuality are many. People usually talk about romantic relationships or marriages; use this as a point to introduce the topic with a general question, such as "How has the relationship developed sexually?" or "Can you tell me about your sexual experience with this person?" When a patient talks about menstrual functioning, energy level, depression, or other general complaints, you can turn to the subject of sex with a question like, "How does this symptom affect your sexual relationships?" With some patients (e.g., adolescents or severely isolated individuals) who you suspect may have very limited sexual experience, you might begin with a general inquiry, e.g., "What have your sexual experiences been like?"

People are commonly concerned that some aspect of their sexuality is abnormal. It will be helpful to frame your questions so that you imply that many people have similar feelings and attitudes. For example, in inquiring about previous homosexual experiences, you might phrase your question as follows: "Many people have sexual experiences with members of the same sex at some point in their lives. Have you had any experiences with other men (women)?" Or concerning common practices that may be a source of embarrassment, you might word a question as follows: "How old were you when you began masturbating?" rather than "Have you ever masturbated?"

When inquiring about sexuality, take your language cues from the patient. This is particularly important in talking with gay and lesbian patients. If you assume a heterosexual orientation (e.g., asking a man about girlfriends), you may make it more difficult for your patient to tell you about homosexual experiences. Thus, when talking about romantic relationships, use neutral terms such as "lover" until your patient offers specific names or pronouns that make sexual object choice clear.

Also, be sure to use your patient's terms whenever possible to describe sexual experiences and anatomy. Some patients use slang (e.g., "cock" for penis, "screwing" for intercourse), while others would find such terms offensive. Use your judgment, but remember that many words carry different connotations for different people. When in doubt, use the most neutral and widely accepted terms until you discover a common language with your patient.

Your Own Attitudes About Sex

Your comfort or discomfort in discussing sexual matters will undoubtedly be communicated to your patients. Many of us were raised in environments in which sex was never discussed, or only mentioned among intimates. It is no small task to learn to speak openly with patients about sexual functioning. You may find that you are embarrassed by or uncomfortable with some of what you encounter as a beginning clinician.

Unresolved conflicts about your own sexual life may hamper your ability to listen and evaluate sensitively. For example, an interviewer who is frightened by his or her own homosexual feelings may have difficulty in evaluating patients' homosexual concerns. Clinicians who believe that sex is "no one else's business" may be reacting to guilt feelings about their own unacknowledged sexual curiosity, and may refrain from asking necessary questions. Or, such people may overcompensate, asking intrusive and overly detailed questions about matters irrelevant to the patient's complaints.

Those who are achievement-oriented may tend to think of sex as a performance. Frequency of intercourse, number of orgasms attained, and the extent of the partner's visible satisfaction during lovemaking are all aspects of sexuality that can come to represent tests of competence. Such notions about sex can greatly distort not only your own sexual experiences, but your understanding of your patient's experiences.

Your job is to remain nonjudgmental and professional in your attitude toward your patient's sexual life. If you find yourself becoming anxious or imposing your personal values on a patient, you must stand back and (with the help of a colleague or supervisor) attempt to understand the source of the problem. Only then will you be able to be effective in helping patients to deal with sexual concerns.

Sample Interview Questions

Proceed from general questions to more specific ones in obtaining a sexual history. The following are suggestions for "openers":

"Tell me about your romantic life."

"How would you describe your sex life at this time?"

"Is there anything troubling you about your sex life?"

"Have you had any sexual thoughts that concern or disturb you?"

The following questions on three more specific areas may help you to focus in on the particular concerns of your patient:

Orientation

"Are you primarily attracted to members of the opposite sex? Your own sex? Both men and women?"

Current functioning

"How frequently do you have sexual contact? What does this involve? Are you (or your partner) concerned about the frequency with which you have sex?"

"How often do you masturbate?"

"What sort of sexual activities have been most (least) satisfying?"

"Have you had any difficulties in achieving orgasm or in helping your partner to achieve orgasm?"

"Are you involved in any sexual activities that worry you or others, or that you must keep secret from others?" (See the deviations described below.)

History

"What were your parents' attitudes toward sex?"

"How would you describe your parents' sexual relationships?"

"From whom did you learn about sex?"

"Did you have any sexual experiences as a child with older people, e.g., parents, siblings? If so, what were the circumstances?"

"Who prepared you for the onset of puberty/menstruation?"

"When did you begin masturbating?" (Ask about feelings, fantasies.)

"What was your sexual experience like as a teenager? As a young adult?"

"How have you felt about yourself as a man/woman?"

"Would you say that you are comfortable with yourself as a sexual person?"

THE SEXUAL RESPONSE CYCLE

In evaluating your patients' sexual functioning, keep in mind the normal cycle of sexual response. Many texts (e.g., Masters and Johnson,

1966) have excellent detailed discussions of this cycle. The brief discussion included here is only meant to provide an introductory overview.

Sexual stimulation produces characteristic responses in men and women that can be conceptualized as a four-phase cycle. These phases were described by Masters and Johnson in their research on human sexuality, and have been useful to clinicians in understanding normal and disturbed sexual functioning.

Phase I: Excitement. Sexual excitement may be brought about by psychological stimulation (through fantasy or by the presence of a desired person), or it may be brought about by physical stimulation (e.g., kissing, caressing). Excitement is characterized by erection of the penis in the man and vaginal lubrication in the woman. Excitement may start within 10 to 30 seconds after stimulation has begun, and it may last from several minutes to several hours. Another observable physical response in the excitement phase is nipple erection, more common in women than in men. Women also experience thickening of the labia minora and erection of the clitoris due to venous engorgement.

Phase II: Plateau. Continued sexual stimulation brings the individual to the threshold of orgasm, resulting in further physiologic changes and increasing sexual tension in both men and women. In women, the vaginal barrel constricts along the outer third (the orgasmic platform), while the clitoris elevates and retracts behind the symphisis pubis (but may be stimulated indirectly through traction on the labia minora). Breast size increases, and the labia minora become bright or deep red due to venous engorgement. In males, the testes increase in size (up to 50 percent) and are brought up toward the body as the scrotal sac tightens and lifts. Two or three drops of mucoid fluid containing viable sperm are secreted from the penis at this stage as well, so that pregnancy can occur even if the man withdraws prior to orgasm. In both sexes, heart rate increases, respiration becomes more rapid, elevation of blood pressure is common, and there are voluntary contractions of large skeletal muscle groups. This pre-orgasmic phase is usually brief, lasting from 30 seconds to three minutes.

Table 10-1. The four phases of the sexual response cycle.

Phase I—excitement	Phase III—orgasm
Phase II—plateau	Phase IV—resolution

Phase III: Orgasm. Increasing sexual tension generally culminates in orgasm, which is experienced as intensely pleasurable. In males, the testes, prostate, and seminal vesicles contract and expel sperm and seminal fluid into the entrance of the urethra. This is followed immediately by three to seven contractions of the urethra and muscles of the penis, ejecting the seminal fluid forcibly through the urethra and out of the penis. In females, orgasms consist of three to 15 involuntary contractions of the lower third of the vagina and strong, sustained contractions of the uterus. Both men and women also have involuntary contractions of the internal and external anal sphincters. In both sexes, muscular contractions during the height of orgasm occur at intervals of 0.8 seconds, and orgasm commonly lasts from three to 15 seconds. Other manifestations of orgasm include voluntary and involuntary movements of large muscle groups (e.g., extension of arms and legs), facial grimacing, and muscular spasm. Blood pressure rises by up to 80 mm systolic and 40 mm diastolic, while heart rate may increase to 180 beats per minute, and respirations up to 40 per minute. Some people also experience a "sex flush," a blotching of the skin in variable patterns on the body that disappears within minutes after orgasm.

Phase IV: Resolution. After orgasm, the resolution phase brings the body back to its resting state by gradual disgorgement of blood from the genitals and a return of these organs to their resting size. If orgasm occurs, resolution is rapid, and may take only 10 to 15 minutes. However, if orgasm does not occur, resolution may take 2 to 6 hours (in some cases even up to a day) and may be associated with pelvic discomfort. Resolution after orgasm is characterized by a subjective sense of well-being. For males, there is a refractory period after orgasm in which they cannot be stimulated to another orgasm. This may last from several minutes to several hours. There is no such refractory period in women; they are capable of multiple and successive orgasms.

Female Sexual Response

Most women have certain physical responses in addition to those mentioned above. The female vagina enlarges during sexual excitement and naturally accommodates to the size of the penis (or other object) inserted into it. Lubrication occurs internally, so lubrication of the outer labia must usually be accomplished by manual manipulation or through the thrusting of the penis.

At the moment of orgasm, the woman has a tendency to increase her pelvic thrusting, while the man tends to freeze his thrusting activity. Female orgasm seems to be triggered by stimulation of the clitoris—either directly, through masturbation, or indirectly, as when the thrusts of the penis cause traction on the labia minora, with resulting stimulation of the attached clitoris. Thus, female orgasm is triggered by clitoral stimulation and manifested by vaginal contractions.

Male Sexual Response

Men tend to show less variation in their sexual response cycles than women do, although there is some variation in the duration of each cycle phase. The man cannot successfully accomplish intercourse without first obtaining an erection that is sufficiently rigid to allow him to penetrate the vagina. Once erection is achieved, it will normally wax and wane if the excitement phase is prolonged; this normal response should not be a cause for concerns about potency.

Men experience two stages of orgasm. The first is a moment of *ejaculatory inevitability*, when the testes, prostate, and seminal vesicles expel sperm and seminal fluid into the entrance of the urethra. The man "feels the ejaculation coming," and at this point can no longer interrupt the process voluntarily. The second stage is *ejaculation*, during which the semen is forcibly ejected out of the penis via the urethra. At the moment of orgasm, the man tends to stop his thrusting activity and hold the ejaculating penis in deep penetration.

Sex and Aging

Some of the most common misconceptions about human sexual response relate to the aging process. As the number of people over age 65 increases in this society, more attention is being focused on all aspects of geriatric life, including sexuality. People vary in their capacity for and interest in an active sexual life beyond middle age. Physical health is important but, barring major physical illness, other factors seem to loom larger in determining sexual activity in later life—most obviously, the availability of a sexual partner. Also, people who have been sexually active in earlier years are more likely to remain so in later life, as are those who live in an environment that is accepting of their sexuality.

Changes in sexual responsiveness do occur with aging. In aging women, the vasocongestive response is diminished, and the elasticity and secretory capacities of the vagina decrease. However, women who continue to have intercourse regularly can minimize these changes and function effectively in spite of them. The aging man takes longer to achieve an erection, and erection may be less complete, although adequate to penetrate the vagina. The expulsive force of the ejaculation also diminishes, refractory time between orgasms is longer, and greater stimulation is required to achieve erection in the first place. For men, erectile difficulty is the only sexual dysfunction that correlates with advancing age. Some of this erectile failure is psychogenic in origin and can be treated (see below); in other cases, impotence is due to neurologic or vascular disease.

Sexual interest and activity are the rule rather than the exception among people in their fifties and sixties; some people continue to be sexually active even in their eighties. One does not become "used up" sexually; indeed, surveys suggest that a lifelong history of active sexual functioning is a good predictor of sexual activity in old age—"If you use it, you don't lose it."

SEXUAL DISORDERS: DEVIATION VERSUS DYSFUNCTION

Sexual deviation (also called "perversion") involves a disturbance of sexual *aim*. Sexual dysfunction denotes a disturbance of sexual *function*. The difference is thus that deviations are characterized by good and pleasurable sexual functioning, while dysfunctions are not. The sexual deviant's choice of sexual object differs from the norm, and he or she is aroused by stimuli that are not exciting to most people—e.g., a child, an animal, or a shoe. He or she may be excited by bondage or by receiving punishment, by looking at or by exposing the genitals, or by inflicting pain. But arousal and orgasm are physiologically normal and bring the sexual deviant pleasure. Sexual deviations are treated with certain types of behavior and insight-oriented therapy, as discussed below.

Sexual dysfunctions are psychosomatic disorders that make it impossible for the person to enjoy sex or, in some cases, to have sex at all. They involve inhibition of normal physiologic responses—i.e., venous engorgement of the sexual organs, and/or the orgasmic response itself—that makes the experience of sexual activity in some way unpleasurable. Sexual dysfunctions are quite common, and they respond to particular types of sex therapy and to a combination of sex therapy and insight-oriented psychotherapy.

You will encounter patients with sexual dysfunctions in almost any area of medical practice you choose, and you may encounter sexual deviations as well. Your receptivity to hearing about such issues, and your awareness of the possibilities for treating these disorders, can be crucial to helping people who are often confused and embarrassed about problems they do not understand.

Female Sexual Dysfunction

General sexual dysfunction (frigidity).. General sexual dysfunction is commonly called *frigidity*, but this is a nonspecific term that carries a pejorative connotation. General sexual dysfunction refers to an inability to derive erotic pleasure from sexual stimulation. Women with this disorder may show little or no physiologic response to sexual stimulation (e.g., no vasocongestion or vaginal lubrication), and may experience themselves as essentially devoid of sexual feelings. Many of these women consider sexual activity an ordeal that they must endure to preserve a relationship, or sex may be so repugnant to them that any activity is impossible. Some women with this disorder are able to enjoy the nonerotic aspects of sexual contact (e.g., touching, physical closeness), despite their lack of sexual responsiveness. Among the factors that seem to foster general sexual dysfunction are strict parental prohibitions against sexual expression in early life, overwhelming anxiety rooted in childhood conflicts or in current concerns, and hostility directed at, but not directly expressed to, the partner or men in general.

Orgastic dysfunction. Orgastic dysfunction is a more limited disorder that denotes a specific difficulty in reaching orgasm. Women who suffer from this disorder frequently have a strong sexual drive and may reach high levels of sexual arousal. The disorder is termed *primary orgastic dysfunction* if the woman has never experienced orgasm by any means of stimulation, and *secondary orgastic dysfunction* if she previously experienced orgasm and subsequently developed this difficulty. The difficulty in reaching orgasm may be present regardless of the setting, or it may depend on the situation—e.g., some women can have orgasms with masturbation but not during coitus, while for others the situation is reversed. Some women rarely

Table 10-2. Types of female sexual dysfunction.

Type	Definition
General sexual dysfunction	Inability to derive erotic pleasure from sexual stimulation
Orgastic dysfunction	Specific difficulty in reaching orgasm
Primary	Never experienced orgasm by any means of stimulation
Secondary	Experienced orgasm but subsequently developed this difficulty
Vaginismus	Impenetrability of the vagina because of involuntary spasm of the vaginal muscles
Dyspareunia	Pain on intercourse

have orgasms with any partner and are surprised when they do, while others only experience difficulty with a particular partner. The diagnosis of a disorder is not always easy, since female response varies greatly. Failure to ever have an orgasm constitutes a disorder in almost all cases. However, not reaching orgasm during coitus (but being able to have orgasms during masturbation) is not necessarily a disorder but may be a normal variation of female functioning.

Women differ greatly in their thresholds for reaching orgasm and require varying amounts of clitoral stimulation, probably due to a combination of physiologic and psychological factors. Coitus actually provides only mild clitoral stimulation (compared with masturbation and other more direct techniques), so only women who can be orgasmic with relatively mild stimulation will have orgasms in this way.

In this and other situation-specific cases, the diagnosis of a disorder depends to a large extent on whether the patient (and/or her partner) is disturbed by the situation and feels the need for treatment. If not, there is no reason to label the inability to reach orgasm during coitus "disordered." Many women are satisfied with other means of reaching orgasm and do not seek treatment.

Orgastic dysfunction is the most common complaint among women who *do* seek treatment for a sexual disorder. When a woman wants to have orgasms and cannot, the cause is often her involuntary inhibition of the response. She may unwittingly do this because the orgasm has acquired some symbolic meaning (e.g., losing control), because its intensity frightens her, because she is in conflict over her erotic feelings, or because she is uncertain about her commitment to her mate or even hostile toward her mate.

Vaginismus. Vaginismus refers to a very specific syndrome in which penetration of the vagina is impossible because of involuntary spasm of the muscles surrounding the vaginal entrance. Whenever penetration is attempted, the vaginal introitus literally snaps shut, so that coitus cannot take place. Even pelvic examinations must often be carried out under anesthesia. In addition to primary spasm of the sphincter vaginae and levator ani muscles, vaginismus may also involve a phobia of coitus and vaginal penetration that prompts avoidance of any situation in which coitus might occur. Some women with this disorder are quite sexually responsive as long as sexual contact does not lead to intercourse.

The diagnosis of vaginismus is made relatively rarely, and can only be made definitely when involuntary spasm is noted on pelvic examination. Among the factors that seem to be associated with this disorder are a history of sexual trauma, stern parental prohibitions against sexuality, confusion about choice of sexual object, and a partner's sexual dysfunction (particularly primary impotence).

Dyspareunia. Dyspareunia refers to pain in the genital area during coitus. While it occurs occasionally in men, it is more common in women. Obviously, there are numerous physical causes of pain on intercourse (e.g., in various medical conditions and after surgical procedures), but *functional dyspareunia* refers to pain with no demonstrable physical cause. It is essentially a somatoform disorder (see Chapter 8), and is thought to be due to underlying fears of or conflicts over sexual activity.

Male Sexual Dysfunction

Impotence (erectile dysfunction). Because a great deal of male self-esteem is invested in the capacity for penile erection, there is probably no other medical condition that is as potentially frustrating or humiliating for a man. Impotence is simply an impairment of penile erection, due to failure of the vascular reflex mechanism to pump sufficient blood into the cavernous sinuses of the penis to render it firm. Probably more than half of the male population has experienced occasional transient episodes of impotence, and these episodes are within the limits of normal sexual behavior.

The diagnosis of impotence is made when erectile dysfunction is recurrent and persistent. Men with *primary impotence* have never been potent with a partner, although they may have full erections when masturbating and may have spontaneous erections. *Secondary impotence* describes a condition in which a man has functioned well in the past but at some point developed erectile dysfunction. The impotent man may feel aroused and excited in a sexual situation and want to make love, and may even ejaculate, but his penis remains flaccid.

Psychological factors play a central role in an overwhelming majority of cases of impotence. Erectile function is impaired in most men when they become anxious. Thus, normal sexual functioning usually occurs only when the man does not feel threatened. There are great variations in the patterns of impotence among men with this complaint, because the precise aspect of the sexual act that arouses anxiety differs. Some men are impotent only upon entering the vagina. Some are impotent with one partner but not another, or are only impotent when they feel the expectation to perform. The source of anxiety may be in the man's current life, or it may stem from early childhood fears and experiences.

Why are some men more prone than others to become impotent when they are anxious? Some clinicians postulate that certain men have a physiologic vulnerability to erectile dysfunction (perhaps because of a highly reactive vasocongestive system) while others do not.

There are numerous medical conditions that cause impotence. Although these are much less common than psychological factors, they must not be overlooked; any man who complains of impotence should have a medical and neurological work-up in addition to a psychological evaluation. Among the most prevalent somatic causes of impotence are fatigue, early undiagnosed diabetes mellitis, low androgen levels, thyrotoxicosis, uremia, liver disease, nonspecific debilitating illness, heart or respiratory illness, and abuse of narcotics, alcohol, or estrogenic and parasympatholytic medications. Neurological diseases that produce impotence include multiple sclerosis, lower spinal cord lesions, and hypothalamic and temporal lobe lesions.

Premature ejaculation. This is a condition in which the man is unable to exert voluntary control over his ejaculatory reflex, so that when he is sexually aroused, he reaches orgasm more quickly than he and/or his partner would like. Men who suffer from premature ejaculation cannot tolerate high levels of sexual tension and stimulation without ejaculating, and their partners are often left unsatisfied when

Table 10-3. Types of male sexual dysfunction.

Type	Impotence
Impotence (erectile dysfunction)	Impairment of penile erection that is recurrent and persistent
Primary	Never potent with a partner
Secondary	Potent in the past but subsequently developed erectile dysfunction
Premature ejaculation	Inability to exert voluntary control over the ejaculatory reflex
Retarded ejaculation	Inhibition of the ejaculatory reflex
Primary	Never ejaculated with a partner
Secondary	Ejaculated normally in the past but subsequently developed this difficulty

orgasm occurs too soon and lovemaking ceases. The premature ejaculator may become anxious about reaching orgasm too soon, and begin to avoid sexual activity so as not to face the difficulty.

When is ejaculation premature? The definition has been difficult, for no one criterion seems to suffice. The number of thrusts a man can tolerate before ejaculating, the number of seconds of coitus he can endure before ejaculation, and the satisfaction of his partner have all been put forward as criteria for the diagnosis, but all are relative and arbitrary. In fact, the crucial aspect seems to be the man's inability to voluntarily control his ejaculatory reflex, regardless of how many seconds have passed or how many thrusts he has made, and regardless of whether his partner has reached orgasm. The rapidity of orgasm is the primary complaint, but many premature ejaculators also have diminished perceptions of their erotic sensations as they become intensely aroused, and therefore are not aware when orgasm is imminent.

Many psychological theories have been put forward to explain the causes of premature ejaculation. Covert hostility toward women has been proposed by traditional psychoanalytic theorists, but it has become clear that the determinants of this disorder are more varied and complex. Many men with this disorder have otherwise good and satisfying relationships with wives or lovers. Other clinicians postulate that early hurried sexual experiences (e.g., with prostitutes, or in the back seats of automobiles) play a role. However, many men with a history of such experiences do not go on to develop this disorder.

Clearly, anxiety plays a role in premature ejaculation, since it does not allow the man to perceive erotic sensations correctly. Also, marital difficulties and underlying psychiatric illness have been implicated in some, but not all, cases of premature ejaculation. Among the factors that do *not* seem to play a role are masturbatory practices and familial patterns.

Premature ejaculation is very rarely caused by somatic factors. Among the physical conditions that may contribute to premature ejaculation are local disease of the posterior urethra (e.g., prostatitis), spinal cord lesions, multiple sclerosis, and other degenerative neurologic disorders.

Retarded ejaculation. In this disorder (also called **ejaculatory incompetence**), the ejaculatory reflex is inhibited, although erection is usually not impaired. This may be primary, if the man has never ejaculated with a partner, or secondary, if the condition arose after an initial period of adequate functioning. The disorder may be so severe that the man cannot ejaculate when masturbating by himself, but in most cases extravaginal ejaculation is possible. This disorder may prompt the man to prolong intercourse for a very long period (e.g., more than an hour) or to fake orgasms with his partner and then either remain frustrated or achieve release only through masturbation following intercourse.

The causes of this disorder are rarely physical. Among the somatic illnesses that occasionally play a role are depressed androgen levels, undetected diabetes, spinal cord lesions, and drugs that impair the adrenergic mechanism of the sympathetic nervous system, which controls ejaculation (e.g., certain antihypertensive drugs). Thioridazine (Mellaril) can cause retrograde ejaculation (a point to bear in mind when choosing an antipsychotic for male patients).

The most commonly reported psychological factors that seem to underlie ejaculatory incompetence include a strict religious upbringing that engenders sexual guilt, strongly suppressed anger, ambivalence toward a partner, fears of abandonment by a lover, and childhood fears of parental retaliation for sexual urges.

TREATMENT OF SEXUAL DYSFUNCTION

Whenever a patient presents a sexual complaint, you should proceed with a thorough work-up to determine which type of therapy is indicated. Some patients present with complaints of sexual dysfunction but, in the course of giving you a psychiatric history, will reveal serious psychopathology (e.g., depression, psychosis) that requires treatment before sexual concerns can be addressed. In addition to a careful psychiatric evaluation, be sure that a thorough medical evaluation is carried out, including a medical history and physical examination and, where indicated, a neurologic, urologic, or gynecologic examination and appropriate laboratory studies.

Once you have ruled out organic pathology and serious psychopathology, you have a variety of treatment modalities from which to choose.

Dual-Sex Therapy (Masters and Johnson Techniques)

The new sex therapy originated with the work of William H. Masters and Virginia E. Johnson. This type of therapy relies on behavioral techniques and makes the couple, rather than the dysfunctional individual, the focus of therapy. This is based on the premise that there is no such thing as a partner who is uninvolved in the sexual problem, nor is there one "sick half" in a couple. Both people are expected to participate fully in the therapy, and to learn to focus on their own sexual feelings and desires, as well as to learn those of their partner and to improve communication within the dyad.

Treatment is based on the observation that performance anxiety and demands for sexual performance intensify and perpetuate sexual dysfunction. Using a man-woman team of co-therapists, sessions focus on correcting misinformation or ignorance about sexual functioning, providing support and reassurance, improving communication, and removing the demand to perform sexually.

After a thorough evaluation of the couple, sessions begin with "homework assignments"—exercises the couple carries out in private. All sexual activity, including intercourse, is prohibited until the therapists feel that the couple is ready. This enforced abstinence is the first step in removing the pressure for sexual performance. The first exercises are **sensate focus** exercises, designed to increase sensory awareness of oneself and one's partner. Each partner takes turns "pleasuring" the other, first touching all areas except breasts and genitals, and later including these areas.

Sessions focus on the couple's experiences in carrying out the exercises—these provide crucial information to the therapists about where there is resistance to sexual activity (e.g., the man who is always too tired to do the exercises, or the woman who develops a headache whenever exercises are initiated). Fears and misunderstandings can be clarified in the therapy sessions, and exercises repeated until they are pleasurable for both partners. Once this pleasuring is mastered, couples are usually communicating with each other more effectively than when they began treatment, and sessions move onto specific exercises directed at the particular dysfunction.

General sexual dysfunction is treated with sensate focus experiences to help the woman focus on erotic sensations, followed by genital stimulation by herself and with her partner. Intercourse is initiated when she chooses to do so, and with no pressure to achieve orgasm. As she feels more secure in experiencing sexual feelings with her partner, the woman who suffers from this disorder is likely to be able to achieve considerable pleasure and even achieve orgasm during sexual activity.

Orgastic dysfunction is treated with exercises that heighten the woman's arousal prior to coitus, to increase her awareness of and pleasure in her vaginal sensations, and to maximize clitoral stimulation. This is done by using masturbatory techniques (and in some cases a vibrator), as well as teaching specific coital positions in which the partner can maximally stimulate the woman. All this is done in situations in which the pressure on the woman to reach orgasm is minimized.

Vaginismus is treated by teaching the woman and her partner to use fingers to gently dilate the vaginal opening, and to use mechanical dilators to accomplish the same purpose. Once vaginal dilation has been comfortably accomplished by these means, it is usually possible for the male to insert his penis into the vagina easily and without discomfort to his partner.

Premature ejaculation has been very successfully treated by using exercises that repeatedly stimulate the man to the point of near ejaculatory inevitability and then cease stimulation before inevitability occurs, thereby preventing ejaculation (the *"stop-and-go" technique*). This allows the man to experience intense sexual excitement repeatedly without ejaculating. This technique is accompanied by the forcible prevention of ejaculation when inevitably occurs by using the *"squeeze" technique*, which involves squeezing the head of the penis with the thumb and first and second fingers. The squeeze technique has had almost universal success in treating premature ejaculation.

Ejaculatory incompetence is dealt with in the opposite manner. Exercises are aimed at achieving intravaginal ejaculation, since in most cases ejaculation during masturbation is not impaired. The woman stimulates the man manually to orgasm in her presence, with the penis in gradually closer proximity to the vaginal opening. Eventually, she stimulates her partner to the point of ejaculatory inevitability and inserts the penis into her vagina without interrupting the ejaculation process. A single episode of intravaginal ejaculation often breaks the male's block against intravaginal ejaculation.

Impotence has been alleviated by creating nondemanding sexual situations in which the man can experience erections without the pressure to have intercourse. Exercises include masturbation, stimulation of the penis to erection by the partner, and gradual introduction of the penis into the vagina by the partner in the woman-on-top position. Even when the penis is inserted into the vagina, no thrusting is allowed at first, or only minimal movements to maintain the penis in a stimulated state. Thrusting is allowed in subsequent exercises, and orgasm naturally ensues. Relieved of the demand to perform, the man who can gradually achieve erections and achieve vaginal penetration usually proceeds at his own pace to have effective coitus.

Masters and Johnson have reported high rates of success for these treatment approaches, with an overall rate of 80 percent success for all dysfunctions combined. They report the greatest success with premature ejaculation (97 percent), and the most limited success with primary impotence (59 percent). Although some critics argue that results are temporary, these behavioral techniques have proved valuable in the treatment of sexual dysfunction.

Psychodynamically Oriented Sex Therapy

Combining psychodynamic psychotherapy and sex therapy enables clinicians to treat patients whose sexual complaints are associated with other psychiatric disorders. This therapy may continue for longer than the usual 10-15 sessions involved in sex therapy alone, and it may involve individual work with each partner as well as work with the couple. This approach is particularly useful for couples who have difficulties in their relationship that clearly extend beyond the realm of sex. Couples are given "homework assignments" as described above, but sessions also focus more intensively on the psychological conflicts and distortions that hamper the relationship—often problems that origi- nated for each partner in early childhood relationships.

When one partner is more obviously in need of psychological support and help than the other, individual sessions can be tailored to that person's needs and carried out in addition to the couple's therapy sessions. For example, if a woman who complains of general sexual dysfunction discovers in couple's therapy that she harbors deeply rooted hostility toward men, she may want to work with the therapist individually to understand more about the origins of this anger, while continuing in joint meetings to explore the ways in which she unwittingly distances her husband.

The combination of psychodynamic and sex therapy is commonly used in general mental health facilities, while sex therapy alone is often used in clinics that limit their work to the treatment of sexual dysfunctions.

Hypnotherapy

Some clinicians have found hypnotic suggestions useful in alleviating anxiety (e.g., in a man with secondary impotence) and in removing psychological impediments to vaginal lubrication, erection, and orgasm. This is not a couple's approach, and is aimed at specific symptoms rather than an individual's general ability to experience and communi- cate his or her sexual feelings in a relationship.

Behavior Therapy

This therapy was initially developed to treat phobias, but the technique of systematic desensitization has also been applied to sexual situations that arouse anxiety (see Chapter 14). The patient identifies situations that arouse anxiety and foster symptoms (e.g., when vaginal penetration results in impotence), and the therapist gradually desensitizes the patient to these anxiety-provoking situations. Like hypnotherapy, this approach is generally for individuals rather than couples.

Group Therapy

Groups have been useful in treating people with sexual dysfunction, since they can impart sexual information, provide reassurance, and offer mutual support to people who suffer from similar difficulties.

Some groups consist of people of one sex who have the same disorder; others are composed of couples. Groups are particularly useful for people who need to explore interpersonal difficulties, as well as specific sexual problems.

Individual Psychotherapy

Classical psychodynamic theory holds that sexual dysfunctions have their roots in early childhood experiences and conflicts that therapy can help to elucidate. When irrational fears and fantasies are brought to light and understood, the symptoms of sexual dysfunction often lessen. However, the psychodynamic approach is less effective than the behavioral approach of Masters and Johnson in rapidly removing specific sexual symptoms. Individual psychotherapy is most useful for people whose sexual dysfunction is part of a larger constellation of psychological difficulties and who have other symptoms for which psychotherapy is indicated.

SEXUAL DEVIATIONS

Sexual deviations (also called *perversions* and *paraphilias*) are disorders that involve unusual sexual object choices or sexual acts. The person who suffers from a perversion generally requires these specific acts or objects or images in order to be sexually aroused and to achieve orgasm. He or she must repeatedly recreate the needed situation or fantasy. Perversions most often involve the use of a nonhuman object for sexual arousal (excluding vibrators and other objects designed for that purpose), the experience of suffering on the part of the individual or of his or her partner, or sexual activity with a nonconsenting partner.

Many people with perversions do not regard themselves as ill, and only come to mental health facilities for help when their behavior has brought them into conflict with society (e.g., with their families or with the law). People with sexual perversions are grossly impaired in their ability to participate in mutually gratifying sexual relations with consenting adults, and marital difficulties are common.

Perversions are much more common in men than in women, but the reasons for this are not clear. Environmental factors (particularly early childhood experiences) appear to play a major role in the genesis of sexual perversions, and sons often develop the specific perversions of

Table 10-4. Types of sexual deviations.

Type	Definition
Transsexualism	Persistent sense of discomfort about one's anatomic sex and strong desire to change one's genitals and secondary sex characteristics
Transvestitism	Dressing in clothes appropriate to the opposite sex for purposes of arousal
Fetishism	Use of a nonhuman object as the preferred method of achieving sexual excitement
Zoophilia	Repeated sexual arousal through contact with an animal
Pedophilia	Sexual contact with prepubertal children as the preferred means to sexual excitement
Exhibitionism	Exposure of the genitals in public to unsuspecting strangers to achieve sexual excitement
Voyeurism	Repeatedly looking at unsuspecting people who are disrobing or engaging in sexual activity
Sexual masochism	Obtaining sexual gratification through mental suffering or bodily pain
Sexual sadism	Inflicting physical or psychological pain on another to achieve sexual excitement

their fathers. Since these disorders are relatively uncommon, they will be discussed only briefly.

Transsexualism

This disorder involves a persistent sense of discomfort and inappropriateness about one's anatomic sex and a wish to change one's genitals and secondary sex characteristics in order to live as a member of the opposite sex. Transsexualism must be distinguished from transvestitism and homosexuality (see below), neither of which necessarily involves a desire to change one's sexual anatomy. Cross-dressing and homosexual behavior are common among transsexuals, but the eventual goal for these people is often surgical and hormonal treatment leading to reassignment of gender. Surgical procedures to change external anatomy from male to female are more common than the reverse procedure.

　　Transsexualism is often associated with moderate to severe personality disturbance. Surgical correction does not bring about a satisfactory sexual adjustment for some transsexuals, and depression and suicide attempts are frequent complications of this disorder. Thus, careful and detailed psychiatric evaluation must be a prerequisite to surgical procedures for anyone wishing to change his or her sex.

Transvestitism

Transvestitism involves dressing in clothing appropriate to members of the opposite sex for purposes of arousal and as an adjunct to masturbation or coitus. This generally occurs among *heterosexual* males, and may range from occasional cross-dressing to intense involvement in an elaborate transvestite subculture. When not cross-dressed, the transvestite usually appears and acts masculine. Homosexual experiences are reported in this population, but sexual preference is generally for members of the opposite sex.

Cross-dressing often begins in adolescence, but may start earlier, and is often used to alleviate anxiety in addition to providing erotic stimulation. Transvestitism must be distinguished from cross-dressing by homosexuals, which is often carried out in order to attract homosexual partners; and transsexualism, which involves a conscious desire to change one's anatomy in order to become a member of the opposite sex.

Fetishism

Fetishism involves the use of a nonhuman object as the preferred (or only) method of achieving sexual excitement. These objects tend to be shoes, corsets, gloves, or other items of apparel closely associated with the human body. Fetishes may also involve body parts (e.g., feet, hair) rather than inanimate objects. The object may be the sole focus of sexual activity (e.g., masturbation into a shoe) or may be integrated into sexual activity with a partner (e.g., the demand that the partner wear high-heeled shoes).

The fetish differs from simple experimentation to achieve sexual arousal, since people with true fetishes *require* the presence of a specific object (at least in fantasy) for arousal to occur, and the object is preferred over human beings. The desired object is usually linked to someone important from the individual's childhood, and serves to help maintain some special relationship in fantasy with that person.

Zoophilia

Zoophilia involves repeated sexual arousal through contact with an animal. Sexual contact with animals (masturbation or coitus) is not uncommon among adolescents, particularly those raised in rural settings. However, true zoophilia involves preference for sexual contact with an animal even when other sexual outlets are possible.

Pedophilia

Pedophilia involves sexual contact with prepubertal children as the preferred or only means of achieving sexual excitement. Pedophiles tend to fall into two distinct groups: those who choose children of the opposite sex (*heterosexual pedophiles*) and those who choose children of the same sex (*homosexual pedophiles*). Virtually all pedophiles who come to the attention of mental health professionals are men.

Heterosexual pedophiles tend to be socially maladjusted men, often alcoholics with troubled marriages. The incidence of heterosexual pedophilia peaks among late adolescent boys and among men in their forties and sixties. They generally prefer to engage in sexual activity with 8- to 10-year-old girls.

Homosexual pedophiles tend to be men who have never married, and they tend to prefer prepubertal or pubescent boys as the objects of sexual activity. Many of these men were themselves sexually abused by older men when they were children.

There are few reliable statistics on the relative incidences of homosexual and heterosexual pedophilia, but a great majority (some estimates are as high as 90 percent) of incidents are perpetrated by heterosexual men. Especially common is sexual activity between fathers (or step-fathers) and their preadolescent or early adolescent daughters. Thus, contrary to popular myth, homosexual men do not pose the most significant sexual threat to children in our society.

Exhibitionism

Exhibitionism involves exposure of the genitals in public to unsuspecting strangers as a means of achieving sexual excitement, with no attempt at further sexual activity with these strangers. The exhibitionist is usually aware of the desire to shock observers. Exhibitionists are exclusively men, and they generally expose themselves to women and girls. They may begin this practice at any time after the onset of puberty, but the disorder most commonly begins in the mid-twenties. These men are frequently arrested for their behavior, but they generally do not constitute a danger to those to whom they expose themselves.

Voyeurism

Voyeurism involves repeatedly looking at unsuspecting people (usually strangers) who are disrobing or engaging in sexual activity. This activity is the voyeur's preferred means of achieving sexual excitement. No sexual activity with the person is sought, but the voyeur often achieves orgasm through masturbation during the voyeuristic activity or afterwards, while recalling the activity.

Such people (usually men) are generally isolated, withdrawn individuals who prowl neighborhoods looking for opportunities to "peep." This behavior often gets the voyeur into minor legal difficulties.

Voyeurism differs from sexual excitement achieved by watching a partner undress or by viewing pornography, in that sexual partners and pornographic entertainers are willing participants and are aware of being watched.

Sexual Masochism

Masochism consists of sexual gratification obtained through mental suffering or bodily pain. The individual prefers to be excited or can only be excited by being bound, beaten, humiliated, or tortured. The diagnosis is made on the basis of one or more episodes in which an individual achieves excitement through suffering.

Masochistic sexual behavior occurs among heterosexuals and homosexuals. It may begin at any time, but most commonly begins in early adulthood. It may be quite dangerous, particularly if the individual must engage in increasingly harmful activities in order to be aroused. Permanent bodily injury, castration, and even death may result from such activity. Masochistic individuals often engage in sadistic sexual practices as well. Sexual masochism is distinct from masochistic personality in that masochistic personality traits are not associated with conscious sexual excitement.

Sexual Sadism

Sexual sadism involves inflicting physical or psychological pain on another person as a means of achieving sexual excitement. The partner may be consenting or nonconsenting, and this mode of sexual arousal is both repeated and preferred over others. Sexual sadism occurs among both heterosexuals and homosexuals, and most commonly begins in early adulthood. The harm inflicted on a partner may be mild and may not escalate over time, or harm may be quite severe and result in death or permanent disability or disfigurement of the victim. Severe sadistic practices can result in legal action and imprisonment. Sexual sadists sometimes engage in masochistic activities as well.

Treatment of Sexual Deviations

Sexual deviations are thought to be psychologically based and rooted in early childhood experiences. Thus, many clinicians have found psycho-therapy to be the treatment of choice in these disorders. Psychoanalysis attempts to elicit and resolve early childhood conflicts that are responsi-ble for the perversion, but many disturbed patients (e.g., those with severe personality disorders or psychoses) cannot tolerate such intense treatment. Individual psychotherapy can be useful to help patients identify the feelings and fantasies that prompt deviant sexual behavior, to help them find more acceptable means of obtaining sexual gratifica-tion, and to help them diminish the extent to which perverse behaviors interfere with other aspects of their lives.

Antiandrogen agents such as medroxyprogesterone (Depo-provera) have been used in men with sexually hyperactive perversions (e.g., in those who are involved in compulsive sexual assaults) to decrease sexual activity and thereby decrease dangerousness to self and others.

HOMOSEXUALITY

Imagine a textbook discussion on heterosexuality as a clinical entity. Most of us take heterosexuality for granted in our dealings with other people; it is considered the norm. Yet a large portion of the population consists of men and women who prefer same-sex partners for sexual activity. You undoubtedly have encountered and will continue to encounter gay people in your personal and professional life. Whether your gay friends, colleagues, and patients feel they can tell you about their sexual orientation will depend in large part on your sensitivity and receptivity to nonheterosexual orientation and life styles.

It has been said that gay people have as much in common as coffee drinkers. There is tremendous diversity in personality traits, life styles, and sexual practices among people whose primary orientation is homosexual. It is difficult even to define the gay population. How would one classify the many people who are heterosexual in practice and homosexual in fantasy, or those who are sexually active with both men and women, or others who make abrupt mid-life changes in their sexual-object choices?

Prevalence

Homosexual behavior occurs in virtually all societies. The prevalence of homosexuality is difficult to determine, in part because of problems in defining what constitutes homosexuality and in part because much homosexuality goes unreported because of societal prejudices and pressures against open disclosure of a homosexual orientation. The best data probably remain those of Kinsey and his co-workers, who in their 1948 and 1953 studies of sexual behavior in men and women interviewed more than 11,000 men and nearly 8,000 women. Kinsey found that 4 percent of men were exclusively homosexual throughout their adult lives, while another 13 percent were predominantly homosexual for at least three years between the ages of 16 and 55. Most surprising to the American public was the disclosure that 37 percent of the men in Kinsey's sample reported at least one sexual experience with another man leading to orgasm during their postpubertal years. His findings showed the prevalence of homosexuality among women to be roughly one-third that found among men. About 28 percent of the women in his sample reported some homosexual experience or arousal at some time from the onset of puberty, with 13 percent experiencing associated orgasm. He estimated the prevalence of exclusive homosexuality among women in his sample to be between one-half and one-third of that among men.

Causes

Why do some people grow up with a heterosexual orientation and others with a homosexual one? There are no clear-cut answers. In attempting to elucidate the causes of homosexuality, researchers have explored a variety of psychological and biological hypotheses.

Traditional psychoanalytic theory views homosexuality as an arrest of psychosexual development. For men, the disturbance is thought to result from early childhood experiences with a close-binding, intimate mother and a passive, hostile, or absent father. For women, no such clear-cut family pattern has been hypothesized, but traditional theorists believe that female homosexuality involves unresolved developmental difficulties. These psychoanalytic hypotheses have not been consistently validated in clinical studies of gay men and women. And this research is significantly flawed, for most of it has been conducted by using populations of gays who have consulted a psychiatrist for emotional difficulties, thus biasing the sample toward those who are psychologically troubled.

Genetic theories of the origins of homosexuality have been supported by twin studies that show a substantially higher rate of concordance for homosexuality among monozygotic than among dizygotic pairs of twins. However, some cases of discordance among monozygotic twins have been reported, and studies of twins reared together versus those reared apart (which would better separate genetic from environmental factors) have yet to be carried out. Thus far, it has been impossible to prove or disprove that genetic factors play a role in homosexual orientation.

Neuroendocrine studies of possible causes of homosexuality have focused on the hypothalamic-pituitary axis. Studies of serum testosterone levels have not consistently shown differences between homosexual and heterosexual populations. However, new research is focused on the hypothesis that *in utero* variations in androgen levels may program the developing fetus for a heterosexual or homosexual orientation. To date, no conclusive data have emerged from this research.

In summary, the numerous theories about psychological and biological causes of homosexuality remain unproven. It is likely that both developmental and biological factors play a role in the genesis of homosexuality, as they do in the genesis of heterosexuality.

Lifestyle

Much publicity has been given to the gay lifestyle, which stereotypically involves frequent anonymous sexual contacts and little sustained emotional attachment. The subculture of gay bars and baths that facilitates such impersonal contacts has come increasingly into the public eye in recent years, as homosexuality has been more openly discussed. To be sure, such stereotypes do hold for some gay people, more commonly for men than for women. However, the pattern of frequent anonymous sexual contacts is typical of only one subset of the gay population; those who are involved in stable, intimate relationships are often less visible.

Some clinicians cite fleeting relationships as evidence that gay men in particular cannot sustain intimate emotional ties; others argue that our society provides no social supports that encourage gay people to form lasting relationships in the way that the institution of marriage is socially sanctioned.

It is also true that, as the divorce rate climbs to nearly 50 percent and singles bars become a more prominent part of heterosexual culture, heterosexuals and homosexuals come to look increasingly similar with respect to the frequency with which they sustain intimate relationships. In dealing with either heterosexual or homosexual patients, you must never make assumptions about lifestyle or sexual behavior until your patient shares that information with you.

Psychopathology

There continues to be considerable controversy within our society and within the mental health profession about whether homosexuality per se is a mental disorder. Although Freud did not believe it to be so, many later psychiatrists have adhered to the notion that homosexuality is pathological. Recent studies of large nonpatient populations of heterosexuals and homosexuals do not support the thesis that homosexuality is associated with pathological personality traits or increased emotional distress or social dysfunction. Thus, the American Psychiatric Association has removed homosexuality from its *Diagnostic and Statistical Manual of Mental Disorders* (DSM-III).

Obviously, the range of psychopathology found among homosexuals is as broad as that found among heterosexuals. But homosexuality per se is only cited as a disorder in DSM-III when it is ego-dystonic, i.e., when an individual strongly desires to change his or her homosexual orientation to a heterosexual one in order to lead a heterosexual lifestyle.

Treatment

Many different treatments have been employed to help people who want to change their homosexual orientation. Psychotherapy, psychoanalysis, and behavior therapy have been the modalities most commonly employed, and all have met with limited success. Some clinicians estimate that one-third of gay men who enter treatment with this goal in mind achieve a heterosexual orientation through therapy. However, others are more pessimistic about the possibility of achieving a lasting reorientation of sexual preference through any form of treatment. For men, factors reported to weigh in favor of achieving a heterosexual reorientation include youthfulness (under 35), some experience of heterosexual arousal, and high motivation. Few data are available for homosexual women.

Many gay people who are troubled by their sexual orientation have been treated at counseling centers that do not aim to change one's sexual perference, but instead direct treatment interventions toward enabling the person to be more comfortable with a gay lifestyle—decreasing the shame, guilt, and anxiety that are too often associated with homosexuality.

Advice to the Clinician

Unfortunately, many health care professionals are either insensitive or openly hostile to the concerns of those with a bisexual or homosexual orientation. You can do a great service to *all* of your patients by paying attention to some simple interviewing techniques:

• Do not assume that you know your patient's sexual orientation until you are told.

• Do not assume that you understand your patient's sexual practices or lifestyle until he or she tells you.

• Do not assume that a patient who is homosexual is troubled by his or her sexual orientation.

• When you are taking a sexual history, use neutral terms like "lover" and "relationship" until your patient tells you whether sexual relationships have been with men or women or both.

• Use your patient's words for his or her sexual behavior—some people call themselves "homosexual," but for others this term carries negative connotations and "gay" is more comfortable.

REFERENCES

Diagnostic and Statistical Manual of Mental Disorders, 3rd ed. Washington, DC, American Psychiatric Association, 1980.

Freund K: Should homosexuality arouse therapeutic concern? J Homosexuality 2:235-240, 1977.

Group for the Advancement of Psychiatry: Assessment of Sexual Function: A Guide to Interviewing. New York, GAP Publications, Vol. 8, Rep 88, 1973.

Kaplan HS: Disorders of Sexual Desire and Other New Concepts and Techniques in Sex Therapy. New York, Brunner/Mazel, 1979.

Kaplan HS: The New Sex Therapy. New York, Brunner/Mazel, 1974.

Kinsey AC, Pomeroy WB, Martin CE: Sexual Behavior in the Human Male. Philadelphia, WB Saunders, 1948.

Kinsey AC, Pomeroy WB, Martin CE, Gebhard PH: Sexual Behavior in the Human Female. Philadelphia, WB Saunders, 1953.

Masters WH, Johnson VE: Human Sexual Response. Boston, Little, Brown, 1966.

Meyer JK: Paraphilias, Comprehensive Textbook of Psychiatry, 3rd ed. Edited by Kaplan HI, Freedman AM, Sadock BJ. Baltimore, Williams and Wilkins, 1980, pp 1770-1783.

The psychiatric aspects of sexuality, in Psychiatry, 1982. Edited by Grinspoon L. Washington, DC, American Psychiatric Press, 1982, pp 7-73.

Saghir M, Robbins E: Male and Female Homosexuality. Baltimore, Williams and Wilkins, 1973.

11

Alcohol and Drug Abuse

Drug ABUSE AND DRUG DEPENDENCE are major social problems in our culture, yet it is difficult to define exactly what sort of behavior constitutes abuse. The use of mind-altering substances is sanctioned in almost every group in Western society. Which substances, then, are not permissible? And among sanctioned substances, how much is too much? It may be useful to begin with some definitions.

The World Health Organization defines *drug abuse* as excessive drug use that is inconsistent with acceptable medical practice. Some drug abuse results in *tolerance*, which is an altered physiologic state caused by continuous use of a drug, resulting in a diminished response to the same dose of the drug over time, so that progressively larger doses are required to produce the same drug effect.

Drug dependence refers to the psychological or physical compulsion to take a drug on a continuous or periodic basis in order to experience its psychic effects or to avoid the discomfort of its absence. Clinicians often speak of two types of drug dependence: *physical dependence* involves an altered somatic state due to continued drug use that results in physiologic symptoms (abstinence syndrome) when the drug is abruptly discontinued; *psychic dependence* is a less specific term

Table 11-1. Effects of some commonly abused substances.

Drug	Tolerance	Psychic dependence	Physical dependence
Alcohol	+	++	++
Amphetamines	++	++	O?
Barbiturates	++	++	++
Caffeine	+	+	O
Chlordiazepoxide	++	++	+
Cocaine	+	++	O
LSD	++	+	O
Marijuana	+	+	O
Nicotine	+	++	+
Opiates	++	++	++

Key: O = no effects, + = mild effects, ++ = marked effects.
Source: Vaillant GE: Alcoholism and drug dependence, in *The Harvard Guide to Modern Psychiatry*. Edited by Nicholi AM Jr. Cambridge, MA, Harvard University Press, 1978, p 568.

used to refer to drug dependence without any apparent physical component. Psychic and physical dependence often occur together, so that treatment must address *both* somatic and psychological cravings. Table 11-1 lists some of the more commonly abused substances and their effects.

Obviously, not all drug abuse results in drug dependence, nor does every instance of drug abuse imply the presence of an illness. When does the use of mind-altering substances constitute a disorder that requires treatment? *Drug use is pathological when it in any way impairs an individual's family and social relationships, health, job efficiency, or ability to avoid legal difficulties.* This definition is deliberately broad, in order to include the almost infinite variety of ways in which drugs can hamper people's lives.

Alcoholics and polydrug abusers. What sorts of people use particular drugs? Although drug abusers are often classified by clinicians according to the substances they abuse, such categorization actually tells us very little about the people involved. One common myth is that alcoholics tend to remain "faithful" to alcohol and do not generally go on to abuse other substances, while those who abuse opiates or barbiturates or hallucinogens are likely to abuse other drugs, including alcohol, during the course of their lives. In fact, many patients—

whether primarily categorized as alcoholics or as polydrug abusers—use whatever substances are available to alter their psychic state.

What causes people to abuse drugs and alcohol? Obviously, there is no single factor that accounts for why some people develop these disorders and others do not. The following variables seem to be important in determining patterns of drug abuse:

Availability of drugs. People who work in situations where drugs are readily accessible are more prone to abuse them (e.g., bartenders).

Onset of action of the drug. Drugs that act quickly (e.g., alcohol, fast-acting barbiturates) are more prone to be abused than those that exert their effects more slowly.

Development of tolerance and physical dependence. Withdrawal symptoms are unpleasant and may be life-threatening. The avoidance of these symptoms is a powerful factor in the continued use of drugs that create physiologic dependence (e.g., alcohol, heroin).

Genetic background. The child of an alcoholic, adopted at birth into a nonalcoholic family, is at a greater risk of developing alcoholism than the child of a nonalcoholic who is adopted into a nonalcoholic family. There thus appears to be some genetic predisposition to alcoholism, although the importance of this factor has yet to be fully elucidated. No comparable studies have been done for polydrug abusers.

Childhood environment. In addition to the genetic factors mentioned above, alcoholics (particularly men) are more likely than nonalcoholics to have alcoholic parents and siblings. The process by which drinking habits are "handed down" from one generation to another is thought to be based on the mechanism of *identification*, whereby children unconsciously adopt characteristics of important caretakers and others who are role models as they grow up. No general statements can be made with certainty about the childhood experiences of polydrug abusers. Some writers claim that polydrug abusers tend to come from noncohesive home environments where one or both parents were neglectful of or abusive toward the children, but this hypothesis has yet to be well substantiated empirically.

Culture. Drug abuse is less likely where drug use is prohibited on religious grounds, or where there are clear guidelines for nonabusive drug use. Thus, rates of alcoholism are very low among Moslem and Mormon communities, where alcohol is prohibited, and among Italians and Jews, who allow children to drink in socially sanctioned ways but prohibit drunkenness.

Socioeconomic status. Drug abusers often fail to conform to popular stereotypes. To be sure, there are sociopathic addicts who live on the street and steal to finance a heroin habit. But other "hard-core" addicts and alcoholics include physicians, teachers, housewives, and students—people from all backgrounds and socioeconomic groups.

Psychiatric illness. Many people who abuse drugs and alcohol suffer from mental disorders. It is often difficult to distinguish between psychiatric symptoms that result from substance abuse and those that prompt it. However, it is clear that many patients begin to abuse drugs to "medicate" pre-existing emotional disorders such as depression, anxiety, and psychosis (e.g., the depressed homemaker who becomes addicted to Valium). Disorders that commonly underlie drug abuse include affective disorders, anxiety disorders, somatoform disorders, and personality disorders (e.g., borderline, narcissistic, and antisocial personality disorders). No one personality type has been found among substance abusers. People who become alcoholics have often been stereotyped as passive, dependent, and depressed; polydrug abusers are thought to be primarily sociopathic. But these generalizations are not valid. Alcoholics and polydrug abusers vary greatly with respect to personality type and underlying psychopathology.

Psychiatrists are often consulted for treatment of emotional problems by people who minimize the extent to which their drug use affects their mental health. It is virtually impossible to get an accurate picture of a substance abuser's baseline state of mental health while the patient continues to use drugs. Thus, accurate psychiatric assessment and effective treatment of psychiatric illness are not possible until substance abuse has ceased.

ALCOHOLISM

It is estimated that 5 to 10 percent of the adult population in the United States is afflicted with alcoholism. It is more prevalent among men than women, but the incidence among women is increasing. Not surprisingly, it is also more prevalent among the urban poor and deprived minority groups, although it cuts across all class, ethnic, and geographical lines. A public health problem of major proportions, alcoholism is also significantly underdiagnosed—perhaps as many as half of the alcoholics seen by physicians go entirely undiagnosed. This occurs in part because alcoholics tend to strongly deny that they have a problem; in many cases, only family and friends can supply accurate information about drinking habits and resulting impairment of functioning. The alcoholic is likely to rationalize job difficulties and interpersonal problems as the *causes* rather than the *results* of drinking. And physicians do not generally suspect alcohol abuse among patients who do not conform to the stereotype of the skid-row bum.

Alcoholics commonly do not seek treatment until they are forced to by others. This often involves some sort of confrontation or coercion. For example, an exasperated spouse may threaten to leave if the alcoholic does not stop drinking. Or an irate employer may give the alcoholic one last chance to sober up or be fired. Unless the alcoholic's way of life seems significantly threatened, he or she is not likely to view drinking as a problem that requires treatment.

You will most often deal with alcoholics who want to hide the severity of their drinking problem from you, from friends and family, and from themselves. They will tend to minimize the extent to which they abuse alcohol, and see their current physical or psychiatric symptoms as unrelated to drinking.

You will not diagnose alcoholism if you do not look for it. A drug and alcohol history is part of every psychiatric evaluation. You must be particularly diligent about pursuing any clues or intuitions you have about the presence of alcohol abuse, or you may miss a problem that is primary to your patient's complaints.

Diagnosis

Ask every patient about the amount and frequency of alcohol use. *Assume* alcohol use and begin with such questions as "How much do you drink? In what situations? How often do you take a drink?"

Give patients who are vague about amount and frequency some suggestions that are more likely to *overestimate* drinking than to underestimate it—e.g., "Do you have several drinks each day?" When you suspect a problem, the following questions may help you clarify the situation. They are grouped roughly according to the severity of the symptoms they are designed to elicit.

- Do you sometimes feel a little guilty about your drinking?
  Do you often find that you want to continue drinking after your friends say they have had enough?

Are you irritated when your family or friends comment on your drinking?

Have you ever argued with someone close to you about your drinking?

- When drinking with others, do you try to have a few extra drinks when others will not know it?

Did you ever wake up "the morning after" and discover that you could not remember part of the evening before, even though your friends tell you that you did not pass out?

When you are sober, do you ever regret things you have done or said while drinking?

Have you failed to keep promises to yourself about controlling your drinking?

Do you try to avoid family or close friends when you are drinking?

- Are you having more financial or work problems lately?

Do you eat little or irregularly when you are drinking?

Have you ever been in a car accident after you have been drinking, or have you ever been arrested for drunk driving?

Do you sometimes have "the shakes" in the morning and find that it helps to have a little drink?

Do you sometimes drink steadily for several days at a time?

After periods of drinking, do you sometimes see or hear things that aren't really there?

Positive answers to any of the questions at the beginning of this list should make you think seriously about alcoholism and explore the matter further. If you suspect that your patient is denying the seriousness of the problem, ask to speak with family members, and do so with the patient in the room. This should help you assess the extent to which alcohol has impaired work, home life, or health, and whether it constitutes an illness requiring treatment. In particular, be alert to a history of withdrawal symptoms ("the shakes," delirium tremens) or "blackouts" (memory loss while intoxicated), for these are clear signals that the problem is significant and may result in serious withdrawal reactions in the future.

Treatment

Once you have diagnosed alcohol abuse, you must decide what forms of treatment are indicated and assess your patient's motivation for treatment. Obviously, emergency situations must be treated first. Anyone presenting with severe intoxication that threatens to compromise respiratory functioning, or with severe withdrawal symptoms like delirium tremens or seizures, should be admitted immediately to a medical ward or intensive care unit. For information on the management of these situations, consult a general medical textbook.

Patients who present for psychiatric evaluation are generally those for whom there is no medical emergency, but they may nevertheless require careful medical and psychiatric treatment in order to avert consequences of alcohol abuse or withdrawal.

Detoxification. Detoxification is the first step in the treatment of those who are addicted to alcohol and have experienced significant withdrawal symptoms when they have stopped drinking in the past. Detoxification is generally carried out on a medical or psychiatric inpatient unit, in order to allow careful monitoring of the patient's physical status and to prevent potentially lethal withdrawal reactions. Inpatient treatment also allows the patient to begin other types of therapy (discussed below), which can be continued on an outpatient basis.

Physiologic withdrawal from alcohol usually begins 6 to 24 hours after the patient has stopped a period of heavy drinking, and may begin as late as 36 hours after the patient's last drink. The early signs and symptoms of alcohol withdrawal are shown in Table 11-2.

The later complications of alcohol withdrawal include the following:

Worsening of early symptoms noted in Table 11-2, especially tachycardia, sweating, agitation, and tremor

Seizures
Most likely in the first 24-48 hours after the last drink

Table 11-2. Early manifestations of alcohol withdrawal.

Signs	Symptoms
Tachycardia (increasing pulse rate)	Irritability
Elevation of systolic blood pressure	Agitation
Sweating	Difficulty concentrating
Fever	Insomnia
Hyperventilation	Abdominal pain
Hyperreflexia	Nausea, vomiting
	Diarrhea
	Tremulousness ("shakes")

Usually nonfocal and generalized

Self-limiting

Generally precede agitation, delirium, and hallucinations

Alcoholic hallucinosis

Most common in the first 24-48 hours after the last drink

May involve visual or auditory hallucinations, or both

Delirium tremens (DTs)

Usually occur 50-100 hours after the last drink; may last up to 2
   weeks

Hallucinations, delusions

Hypermetabolic state: hyperpyrexia, dehydration,
  electrolyte imbalance

Mortality as high as 15 percent

Major withdrawal syndromes can usually be prevented by treating
earlier manifestations before they become severe. The key is early and
aggressive treatment, for it is much more difficult to "catch up" once
withdrawal has progressed beyond the preliminary stages.

   Treatment of early signs of alcohol withdrawal.
Chlordiazepoxide (Librium) is an effective pharmacologic substitute for
alcohol that has a wide margin of safety, little respiratory depression,
low addiction potential, anticonvulsant effects, and a long half-life (24-
30 hours). It both alleviates the signs and symptoms of early withdrawal, and prevents progression to more severe syndromes (DTs,
seizures).

   *Treatment should be begun as soon as patients show any of the
early signs of withdrawal: evaluated pulse rate (over 110 beats per
minute), elevated systolic blood pressure, sweating, or elevated temperature.* These signs are more reliable indicators than subjective symptoms
like anxiety and agitation, which may be present for many reasons
other than withdrawal.

   1. Give 50-100 mg of chlordiazepoxide orally at the first signs of
withdrawal (the dose will depend on the patient's physical size and
extent of recent alcohol abuse). For persistent symptoms, the dose may
be repeated in an hour.

   2. Patients experiencing withdrawal can then be put on an ongoing
regimen of 25-100 mg of chlordiazepoxide orally every 4 hours as
needed to keep vital signs stable during the first day. The average patient
will require 300-400 mg/day on the first day; the total daily dosage
should not exceed 600 mg.

   3. Further doses should be given as needed for agitation, hyperten-

sion, or tachycardia. A useful guideline is to medicate so as to keep the pulse rate below 110, provided the patient is alert.

4. After the first 24 hours, if symptoms are controlled, the dosage of chlordiazepoxide may be cut in half each day until it is tapered off within four to five days.

5. If more than 400 mg/day of chlordazepoxide is required to control symptoms in the first day of withdrawal, 50 mg of chlorpromazine (Thorazine) can be added orally to each 100-mg dose of chlordiazepoxide, but this may complicate the treatment, since chlorpromazine lowers the patient's seizure threshold.

Once withdrawal symptoms have been controlled, other forms of treatment may be initiated.

You may be surprised by the onset of alcohol withdrawal among patients you have admitted to the hospital for seemingly unrelated medical or psychiatric reasons but who have a history of recent heavy drinking. These people may only admit to the full extent of their alcohol abuse when, in a setting where alcohol is suddenly unavailable, withdrawal symptoms set in. You must therefore consider the possibility of alcohol withdrawal whenever you hospitalize a patient who has a history of alcohol abuse.

Wernicke's encephalopathy and Korsakoff's syndrome. The medical consequences of alcohol addiction, such as hepatic cirrhosis and polyneuropathy, are well outlined in general medical texts. One neuropsychiatric syndrome deserves special mention here because it is characterized by dramatic psychological symptoms. Chronic alcoholics develop the syndrome, presumably because of a prolonged inadequate diet that results in thiamine deficiency.

Wernicke's encephalopathy is an acute, life-threatening condition characterized by clouding of consciousness, ophthalmoplegia (weakness of the muscles controlling movement of the eyes), and ataxia (a wide-based gait, falling, or inability to walk or stand).

At autopsy, patients who develop this condition are found to have brainstem hemorrhages, particularly in the area of the mamillary bodies. The condition comes on rapidly and requires emergency treatment with thiamine to prevent death and minimize residual brain damage. *Anyone* with a history of chronic alcohol abuse who presents with acute psychiatric or neurologic symptoms should be given 100 mg of thiamine intramuscularly. Symptoms often respond dramatically to treatment, but residual impairment is common.

Korsakoff's syndrome is a chronic condition that remains when Wernicke's encephalopathy is treated. It may also occur after one or more episodes of delirium tremens. The most prominent feature of Korsakoff's syndrome is *recent memory impairment*, although peripheral neuropathy, ataxia, and oculomotor difficulties may also be present. Classically, these patients have been described as using confabulation— i.e., fabricating answers to questions in an attempt to fill in details they do not recall. However, confabulation is actually infrequent and is not necessary to establish the diagnosis. The most common memory impairment involves difficulty in learning new information (e.g., your name). Korsakoff's syndrome improves in about 75 percent of patients who stop alcohol abuse and are maintained on an adequate diet for six months to two years, but only about 25 percent of those with this syndrome achieve full recovery. The only prevention against Wernicke-Korsakoff syndrome is an adequate diet, and, after emergency treatment with thiamine, diet is the only necessary treatment for those recovering from the syndrome.

Long-term treatment of alcoholism. Most clinicians consider alcoholism a disease rather than a moral failing. This viewpoint is useful in helping to alleviate the heavy burden of guilt carried by many alcoholic patients. However, the disease concept does not absolve alcoholics from responsibility for their drinking, nor does it imply that other people can bail them out of their difficulties. The treatment of alcoholism is long and difficult for patients, families, and treaters alike. Alcoholics are asked to give up forever a substance they truly (if ambivalently) love.

Effective treatment involves giving patients a nonchemical substitute for the lost addiction, reminding them continuously that even one drink can lead to relapse, repairing the social and medical damage that has occurred, and restoring their self-esteem. A variety of treatment modalities have been employed to achieve these goals, the most effective of which are listed below.

Alocholics Anonymous (AA). This is the most effective treatment known for alcoholics. It provides continuously available group support by individuals who have themselves suffered from alcoholism. Meetings are held in many cities at every hour of the day and night, so that support is available as frequently as the alcoholic wishes it. These meetings involve peer support and gentle confrontation of the ways in which alcoholics deny their illness. AA techniques also help the alcoholic understand the conditioned and impulsive aspects of drinking. AA replaces drinking companions with a new group of peers with whom the alcoholic can identify. It allows members not only to receive help from other alcoholics, but also to give help to others, thereby enhancing self-esteem.

Many alcoholics are initially reluctant to participate in AA. In recommending this treatment, you should be consistently supportive and, if possible, find a way for other AA members to personally introduce the patient to these meetings. Because alcoholism often takes a devastating toll on the families of alcoholics, you may want to refer them to *Al-Anon*, a self-help group that helps spouses deal with their own emotional difficulties, as well as teaching them about alcoholism and how to avoid interfering with the alcoholic's recovery. *Alateen* is a similar organization that offers support to adolescents who are coping with alcoholic parents.

Psychotherapy. This is not the primary treatment of choice of alcoholism, for it cannot provide the continuous support that is often required. However, when used adjunctively with other modalities like AA, it can be extremely useful—e.g., in helping to uncover family problems that perpetuate the patient's drinking, and in helping the patient to see ways in which drinking provides him or her with certain benefits (*secondary gains*). In most cases, psychotherapy cannot be effective until the patient stops drinking, for only then can the therapy address the uncomfortable feelings and symptoms the alcoholic habitually "medicates" away with ethanol.

Disulfiram (Antabuse). This medication blocks the normal oxidation of alcohol so that acetaldehyde accumulates in the bloodstream and causes unpleasant symptoms, such as tachycardia and vomiting. Obviously, the use of this medication is voluntary (usually in oral doses of 125 or 250 mg/day) and patients must be made aware of its adverse interactions with alcohol. Although Antabuse provides a deterrent to drinking, it does not help with such factors as low self-esteem and the loss of the addicting substance. By itself, therefore, it is of limited use in the treatment of alcoholism. However, many clinicians use it in conjunction with AA or psychotherapy.

Behavior modification. Hypnosis, desensitization, relaxation training, and aversion therapy (coupling alcohol use with noxious stimuli like shocks or emesis) have been somewhat successful in treating alcoholism. In particular, aversion therapy that couples alcoholism with emesis has shown some promise.

Adjunctive services. Halfway houses, vocational rehabilitation programs, and other social institutions that give alcoholics support and help them recover lost skills have been useful as part of a treatment plan that includes other modalities like AA.

OPIATES

Opium is an ancient drug around which entire cultures and economies have revolved. Today, many opium-related compounds are used illegally in this country. In addition to the natural alkaloids of opium— morphine and codeine—there are important synthetic derivatives— such as heroin, dihydromorphinone (Dilaudid), and oxymorphone (Numorphan)—as well as purely synthetic opioids, such as meperidine (Demerol), methadone (Dolophine), phenazocine (Prinadol), pentazocine (Talwin), and dextropropoxyphene (Darvon).

All of these drugs are sedating; more importantly, they are the strongest pain-killers known. Thus, they are highly useful for medical purposes. However, they have strong potential for the development of tolerance, as well as psychological and physiological dependence. Although the majority of narcotics addicts live in the slums of large cities and obtain drugs on the street, addiction cuts across all class and social lines. Some health care professionals who have ready access to narcotics become addicted to them. Men outnumber women by almost four to one among narcotics addicts.

Many addicts seek treatment for their addiction in outpatient settings, but you may also encounter them in emergency rooms when they are experiencing acute symptoms of overdose or withdrawal.

Overdose

Overdose with narcotics often occurs because the user is unaware of the strength of the illicit supply he or she has purchased. Also, one's tolerance to a given dose of narcotic varies according to how much one has used recently; addicts may overdose even on their usual "fix" if their tolerance has been lowered by short supply of the drug.

The signs of acute overdose are the following: constricted pupils, diminished pulse rate, diminished respiratory rate, pulmonary edema, and stupor or coma. Acute overdose requires emergency treatment. First, support the patient's vital functions, and administer glucose intravenously. Then use an *opioid antagonist*. Although there are several drugs that block the action of opiates, naloxone (Narcan) is the drug of choice, since it is pharmacologically inert in the absence of opiates. The usual initial adult dose is 0.4 mg intravenously, although up to 1.2 mg may be required to reverse coma and respiratory depression. Comatose patients should be put into physical restraints before Narcan is given, since they may be combative as they emerge rapidly from coma. Narcan will reverse the signs of acute overdose within minutes, but its effect may wear off within 30 to 120 minutes, at which time the narcotic will again produce symptoms of overdose. Thus, patients who emerge from coma must not be allowed to leave the hospital but must be monitored carefully for up to 48 hours, repeating the administration of Narcan as needed.

Withdrawal

Withdrawal from opiates has been given much publicity in films and on television, and the abstinence syndrome associated with narcotics is very unpleasant. However, abrupt withdrawal is *not* life-threatening in otherwise healthy patients, as it may be from severe alcohol or barbiturate addiction. In fact, in terms of discomfort and medical danger, opiate withdrawal has been compared to a one-week bout with influenza. The symptoms are listed in Table 11-3.

Table 11-3. Symptoms of opiate withdrawal.

Early (12-36 hours after last dose)	Late (48-72 hours after last dose)
Yawning	Abdominal cramps
Sweating	Diarrhea
Gooseflesh (piloerection)	Vomiting
Insomnia	Elevated blood pressure
Dilated pupils	Increased respiratory rate
Anorexia	Increased heart rate
Muscle cramps	Fever
Tremor	

Treatment of Opiate Withdrawal

Methadone substitution. Methadone is a synthetic opiate that has proved to be effective in treating withdrawal from narcotics because it is long-acting and produces little euphoria (even so, it is commonly abused by recovering addicts). It is used for withdrawal primarily on an inpatient basis and in certain specialized outpatient clinics. It is given orally, beginning with 10 mg every 4-6 hours as needed for signs of withdrawal, and generally no more than 40 mg in a 24-hour period. The dose is adjusted to the minimum level that will suppress symptoms, and is then decreased by 5 mg (or 20 percent) every day until it is discontinued. It is important to use objective signs (blood pressure, temperature, heart rate) to assess the patient's condition, rather than relying on subjective complaints.

Clonidine. Recent studies have demonstrated that clonidine is very effective in alleviating the signs and symptoms of withdrawal from opiates, presumably by suppressing the noradrenergic hyperactivity that appears to mediate the withdrawal process. Clonidine is nonaddicting and produces no euphoria, so it is not likely to be abused. New research suggests that it may be the most effective treatment available for withdrawal from methadone, heroin, and other opiates.

Outpatient methadone maintenance. This is a controversial treatment designed to provide addicts with methadone as a long-term substitute for street drugs, in order to reduce the craving for these drugs. Methadone is given in doses of up to 120 mg orally per day, and addicts are monitored carefully with urinalyses and other control measures. However, abuse of methadone and its illicit sale on the street have been complications of such programs. Methadone maintenance must be carried out in conjunction with other support services that address the social aspects of addiction.

Long-acting opioid antagonists. These agents, such as naltrexone, prevent addicts from experiencing the effects of narcotics, and thus are thought to act as deterrents to drug abuse. The long-term use of opioid antagonists is still an experimental form of treatment, but some clinicians have achieved promising results with low rates of relapse.

CENTRAL NERVOUS SYSTEM DEPRESSANTS

Sedatives, hypnotics, and antianxiety agents all depress the central nervous system (CNS). They are often referred to as *downers*. Most are prescription drugs that are either obtained illegally or obtained legally from physicians but misused. The pharmacologic properties of these drugs are described in Chapter 15. Downers are commonly abused along with alcohol and opiates, and both abuse and overdose frequently involve combinations of drugs. Individuals who use barbiturates and other sedative-hypnotics are very prone to develop psychological dependence, followed by increasing tolerance and physical dependence.

Overdose

The symptoms of intoxication and overdose resemble those of drunkenness—drowsiness (coma in severe overdoses), slurred speech, lack of coordination, memory impairment, confusion, nystagmus, tremor, decreased muscle tone, agitation, paranoia, and inappropriate affect.

Management of overdose. If the patient is *awake*, induce vomiting or perform gastric lavage to clear the stomach of any unabsorbed substance. Send blood and urine samples and gastric contents for toxicologic analysis. Monitor and support respiratory and cardiac functions for at least 24 hours.

If the patient is *comatose or semicomatose*, attempt gastric lavage if the drug was taken less than 12 hours before. Alkalinize the urine to increase excretion. Support basic life functions through intubation, administration of oxygen, plasma expanders, and vasopressors.

Obviously, severe overdose with CNS depressants requires immediate medical attention and necessitates admission to a facility where intensive care can be provided.

Withdrawal

Withdrawal from CNS depressants can be quite dangerous if it occurs abruptly. In particular, withdrawal can result in seizures and cardiovascular collapse, and it carries a significant risk of death. The possibility of withdrawal must be considered for every patient who presents with a history of abuse of or dependence on CNS depressants. The withdrawal symptoms are listed in Table 11-4.

Table 11-4. Symptoms of withdrawal from CNS depressants.

Mild	Severe
Agitation	Seizures
Anxiety	Delirium
Anorexia	Hypothermia
Vomiting	Cardiovascular collapse
Increased heart rate	
Postural hypotension	
Hyperreflexia	
Tremor	

Treatment of withdrawal

Treatment is conducted on an inpatient basis and relies on substitution of pentobarbital for the abused CNS depressant. Pentobarbital is a short-acting barbiturate that is used to alleviate withdrawal symptoms and subsequently tapered over many days. Treatment begins with a pentobarbital tolerance test on day 1, to determine how much pentobarbital must be given initially to prevent severe withdrawal.

Pentobarbital tolerance test. First, a 200-mg test dose of pentobarbital is given orally. If intoxication results (with nystagmus and/or ataxia), then tolerance is not presumed to be great, and the patient is maintained on 150-200 mg of pentobarbital orally every six hours for the first day of treatment.

If no intoxication results from the 200-mg test dose, the patient is given 100 mg orally every 2 hours until intoxication develops. The total dose required to produce intoxication is then given every six hours for the first 24 hours of treatment. That is, if intoxication develops after 400 mg has been given, the dose for day 1 is 400 mg orally every six hours.

After the first 24 hours, the dose of pentobarbital is reduced by 10 percent each day and withdrawn gradually over a period of about three weeks. Patients are monitored carefully for signs of intoxication or withdrawal, with subsequent adjustments in dosage.

Some clinicians use phenobarbital instead of pentobarbital in the treatment of withdrawal, because there is less fluctuation in blood levels of phenobarbital and because it has antiseizure activity. In this procedure, substitute 30 mg of phenobarbital for each 100 mg of pentobarbital, in three divided doses, and decrease the dose by 30 mg/day.

If a patient is dependent on both opiates and barbiturates, barbiturate withdrawal is carried out first.

CENTRAL NERVOUS SYSTEM STIMULANTS

Amphetamines

Amphetamines are prone to abuse by a wide variety of people, including students who want to be able to stay up for many hours preparing for examinations or writing papers. However, amphetamine use in large doses can produce acute delirium and psychosis. Overdose is potentially lethal. The symptoms of amphetamine intoxication and overdose are listed in Table 11-5.

Treatment of acute intoxication involves decreasing CNS irritability and controlling psychotic symptoms. Toward this end, support and reassurance in a quiet setting may suffice in mild intoxication. In more severe cases, 25-50 mg of chlorpromazine (Thorazine) administered orally every six hours will ease agitation and diminish psychosis.

Amphetamine psychosis occurs in a more chronic form after prolonged use of the drug. The psychotic symptoms can be difficult to distinguish from schizophrenia. Symptoms include talkativeness, hyperactivity, stereotyped or repetitious behavior, bruxism (grinding the teeth), picking movements, suspiciousness, and (in more severe cases) persecutory delusions, hallucinations, ideas of reference, and hypersexuality. Management of amphetamine psychosis is also carried out with antipsychotic medication (e.g., chlorpromazine in the doses noted above) to decrease agitation and diminish psychotic symptoms.

Table 11-5. Symptoms of amphetamine intoxication and overdose.

Mild	Severe
Restlessness	Confusion
Irritability	Delirium
Weakness	Hallucinations
Confusion	Paranoia
Talkativeness	
Anxiety	
Tremor	
Hyperreflexia	
Insomnia	
Euphoria, with lability of mood	

Although physical addiction to amphetamines does not develop, a sudden withdrawal of the stimulant after prolonged use or administration of high doses results in a marked decrease in CNS activity known as "crashing," which is characterized by somnolence, fatigue, apathy, and severe depression that may lead to suicidal ideation. Patients need sleep, as well as physical and emotional support, until CNS activity returns to normal.

Cocaine

Cocaine use has increased dramatically in the United States in recent years. It enjoys a special status as the recreational drug of the affluent. Its use results in an initial stimulation of the CNS like that seen in amphetamine use, followed by CNS depression. The drug is commonly absorbed via the nasal mucosa after "snorting," but smoking and intravenous use are also common and are more likely to be the routes in severe overdoses. Overdose may result in psychosis and even cardiac arrest.

Antipsychotic drugs help to diminish psychosis in cases of cocaine overdose, and propranolol is used to decrease cardiac excitation. Although cocaine does not create physical dependence, it can create a psychological dependence resulting in chronic use.

HALLUCINOGENS

Hallucinogens include a wide variety of substances grouped together somewhat arbitrarily based on their ability to induce altered states of awareness that resemble those of natural psychoses. Some hallucinogens, like psilocybin (mushroom) and mescaline (peyote cactus), come from natural sources, while drugs like D-lysergic acid diethylamide (LSD) and dimethyltryptamine (DMT) are synthetic.

Signs and symptoms of hallucinogen intoxication include alteration of mood (often euphoria), vividness of real or fantasied sensory illusions and hallucinations, synesthesia ("overflow" from one sensory modality to another), and confusion. Many other psychological manifestations may be present, including a sense of time slowing, a loss of body boundaries, and feelings of grandiosity or omnipotence.

Although each hallucinogen has slightly different characteristics and produces somewhat different signs and symptoms, they all produce adverse reactions in some people. These reactions include acute panic attacks, psychosis, flashbacks, and precipitation of underlying psychosis (e.g., in people with latent schizophrenia). Whether a person has an adverse reaction to a hallucinogen (a "bad trip") depends on such factors as the dose of the drug, the setting in which it is used, and the personality characteristics of the user. LSD intoxication is particularly common, and is manifested by such physical signs as pupillary dilation, hyperreflexia, muscle weakness, increased blood pressure, increased heart rate, and fever.

Treatment of hallucinogen intoxication generally involves support, reassurance, and diminishing stimulation around the patient until the drug wears off. In many cases, putting the patient in a quiet, dimly lit room and talking to help him or her distinguish psychotic symptoms from reality will suffice to weather the crisis. However, severe panic may be treated effectively with oral or parenteral diazepam (Valium). Unless psychosis is unusually severe and prolonged, it is best to avoid using antipsychotic medication because of possible adverse anticholinergic reactions.

Phencyclidine (PCP) is unique in action compared with other psychedelic drugs, and it is not a true hallucinogen. A synthetic drug initially developed as a possible anesthetic agent for humans, it is now licensed only for use as an immobilizing agent for nonhuman primates. Often called "angel dust," it is a common drug of abuse. Its psychological effects include changes in body image (e.g., "My head is growing larger"), depersonalization, anxiety, disorganization of thought, depression, and hostility. PCP abusers sometimes behave with great violence under the influence of the drug. Physical signs of intoxication include elevated blood pressure, rapid respiration, and neurological signs such as nystagmus, muscle spasm and rigidity, and ataxia. PCP intoxication can result in coma and death.

Treatment of mild to moderate intoxication is different from that for hallucinogens in that "talking patients down" is not usually helpful and may even increase the patient's anxiety. Instead, placing the patient in a quiet, dimly lit room with a minimum of stimulation is successful in most cases. Diazepam (Valium) is used intravenously if severe myoclonus or seizures result. Antipsychotics are not generally helpful. Most cases of intoxication resolve after several hours of reduced stimulation (e.g., in a secluded room in an emergency ward), but some result in prolonged and severe behavioral disturbances, exaggeration of pre-existing thought disorders, and serious medical complications that require hospital admission.

CANNABINOIDS

Cannabinoids, such as marijuana and hashish, are mild euphoriants with some sedative effects. Many people use these drugs as others use alcohol socially. It is estimated that as many as 30 million Americans have had some experience with marijuana, but only a fraction of that number use the drug heavily on a continuous basis. Signs and symptoms of acute intoxication include disconnected speech, recent memory impairment, emotional lability, depersonalization, and confusion, as well as increased heart rate, conjunctival injection, and decreased body temperature. While adverse reactions such as panic, psychosis, and depression do occur as a result of cannabis intoxication, these reactions are rare.

The effects of chronic use of cannabinoids are the subject of some debate. Chronic psychotic states secondary to cannabis use have been reported in Eastern cultures where doses are presumably much higher, but such reactions have been rare in the West. Some clinicians have identified *amotivational syndrome* of low drive, poor judgment, introversion, loss of insight, poor communication skills, and depersonalization. This syndrome occurs in people who use marijuana heavily on a regular basis for many months or years. At this time, however, it is not clear whether heavy cannabis use causes or results from this condition of low motivation, and adverse effects of intermittent cannabis use have not been clearly identified.

TREATMENT OF POLYDRUG ABUSE

Your first task in dealing with people who abuse drugs is to avoid stereotyping them. As was noted above, polydrug abusers come from all backgrounds—including highly educated professionals and "sweet little old ladies." If you only look for people who come in covered with tattoos and needle marks, you will fail to notice the many cases in which substance abuse is a major problem.

Your second task is to take a nonjudgmental approach to the evaluation and treatment of drug abusers. Clinicians often see addicts as hopeless cases. Your first impulse in dealing with such people may be to try to usher them out of your office as quickly as possible. *Every drug abuser you see deserves a thorough medical and psychiatric evaluation*, with particular attention to possible underlying psychiatric illness (e.g., affective illness, anxiety disorders, personality disorders). You should either do the evaluation yourself with supervision, or you should refer the patient to a psychiatrist who is experienced in the treatment of drug abuse, or to a drug treatment center.

Treatment of drug abuse is difficult. Detoxification and crisis management are only the beginning of a long and difficult course to recovery. Like alcoholism, polydrug abuse involves substituting a substance for human contact. Many addicts' lives revolve around the process of obtaining drugs, and this provides a daily structure and a set of personal contacts that must be replaced even after physical addiction is eliminated. Also, polydrug abusers often "medicate" unpleasant feelings (anxiety, depression) that are likely to persist or worsen when the drug is taken away.

Reformed drug abusers who come from lower socioeconomic groups often find little support among peers who are likely to be antisocial and to encourage drug abuse. Thus, an important part of treatment for many patients consists of helping them to establish new support systems. This may take the form of self-help groups like *Narcotics Anonymous* or *Pills Anonymous* (similar to Alcoholics Anonymous), vocational rehabilitation programs, day care centers, or drug-free residential communities (e.g., Synanon).

Psychotherapy cannot, in and of itself, provide the continuous support and peer group encouragement many recovering substance abusers require. However, as an adjunct to other treatment programs, psychotherapy can help some drug abusers to cope more effectively with feelings and problems that may have promoted drug use in the first place. Family therapy can also be useful in pointing out the family's pathological patterns of coping with stress. Group therapy can be especially useful in providing support, as well as in confronting drug abusers with the consequences of their self-destructive and antisocial behaviors, especially when other group members are themselves recovering or recovered drug abusers. No one treatment modality is as useful as a combination that provides the patient with support, daily structure, and vocational skills that help to increase self-esteem.

REFERENCES

Cohen SE: Cannabis: impact on motivation, part I. Drug Abuse and Alcoholism Newsletter 9(10), 1980.

Gold MS, Redmond DE Jr, Kleber HD: Noradrenergic hyperactivity in opiate withdrawal. Am J Psychiatry 136:100-102, 1979.

Mendelson JH, Mello NK: Biologic concomitants of alcoholism. N Engl J Med 301:912-921, 1979.

Mirin, SM, Weiss R: Substance abuse, in The Practitioner's Guide to Psychoactive Drugs. Edited by Bassuk E, Schoonover S, Gelenberg A. New York, Plenum Press, 1983, pp 221-290.

Showalter CV, Thornton WE: Clinical pharmacology of phencyclidine toxicity. Am J Psychiatry 134: 1234-1237, 1977.

Vaillant GE: Alcoholism and drug dependence, in The Harvard Guide to Modern Psychiatry. Edited by Nicholi AM Jr. Cambridge, MA, Harvard University Press, 1978, pp 567-577.

12

Suicide

THE INTENTIONAL DESTRUCTION of one's own life is an act of enormous power. Suicidal intent and suicidal behavior constitute one of the most emotionally charged of medical emergencies—for patients, for their families, and for clinicians.

Approximately three-quarters of those who commit suicide consult a physician within six months before their death. Each year, the average physician encounters half a dozen patients who are seriously contemplating suicide. Suicide is ubiquitous, and confronts practitioners in every branch of medicine.

The pathways to suicide are many, but virtually all suicidal people have reached a state of intolerable emotion. The rage, defiance, despair, and helplessness that you will encounter in such patients is often frightening and confusing.

Suicidal people invariably arouse intense emotions in those close to them. Families and friends may react to suicide threats with sympathy, anxiety, or hostility. They may feel impotent and overwhelmed; they often blame themselves for the crisis; and they usually feel responsible for its outcome.

You, too, are likely to find your equanimity challenged by the suicidal patient. As a physician-in-training, you are charged with preserving life and promoting health—yet people who are intent on killing themselves often go to great lengths to thwart those aims. They may reject every offer of aid, thereby making you feel what they feel— helpless and angry. Or they may attribute to you unrealistic powers over life and death, and make you believe that you alone will be responsible if they carry out their self-destructive plans. Suicidal patients force you to confront the limitations of how much responsibility you or anyone else can take for another's life. If you are to deliver effective care in such situations, you must learn to tolerate your own fear and anger and frustration without retaliating against the patient.

Often, in the midst of emotional turmoil, you will be called on to make a considered judgment about the lethality of the patient's intentions and actions. You must use that judgment to intervene in a quick and decisive manner. There are no fool-proof formulas for the prediction of suicide risk, and lethality remains a matter of clinical judgment. But the study of suicide has yielded valuable guidelines for emergency assessment, and these guidelines, along with a heightened sensitivity to your own reactions, can make the care of the suicidal patient safer and more efficient.

MYTHS ABOUT SUICIDE

A great many misconceptions about suicide have flourished, even among mental health professionals, and these can hinder clinical work.
Suicidal people are fully intent on self-destruction and have the right to die. Nearly all suicidal people are ambivalent about dying—they want to die and at the same time wish to be saved from death. For many, the fact that they have reached a physician is evidence of these mixed feelings.

Once decided upon, suicide is inevitable. Strong suicidal intent usually represents an acute condition, and intent generally falls sharply when the immediate circumstances compelling the event are survived.

People who talk about killing themselves are not the ones who actually do it. In more than 80 percent of cases, people who succeed at suicide have given definite warnings of their intent to die.

Improvement following a suicidal crisis means

that the period of risk is over. Most completed suicides occur within three months after an acute crisis, when "improvement" affords the suicidal person more energy with which to put his or her intentions into effect.

Discussing suicidal thoughts and plans with the patient will fix ideas of suicide more firmly in his or her mind. In fact, the careful eliciting of such thoughts and plans can be enormously relieving to people who have been unable to share their feelings of desperation. Sensitive and open discussion may well ease the crisis, and will rarely if ever exacerbate it.

EPIDEMIOLOGY OF SUICIDE

Suicide is among the ten leading causes of death in the United States (ninth as of 1978).

Roughly 1 out of every 10,000 people kill themselves each year in the United States (in 1980, 12.7 per 100,000 population).

Estimates of the total number of suicides in the United States each year range from 25,000 to 55,000. (Many suspected suicides are never proved.)

One out of every 10 people in the general population have at some time had suicidal feelings that *they* would label "serious."

For every completed suicide, there are between 10 and 40 attempts. (Many attempts are never reported.)

The rate of suicide is increasing for all age groups in the United States.

RISK FACTORS

Suicidologists have long searched for "suicide profiles." They have looked at everything from the phases of the moon to birth order in the family in an effort to solve the mystery of why certain people resort to suicide. The following is a list of the risk factors most consistently identified in recent studies:

Age. The risk of suicide increases with age, and peaks among people in their late seventies. However, in the last 25 years there has been a more than threefold increase in the rate of suicide among adolescents and young adults.

Sex. Men commit suicide three times more frequently than women. However, women *attempt* suicide two to three times as often as men. Men tend to use knives, firearms, and other violent methods of suicide, while women show a preference for self-poisoning.

Race. The suicide rate is higher for whites than for nonwhites. However, the rate among young black adults in ghetto areas has recently increased sharply.

Marital status. Suicide rates are lowest for married people and higher for those who are separated, divorced, or widowed.

Living situation. People who live alone are at a higher risk of suicide than people who live with others.

Employment status. People who are unemployed are at higher risk of suicide than those who are working in or out of the home. Professionals (especially male physicians) are also at a disproportionately high risk.

Physical health. Physical illness, or the perception that one is ill, is more frequent among those who commit suicide. In particular, there is a high correlation between completed suicide and visits to a physician for medical complaints during the preceding six months.

Mental health. Among the mental illnesses that have been correlated with a high risk of suicide are depression, manic-depressive illness, schizophrenia, and personality disorders. In general, the presence of major mental illness should alert the clinician to the possibility of suicide.

Alcohol abuse or addiction. Alcoholism markedly increases the risk of suicide.

Previous suicide attempts. A history of suicide attempts has been estimated to increase the risk of completed suicide by as much as 64 times that of the general population.

The following factors, while less easily quantifiable, have also been associated with completed suicides:

Hopelessness. Several studies have concluded that the specific symptom of hopelessness about one's life situation is more highly correlated with suicide than is the more general category of depression.

Interpersonal loss. There is a high correlation between interpersonal loss and suicide. *Loss* is defined as the separation from, divorce from, or death of a significant other, and may include relatives, friends, lovers, and therapists. The risk of suicide is particularly high among alcoholics who have suffered interpersonal losses within the previous six weeks.

Life stresses. A high frequency of major life events in the previous six months has been found among those who commit suicide. Such events include job changes, moves, births, graduations, financial reversals, marriage, retirement, and menopause. Such changes are important to identify in assessing both the precipitants of a suicidal crisis and the possibilities for therapeutic intervention.

Interpersonal conflict. Longstanding intense interpersonal conflict with family members or other important people is associated with a high risk of suicide and has led some observers to characterize suicide as a fundamentally dyadic event. Such conflict, if unremitting, may continue to jeopardize the life of the patient after a particular crisis has passed.

ASSESSING THE SUICIDAL PATIENT

When to Assess

Like many other potentially lethal conditions, suicidal intent can present itself to the clinician in a variety of subtle and obscure ways. Many suicidal people express their desperation covertly, and the danger to their lives may go unnoticed.

You must ask about suicide *whenever* it crosses your mind, and with each new patient who presents with an emotional complaint. Even this will not be sufficient unless you are attuned to the types of verbal and nonverbal clues that desperate people often give.

Verbal clues. Direct statements about suicide are easy to identify, but patients may couch these in an off-hand or joking manner. *Statements about killing oneself are to be taken seriously until proven otherwise.*

Suicidal people will often speak indirectly about their desire to die. They commonly express frustration with particular aspects of their lives ("My job is too much, doctor—I can't handle it any more") or they describe a general state of unhappiness ("I can't take it—nothing is going right"). Hopelessness is particularly evident among people who are suicidal. Statements such as "I might as well give up because I can't make things better for myself," or "I don't expect to get what I want," may allude to a patient's deep-rooted sense that the future is intolerable. Such declarations often sound like everyday "garden variety" complaints, but it is here that careful inquiry often elicits profoundly self-destructive ideas and plans.

Behavioral clues. People who are unable to verbalize their wish to die may act it out in a number of ways. The patient who abruptly decides to make a will, buy a casket, or give away prized possessions may be putting affairs in order prior to suicide. Nonlethal experimentation with potentially lethal agents (drugs, weapons) may be a prelude to a serious attempt. A new interest in life insurance policies, cemetery plots, or gravestones may seem like prudent planning, and may only in retrospect appear to reflect suicidal intent. Accidents and accident-proneness are very common among suicidal people, who may be genuinely unaware of the ways in which they put themselves in danger so as not to have to acknowledge the existence of suicidal impulses. All of these behaviors should alert you to the possibility of suicide, and should prompt the sort of examination described below.

How to Assess

People on the verge of suicide are desperate. Their usual methods of coping with life have failed, and they may feel very ashamed of their condition. A nonjudgmental, objective concern on the part of the clinician may do much to alleviate these patients' burdens of humiliation, enabling them to be more open about their feelings and plans.

Whenever possible, the suicidal patient should be interviewed in a quiet and relatively private setting. When the patient has made a suicide attempt, it is essential that the interview be conducted only *after* the patient has had a full medical evaluation and is medically stable. Initially, you will usually want to speak to the patient alone, and at some later point speak with friends or family in person or by telephone. You should make it clear to everyone involved how the evaluation will proceed. A calm and organized approach will help to ease the extreme tension that suicide threats inevitably generate in patients and family members or friends. Avoid premature reassurance, for the patient may interpret this to mean that you do not understand the seriousness of the situation.

Obviously, this sort of assessment requires time and thoughtful attention to emotional nuances—and both of these factors are usually in short supply in such places as a busy hospital emergency room. Nevertheless, you must take care to establish a setting in which you can gather the data you need.

What to Assess

Assessment of suicide risk must focus on suicidal intentions, suicide attempts (if any have been made), general psychiatric condition, and potential resources for correcting the situation. An outline is provided in Table 12-1.

Suicidal Ideation

You must entertain the possibility of suicide with every new patient you see in a psychiatric facility, and with every nonpsychiatric patient

Table 12-1. Outline for suicide assessment.

Assessing suicidal ideation
    Pervasiveness of suicidal thoughts
    Extent to which plans have been formulated
    Lethality and availability of proposed method
    Likelihood of rescue from proposed attempt

Assessing a suicide attempt
    Damage done
        Agent used
        Impairment of consciousness
        Extent of physical harm
        Reversibility of physical harm (recovery time)
        Treatment required
    Likelihood of rescue
        Location of attempt
        Person who acted as rescuer
        Probability of rescue
        Patient's participation in rescue
        Delay until discovery

General psychiatric evaluation
    Social situation—important relationships and recent changes in these
    Occupation—change in status or performance
    Psychiatric history—previous suicide attempts, depression, psychosis, current treatment
    Drug and alcohol history
    Medical history—recent change in physical health
    Mental status examination
    Availability of community resources (family, friends, etc.)

who appears depressed. In such cases, you need to ask about suicidal ideation, even when no attempts have been made and the patient has not spoken of feeling suicidal.

The exploration of suicidal thoughts can usually be done most tactfully and yield the most useful information when the interviewer begins with general questions and proceeds to specifics. A sequence of inquiries might go as follows:

- How is your life going?
- How are you feeling in general?
- How bad does it get?
- Do you sometimes feel like giving up?
- Do you ever think you would be better off dead?
- Have you thought of ending your life?
- Do you ever feel close to harming yourself?
- How would you do it?
- Where would you get the means to do it?
- At what time and in what place would you do it?
- How close have you come to killing yourself?
- Do you feel that you will kill yourself in the near future?
- What has kept you from killing yourself until now?
- Does anyone else know of these feelings?

Each question narrows the focus of the discussion. In some cases, you will find that your patient's responses to general inquiries do not point toward suicidal thoughts; more detailed questioning about suicide plans will then be unnecessary. In other cases, the patient will gradually divulge carefully worked-out schemes for self-destruction.

In discussing suicide plans, the *key factors* are the *lethality* of the method, the *availability* of the method, and the *likelihood of rescue*. Tactful questioning does not increase a patient's desire or ability to plan for suicide.

Direct denials of suicidal intent are usually truthful. People often admit to seriously considering suicide, but insist that they would not actually harm themselves, citing children, spouses, jobs, or other factors in their lives that keep them from killing themselves. Such reassurances are usually reliable, at least temporarily. Of course, one can be misled; you must be especially wary of patients who act self-destructively and at the same time deny any suicidal intent. In such cases, judge patients by their actions rather than their words.

Attempted Suicide

Physicians are often called upon to treat people who have survived a suicide attempt. In such a situation, you must make a judgment about the risk of another attempt in the immediate future. This involves a careful evaluation of the suicide attempt itself, since the lethality of an attempt has considerable prognostic significance for later self-destructive behavior. *No one* who has made a suicide attempt should be sent home from a treatment facility without a psychiatric evaluation.

Below are a number of questions you can ask to quickly estimate the lethality of a particular self-destructive act. These questions evaluate the damage caused by the attempt, and the degree to which rescue from this attempt was likely. The possible answers are listed in order of increasing dangerousness.

Physical harm done in the suicide attempt. The following questions can help you evaluate the physical damage done in an unsuccessful suicide attempt. Since superficial wrist scratches will inspire less alarm than a gunshot wound, the management of two such cases would differ greatly.

1. What agent was used?
    a. Least lethal: ingestion, cutting, stabbing
    b. Intermediate: drowning, asphyxiation, strangulation
    c. Most lethal: jumping, shooting
2. Was consciousness impaired?
    a. Alert
    b. Semicomatose, confusion
    c. Coma
3. How much physical harm did the patient do?
    a. Mild: superficial, self-limited (e.g., scratching without significant blood loss)
    b. Moderate: requires a physician's attention, but not life-threatening (e.g., wound that requires sutures, fractures of small bones, damage to small arteries)
    c. Severe: penetration of vital organs or large vessels, skull or large bone fractures, neurologic changes
4. How quickly can the patient recover from the physical effects of the attempt?
    a. Within 24 hours
    b. Within one to six days
    c. Questionable, possible residual damage

5. What treatment is required?
    a. First aid
    b. Hospital admission
    c. Intensive care

The likelihood of rescue from the suicide attempt. A person who has attempted but not completed suicide has obviously been rescued, and it is useful to determine how likely that rescue was. For example, taking an overdose at home in the living room with others nearby is quite different from taking the same dose while alone in a hotel room in a strange city. The likelihood of rescue provides one measure of the lethality of any given suicide attempt, as well as data for judgment about continued suicide risk.

The following five questions will give you some idea about how far the patient went to conceal or publicize the attempt.

1. What was the setting in which the attempt was made?
    a. Familiar: where the subject would be recognized (e.g., home, office, school)
    b. Nonfamiliar but not remote: where the subject would not be recognized, but could be observed to be in trouble by a passerby (e.g., bridges, subways, public buildings)
    c. Remote: where discovery could not be counted on (e.g., deserted areas, alleys, rural roads)
2. Who initiated the rescue?
    a. Key person: someone who knows the subject (friend, relative, therapist)
    b. Professional: someone whose job is such that he or she would initiate rescue (e.g., physician, police officer, taxi driver, telephone operator)
    c. Passerby: someone with no obligation to initiate rescue, who happened on the scene by chance (e.g., hotel maid, pedestrian, washroom attendant)
3. What was the probability that someone would rescue the patient?
    a. High, almost certain: rescuers were nearby or were faced with the attempt immediately (e.g., spouse was expected home)
    b. Moderate, uncertain: (e.g., a rescuer was nearby but would not know of the attempt)
    c. Low, accidental: rescue was by chance (e.g., subject took precautions to avoid discovery)

4. To what extent did the patient participate in the rescue?
   a. Asked for help
   b. Left clues (e.g., staggered, left notes or empty bottles in conspicuous places)
   c. Did not ask for help
5. How much time elapsed before the attempt was discovered?
   a. Less than one hour
   b. One to four hours
   c. More than four hours

General Psychiatric Evaluation

Suicidal ideation and attempts only make sense in the larger context of a person's life. A careful general history will help you to identify risk factors for suicide, as well as problems that might be amenable to change. One question to keep in mind is "Why now?"—what prompted this person to choose suicide at this particular point in life. Another question to ponder as you hear about the patient's current life is "What would this suicide accomplish for the patient?" Explore the following areas:

Social situation. Current living situation, family, recent changes in or losses of love relationships or important friendships.

Occupation. Job, home responsibilities, school; recent changes in status or performance.

Psychiatric history. Previous suicide attempts (method, severity), depressive episodes (depressed mood, sleep or appetite disturbance, diurnal variation in mood), psychotic symptoms (hallucinations, delusions), psychotropic medications, psychiatric hospitalizations, current therapy.

Drug and alcohol history. Patterns of use or abuse; consider psychosis or depression secondary to drug use or drug withdrawal.

Medical history. Ongoing conditions and treatment, recent changes in physical health.

Mental status examination. Focus on presence or absence of depression, psychosis, and homicidal ideation. The wish to kill others is commonly associated with the wish to kill oneself. Also, hallucinations or delusional beliefs may dictate suicide (e.g., a voice commands the patient to leap from a window), and the patient is at serious risk as long as this form of psychosis persists.

Availability of Resources

You must listen to the patient's story with an ear for possible interventions. Hospitalization is indicated for many who are at risk of suicide, but others can be treated as outpatients if they have adequate resources in the community.

Family and friends. The attitude of those closest to the patient provides important information about treatment possibilities. Significant others who are concerned but not panicked, and who recognize both the seriousness of the situation and the need for treatment, are likely to promote the patient's safety and recovery. Such people, if available to stay with the patient, can be instrumental in helping the patient to weather the suicidal crisis. At the other end of the spectrum, a person who has no one to whom he or she is close would leave the emergency room facing the prospect of returning to an impoverished world.

Often, those closest to the patient are overwhelmed with panic and confusion, or with anger. They may be incapable of assisting in follow-up care. It is even more lethal if friends and family are indifferent to the crisis. They may minimize the dangerousness of the situation and discourage the patient from seeking professional help.

Most lethal is the setting in which significant others covertly encourage the patient to commit suicide. The husband who ignores his depressed wife's suicide threats, or who leaves a bottle of tranquilizers lying about, may consciously or unconsciously wish for his wife's death. If the history demonstrates such collusion, you must arrange to get the patient out of this environment until some intervention can be made.

Other resources. "Significant others" whose help can be enlisted in follow-up care include psychotherapists, family physicians, and clergymen. Important people in the patient's life should be identified and considered as possible resources, particularly if you contemplate outpatient treatment. As a rule, any ongoing caretakers (physicians, therapists) should be contacted while the evaluation is taking place.

TREATMENT

Use your judgment about continued risk and available resources to arrive at a plan of action. Do this with the help of the patient, the family, friends, and any ongoing caretakers who are available to collaborate in the process. The options are essentially the following three:

Send the patient home. The patient who has not made a suicide attempt, and who expresses vague ideas but denies any clear self-destructive plan or intent, is probably a candidate for outpatient treatment, consisting of follow-up by you, the family physician, or a clinician at a mental health facility. The choice will depend on the patient's preferences and the cooperation of those to whom the referral is made. A definite appointment within the following day should always be confirmed before the patient is allowed to leave.

For the person who *has* attempted suicide, hospital admission is often the treatment of choice. However, if the patient denies further suicidal intent, the attempt itself indicates low risk, the patient is not locked into a hopeless or frightened position by depression or psychosis, and concerned relatives or friends can stay with the patient, you may consider sending the patient home. Follow-up care by a mental health professional should take place *the next day*. This may be through a community mental health center or other local facility, or with a private therapist. It is essential that a definite follow-up plan be formulated, that the relevant agencies be contacted, and that the patient have an appointed time and place for follow-up care before he or she is allowed to go home.

Outpatient treatment will be based on the patient's needs and diagnosis, and may range from a few sessions of crisis intervention work to long-term psychotherapy and pharmacotherapy. Possibilities include individual treatment, couples or family therapy, or group therapy. For a description of various treatment modalities, see Chapters 14 and 15.

Voluntary admission to a hospital. Many people who have definite plans for suicide, and most who have actually made serious attempts, will need hospital admission. Hospitalization affords a safe place in which to weather the crisis, as well as the chance for intensive evaluation and prompt initiation of treatment. Desperate patients will often agree to hospitalization, especially if family or friends support such a move. If you suspect that the patient may attempt suicide again even in the hospital, arrange admission to a locked psychiatric unit where the patient will be under careful observation.

Forced hospitalization. Unlike most other medical conditions, suicidal intent carries with it a legal mandate for treatment. A person you judge to be at immediate risk of suffering serious bodily harm *must* be hospitalized, according to the law in most states. Thus, the patient who is bent on self-destruction and refuses voluntary admission must be committed to a psychiatric unit. Commitment is generally done by a licensed physician, who must explain this course of action clearly and decisively and, if necessary, use ancillary personnel to detain the patient against his or her will. Because suicidal people often have enormous conflicts about their wishes, present your plan of treatment as clearly and firmly as possible. Decisions about suicide risk should be clearly documented in the patient's chart.

HAZARDS IN TREATING THE SUICIDAL PATIENT

The mirage of health. A patient may look healthiest immediately *after* a suicide attempt, if the attempt has mobilized support from family, friends, and caretakers. Patients who give perfectly rational explanations for their attempts (eliciting sympathy, getting attention) may convince you that they are out of danger. Do not discharge such a patient (from a medical ward or emergency room) after medical treatment without a psychiatric evaluation or follow-up. The probability of a subsequent, more serious attempt is extremely high if the patient's condition and life circumstances remain unchanged.

Debating the wisdom of suicide. You may find yourself drawn into an argument over the pros and cons of suicide. Remember that almost all suicidal people are ambivalent about dying, and they may well opt to live once the crisis has passed. Impromptu existential debates are rarely helpful.

Monitoring your own reactions. You may be quite disturbed by a suicidal patient's despair, or by what you see as the patient's manipulativeness. Some treaters find themselves furious or frightened by talk of suicide. Other clinicians find their patients to be "kindred spirits," and may unwittingly ignore distress signals in an effort to see patients as healthier than they really are.

You must be attuned to your own reactions to suicide, so that your "blind spots" and personal prejudices do not obscure the nature and severity of the illness. When you sense that your feelings are in some way interfering in your work with a suicidal patient, do not hesitate to seek help from a supervisor. No one needs to manage a difficult crisis alone, and knowing when to ask for support is a crucial aspect of good clinical care.

REFERENCES

Havens LL: The anatomy of suicide. N Engl J Med 272:401-406, 1965.

Miles CP: Conditions predisposing to suicide: a review. J Nerv Ment Dis 164:231-246, 1977.

Murphy GE, Wetzel RD: Suicide risk by birth cohort in the United States, 1949 to 1974. Arch Gen Psychiatry 37:519-523, 1980.

Paykel ES, Myers JK, Lindenthal JJ, Tanner J: Suicidal feelings in the general population: a prevalence study. Br J Psychiatry 124:460-469, 1974.

Schneidman ES, Farberow NL, Litman RE: The Psychology of Suicide, 2nd edition. New York, Jason Aronson, 1976.

Sletten IW, Barton JL: Suicidal patients in the emergency room: a guide for evaluation and disposition. Hosp Commun Psychiatry 30:407-411, 1979.

Tefft BM, Pederson AM, Babigian HM: Patterns of death among suicide attempters, a psychiatric population, and a general population. Arch Gen Psychiatry 34:1155-1161, 1977.

Weisman AD, Worden JW: Risk-rescue rating in suicide assessment. Arch Gen Psychiatry 26:553-560, 1972.

13

Violence

THREATENED AND ACTUAL VIOLENCE are ever more pervasive in our culture. Mental health professionals have long been prominent among those who work with "dangerous" individuals, but the issue of which violent acts to attribute to mental illness continues to cause heated debate in both courtrooms and emergency rooms.

Popular wisdom holds that insane people are dangerous people. Yet this notion does not hold up under scrutiny. Although some investigators report slightly higher rates of violent crime committed by released psychiatric inpatients than by the general population, this difference can be accounted for by patients who have a record of criminal activity prior to hospitalization. Psychiatric patients who do *not* have prior criminal records are, if anything, less prone to violent behavior than the general populace. The President's Commission on Mental Health addressed this issue in its 1978 report (p. 56):

> The sporadic violence of so-called "mentally ill killers" as depicted in stories and drama is more a device of fiction than a fact of life. Patients with serious psychological disorders are more likely to be withdrawn, apathetic, and fearful. We do not deny that some mentally ill people are violent, but the image of the mentally ill person as essentially a violent person is erroneous.

Our understanding of violence is sadly limited. The literature abounds with studies that show psychiatrists' poor record in the prediction of dangerousness. Yet psychiatrists continue to be called upon for expertise in evaluating violent individuals and forecasting their future behavior. Psychiatric assessment of "dangerousness" remains central to the decision to commit a potentially violent person to a psychiatric hospital against his or her will. Such opinions are often influential in distinguishing "patients" from "prisoners," and in determining whether a violent person is to be treated or punished. Although the complex relationship between mental illness and criminal justice is beyond the scope of this discussion, it is of critical importance in modern psychiatry.

This chapter deals with violence on a personal level—how it affects you in your clinical work. Although most mentally ill people are not violent, threatening behavior does occur in mental health settings— and indeed in all health care facilities—for we regularly deal with people who are under severe emotional stress. You may be faced with violence where you least expect it (e.g., from an enraged father who cannot accept the death of his hospitalized child), so it is essential that you become familiar with some basic principles of management. As an informed clinician, you can make critical interventions that prevent injury, diminish fear, and deliver much-needed care to people who are on the verge of losing control, or who have already lost it.

SOME BASIC PRINCIPLES

Violence generally denotes an assault on objects or people. Where people are involved, it implies an intrusion that threatens another person's sense of safety or well-being. We often speak of verbal violence as well as physical violence, but "violence" will be used here to denote physical harm done by one human being to another.

Violence is a behavior, not a diagnosis. Violent behavior cuts across all diagnostic categories in psychiatry, and it is common among people who have no diagnosable mental disorder. It is not an illness, but in some cases, it is a symptom of an underlying illness.

Violence or the threat of violence preempts all efforts at treatment. It demands immediate management, for you cannot care for someone competently when you feel that you are in danger. Much like a cardiac arrest, the violent act in a medical setting is an emergency that must be responded to and effectively controlled *before* you can step back and think about underlying causes and possible remedies.

Minimizing or denying your own fear is the most dangerous thing you can do in dealing with people who may act violently. It is also the most common error made by inexperienced clinicians. Your own reaction to a patient constitutes important data about how safe you are and how close the patient is to losing control. It may be your only clue to an imminent attack. If you do not pay attention to your own responses, you put yourself, your patient, and other people in real danger of being harmed, even killed. If this sounds overly dramatic, remember that health care professionals are at times the unfortunate victims of those they treat.

Why are we so prone to deny our fears in working with potentially violent people? As professionals, many of us harbor the unrealistic belief that we should be able to cope with any problem under any and all circumstances. Admitting that we are afraid, or that we need help, is not consonant with that belief. You are not omnipotent if you summon security guards, or end an interview and leave the room after acknowledging to your patient that you are concerned about his or her threatening behavior. You may be accustomed to putting your personal feelings aside until a crisis is over. But in fact, failing to attend to your own fears as you sit with a threatening patient is like failing to monitor the patient's vital signs during a cardiac arrest—you ignore critical data and thereby risk making the situation worse.

CLUES TO VIOLENCE

Potential violence may be easy to ignore, and it often goes unrecognized. Physicians who are hurried, emotionally withdrawn, or overly sympathetic may screen out clues to dangerousness and allow their patients' warnings to go unnoticed. You must be attentive to a variety of verbal and behavioral clues if you are to help people who cannot keep their violent impulses in check.

Threats. Roughly 5 percent of homicidal threats culminate in murder. Even when made in an offhand manner, threats of harm to others must be taken seriously and actively explored. A patient may make casual threats to test your receptivity to the problem, and a concerned response allows the patient to make a more explicit request for help.

Body space. The patient who remains constantly vigilant may be ready to lash out violently in self-defense. Such people reveal their inner terror in a variety of ways:

Shrinking from physical contact—particularly when approached for a physical examination.

Feeling crowded—paranoid people require roughly four times as much space as others do to maintain comfortable conversational distance.

Retreating when approached suddenly.

Protecting the rear—a fear of being approached from behind and surprised by an assailant.

Physical findings. Unusual numbers of scars, lacerations, bruises, old fractures, and missing teeth may indicate that a patient is habitually involved in violent activities.

Your gut response to the patient. This is often the *only* clue to dangerousness. It is better to be overcautious and to overestimate possible danger than to underestimate it and be sorry.

Table 13-1. General guidelines for managing a violent patient.

When there is a possibility of violence	When violence is present or imminent
Show available force	Summon help
Establish a nonthreatening setting for the interview	One staff member should assume leadership
Establish a collaborative tone in the interview	Remove all weapons from the patient
Set verbal limits on threatening behavior	Seclude the patient
Monitor your own reactions	Set physical limits on violent behavior when verbal limits do not suffice
Know when to stop the interview	Administer medication (antipsychotics, benzodiazepines) if needed to ease agitation and combativeness

EMERGENCY MANAGEMENT
OF THE VIOLENT PATIENT

When people become violent or threaten violence in health care facilities, your first priority is to *ensure safety*—the patient's, the staff's, and your own. No effective treatment can begin until treaters and patient feel that the threat of danger has been removed.

Your second task is to *quiet the patient and develop an alliance.* Many violent people assume a hostile and aggressive posture to defend themselves against intense feelings of helplessness and fragility. They are often fearful of losing control over their violent impulses. The following measures will help maintain a safe environment in which some collaboration between you and the patient can take place:

When a Patient Is Potentially Violent but Danger Is Not Imminent

If you are interviewing someone who has a history of violent behavior, or who you sense might become agitated and lose control, you must structure your interview so as to maximize everyone's safety.

Show available force. Before you begin, or at any point when you sense danger, bring security guards and other personnel into the interview room, or station them outside the room within the patient's view. People who fear losing control of their impulses will find outside controls reassuring, and you will feel more comfortable with help nearby.

Establish a nonthreatening setting for the interview. Remain at least at arm's length from the patient. Leave the patient and yourself clear access to an exit, so that either one of you has the freedom to leave at any time (e.g., do not sit between your patient and the door). The door to the interviewing room should remain open at all times. *Never approach the patient from behind.*

Establish a collaborative tone in the interview. The most helpful interviewing style is a straightforward and respectful manner that honors the patient's reasonable requests. You should show empathic concern, but avoid appearing too warm or too friendly at the outset—this may frighten a paranoid patient. Openly inquire about any veiled threats made against you or others, and encourage the paranoid patient to see you as an ally against perceived enemies.

Set verbal limits on threatening behavior. When dealing with someone who is obviously agitated, try to help him or her *verbalize* feelings rather than acting on them. You may want to reassure the patient that you will not allow anyone to be harmed—neither the patient nor others. (Many paranoid people lash out because they are frightened that they will be attacked.)

Monitor your own reactions. Your gut responses to the patient throughout the evaluation and treatment process may be your only clue to the patient's level of hostility and degree of self-control. If you begin to feel unsafe, address this openly with the patient and then remedy it; otherwise, the patient will sense your uneasiness, and his or her own fears of losing control may intensify. You could, for example, ask security personnel stationed outside the interviewing room to come in, so that both you and the patient feel safer to proceed.

Know when to stop. If you have taken precautions as noted above, but the patient continues to be agitated and threatening, do not continue the interview. Instead, let the patient know that you sense his or her difficulty in maintaining self-control, and that you are going to continue the interview at another time, when both of you can feel safer. *Remember*: you have nothing to lose by stopping an interview when you sense danger, and everything to lose by continuing.

When a Patient Behaves Violently or Is on the Verge of Losing Control

Summon help. Call for help at the first sign that a patient may become violent (or before a violent person arrives, if advance warning is given). This help may include security guards, police (where necessary), or anyone capable of helping to restrain an assaultive individual.

Assume leadership. Both staff and patient must feel that you can take charge and direct a team effort. Give your directions clearly and tell the patient what to expect at each step. *No surprises.* Keep your distance from the patient and do not block the doorway.

Remove all weapons. No treatment can be delivered to an armed patient. This include pills and liquor as well as knives, guns, and other instruments of force. Do not take a weapon directly from the patient, but ask that it be placed on a table; then remove it. Explain that it will be held for safekeeping. Police help must be enlisted if an armed patient refuses to cooperate with staff, and the patient may need to be searched for weapons.

Seclude the patient. Take the patient away from large, populated areas (e.g., a waiting room) to a more secluded setting. This will limit potential targets of any violent outbursts and quiet the patient, especially when hostility and hypervigilance are due to fear of others. Seclusion is a common technique for decreasing agitation—a seclusion room diminishes sights, sounds, and voices when the patient's normal ability to screen out such environmental stimuli is impaired.

Set physical limits on violent behavior when verbal limits do not suffice. Remember that severe agitation is very frightening for the patient as well as for others, and physical restraint is often relieving. Physical restraint involves using belts, straps, or other devices to restrict the patient's movements, often by strapping the patient's arms and legs to a bedframe as the patient lies on a mattress. Physical restraints provide concrete external controls when the patient has lost his or her internal controls. Wrist and ankle restraints must not be used punitively, but only when physical harm to self or others appears imminent. The primary clinician generally should not take part in restraining the patient for two reasons: (1) others are usually more skilled in this procedure, and (2) physical struggles between physician and patient may make later work impossible. One person should generally be assigned to restrain each of the patient's extremities; this should be done with a minimum of struggling and as humanely as possible. The use of restraints does *not* replace personal contact.

Medication. The use of medication against the patient's will as a *chemical restraint* is warranted only when there is immediate danger of injury to the patient or to others. However, patients who are acutely anxious will often willingly accept medication if the reasons for treatment and the effects of the medicine are carefully discussed in advance, and the plan of treatment is presented in a firm and confident manner.

Antipsychotics may be given orally or intramuscularly to control agitation and combative behavior. You may, for example, administer 2-5 mg of *haloperidol* (Haldol) orally or intramuscularly every 30 minutes until agitation subsides. This is the drug of choice for many patients, since acute hypotensive reactions are not common. Or you may choose to use *chlorpromazine* (Thorazine), giving 25-50 mg intramuscularly or 50-100 mg orally every 30 minutes until agitation subsides. Chlorpromazine is more likely than the higher-potency neuroleptics (e.g., haloperidol) to precipitate hypotensive reactions and must therefore be used intramuscularly with caution.

Benzodiazepines are particularly useful for those who are agitated but not actively violent and for the elderly, who are more sensitive to hypotensive reactions. Administer 5-20 mg of *diazepam* (Valium) orally or intramuscularly every 4-6 hours, or 50-100 mg of *chlordiazepoxide* (Librium) every 6-8 hours.

For severe alcohol withdrawal, give 10-30 cc of *paraldehyde* orally every four hours.

Amobarbital sodium (Sodium amytal) is another powerful sedative, which may be used in oral doses of 100-200 mg as needed to produce sedation.

PROFILES IN VIOLENCE

There is enormous diversity among those who resort to violence, but certain personal characteristics are common. If you are alert to these correlates of violence, you can use them to put your patient's threats or behavior into perspective and to judge his or her potential to act violently in the future.

Previous violent behavior is the most valid predictor of violent behavior in the future. The probability of future violence increases with each violent act. This includes a history of arrests, assaults on people or property, and a history of accidental or intentional involvement in another person's death.

Age. Violent behavior peaks among teenagers and those in their early twenties. Juvenile violence is increasing at nearly twice the rate of violence among adults. The earlier one is violent, the greater the likelihood that one will continue to be violent.

Sex. Ninety percent of those arrested for violent crimes are male. But much domestic violence (e.g., child abuse) perpetrated by women goes unreported.

Race. Blacks account for 12 percent of the population but 48 percent of all arrests for violent crime in the United States each year. The reasons for this disproportionate representation of blacks among violent criminals are not entirely clear, but social injustices and economic discrimination against blacks in this country are obvious contributing factors.

Drug and alcohol abuse. Substance abuse is highly correlated with violent behavior and predisposes one to violence through a variety of mechanisms (see below).

Socioeconomic status and employment stability.
Violence is markedly increased among members of lower socioeconomic groups and among those with a history of unemployment or irregular employment.

Self-destructive behavior. This factor is often overlooked. Self-mutilation and suicide are disproportionately common among people who act violently toward others.

Other factors that correlate with violent behavior include increased residential mobility ("absent roots"), being single, lower IQ, and lower level of educational attainment.

Childhood Correlates of Violence in Adults

Which children grow up to be violent? We do not know, but the following factors have been found to be particularly prevalent in the childhood experiences of people who behave violently as adults:

Parental deprivation and abuse. Violent people frequently give histories of parental neglect or abandonment, as well as parental abuse (verbal and/or physical). Those who were victims as children commonly become victimizers as adults.

Early exposure to violence. Parental and sibling brutality witnessed in the home provides a model for conflict resolution through violence.

Frequent disruptions in family life. This includes parental separation or divorce, frequent moves, and school changes.

Bedwetting, firesetting, and cruelty to animals. This "triad" is encountered frequently among children who have poor impulse control, but what was once thought to be a clear relationship between this triad and subsequent violent behavior has been challenged in recent studies.

Temper tantrums and frequent fights.

Authority problems. This includes truancy, school problems, and difficulties in the military.

ETIOLOGIES OF VIOLENCE

In evaluating a patient who has acted violently, you must consider the possible causes of this behavior. Many mental disorders underlie violence; some of the most important ones are listed below. But since most violence is perpetrated by people who do not suffer from a major mental disorder, your first task is to determine whether the problem is psychiatric.

You may find it helpful to try to fit your patient's behavior into a broader conceptual scheme of the etiology of violence. Most of us keep our violent impulses in check most of the time. What, then, has prompted *this* person to act on his or her violent impulses in this setting at this time?

Does the patient suffer from an impaired ability to test reality? People who are hallucinating may hear voices commanding them to act violently—for example, a man may hear his dead mother's voice commanding him to kill his father. A patient with visual hallucinations might see you as a vampire who is about to attack.

Paranoid thinking plays a prominent role in many acts of violence. People who resort to the use of violence frequently believe that they are being persecuted, harassed, or unfairly treated; they view the world as hostile and threatening, and they often lash out in "self-defense." Paranoid ideas generally begin with the misinterpretation of real events. The paranoid patient who acts violently often does so because of a distorted view of his or her situation.

Does the patient suffer from an impaired ability to control his or her impulses? We all have violent impulses. On a daily basis, we hear ourselves and others make such statements as "I wanted to wring his neck!" Yet we control these urges, sometimes so rigidly that we push them out of our awareness entirely. We do not attack others whenever we feel like it. People who do not control themselves may not have developed a normal capacity for self-control as children, because of poor parental control, neurologic impairment, a severely disturbed home environment, or other factors we have yet to elucidate. Such people often give histories of impulsivity in many areas of their lives, including sexual behavior, employment, drug abuse, and reckless driving. Other patients lose the ability to control their impulses only temporarily—e.g., under the influence of disinhibiting substances such as opiates or alcohol.

Does the patient show impaired judgment? Judgment is a complex mental function involving a variety of cognitive skills. Obviously, psychosis or drug use can impair one's ability to judge how to behave in a given situation. Other factors that may impair judgment include anxiety, depression, and neurologic impairment (e.g., as a result of head trauma).

Does the patient use violence explicitly to manipulate others? Many people suffer from no impairment in mental functioning, but simply use physical force deliberately and in a calculated fashion to intimidate or to achieve what they want at others' expense. Such people do not require mental health care, but disciplinary action.

Mental Disorders and Violence

Some of the more common mental disorders may foster violent behavior. They are listed in Table 13-2 and described briefly below.

Psychotic illnesses

Schizophrenia: Delusional beliefs and hallucinations become the "motives" for violence.

Mania: Delusions and hallucinations, coupled with uncontrolled rage and hyperactivity, predispose the patient to violence.

Psychotic depression: The hopeless person may kill family members or a lover in the delusional belief that this "spares them grief," and may go on to commit suicide. Elderly people with agitated depression can be surprisingly combative.

Table 13-2. Some disorders that may underlie violent behavior.

Psychotic illnesses	Drug intoxication or withdrawal
Schizophrenia	Alcohol
Mania	Opiates
Psychotic depression	Amphetamines
Brief reactive psychosis	Barbiturates
	Cannabis
Personality disorders, especially:	Cocaine
Paranoid personality disorder	LSD
Borderline personality disorder	Phencyclidine (PCP)
Obsessive-compulsive	
personality disorder	Organic conditions
Antisocial personality disorder	Temporal lobe epilepsy
	Brain damage
Sexual disorders	Dementia
	Adult minimal brain
	dysfunction
	Altered androgen levels
	Delirium

Post-partum depression: This is a special category of depression. Typically, the mother becomes anxious prior to delivery, develops delusions about her husband's infidelity, and becomes depressed after delivery. She is at risk of harming her newborn child.

Personality disorders. Any of the personality disorders may be accompanied by violence, particularly those listed below.

Paranoid personality disorder: Constant, pervasive paranoia may erupt into violence when the paranoid person feels that he or she is under attack.

Borderline personality disorder: Poor impulse control and persistent anger may prompt borderline patients to behave violently toward those who are important to them, but anger turned against the self is more common.

Obsessive-compulsive personality disorder: The highly controlled, obsessional individual may "explode" under severe stress.

Antisocial personality disorder: This disorder is characterized by failure to accept social norms, recklessness, impulsivity, and unstable relationships. Often labeled "sociopaths," people who have this disorder characteristically feel no remorse for antisocial behavior.

Sexual disorders.

Sexual dysfunction: Threats to sexual identity, particularly impotence from any cause, may prompt a show of force to demonstrate virility.

Homosexual panic: Men whose unconscious homosexual strivings come to the surface (e.g., in the military or other situations of forced intimacy) may become acutely anxious and paranoid. In the midst of such panic, the individual in homosexual panic believes others are accusing him of "forbidden" homosexual wishes and practices, and he may pick fights to prove his manhood. Such men frequently brawl in barrooms with "drinking buddies."

Drug-related violence. Drugs may precipitate violence in three basic ways:

Substances with disinhibiting effects can take away an individual's self-control, particularly when that control was tenuous in the first place.

Intoxication may result in delirium or toxic psychosis, in which confusion, delusions, and hallucinations prompt violent behavior.

Drug withdrawal syndromes may include agitation, confusion, and psychosis.

Some drugs commonly implicated in acts of violence are alcohol and opiates (43 percent of all violent crimes are committed by people who are under the influence of opiates or alcohol), amphetamines, barbiturates, cannabis (marijuana, hashish, synthetic tetrahydrocannabinol), cocaine, LSD, and phencyclidine (PCP).

Less common causes of violent behavior, but sometimes encountered among medical and psychiatric patients, are L-dopa, benzodiazepines, and tricyclic antidepressants.

Organic conditions. Some organic conditions may produce violent behavior.

Temporal lobe epilepsy: People who experience psychomotor seizures are at risk for developing impulsive and irritable behavior patterns, characterized by angry outbursts. These outbursts do not occur at random but are often provoked. They do not occur during seizures, do not commonly result in serious injuries, and alternate with prolonged periods of "good behavior." Families often note that the patient seems to have undergone a gradual personality change.

Brain damage: Traumatic lesions most often associated with violence are those involving the frontal or temporal lobes, particularly the limbic system and the area of the amygdala and hippocampus.

Dementia: Alzheimer's disease and senile dementia diminish integrative capacity and produce confusion, which often results in combative states, even among seemingly frail elderly people.

Adult minimal brain dysfunction: This syndrome of aggressiveness, impulsivity, and mood disorder is often found in people with a history of minimal brain dysfunction in childhood.

Altered androgen levels: An uncommon cause of violent behavior, it is found in some cases where violence is associated with sexual activity.

Delirium: Delirium may result from a variety of causes, including metabolic encephalopathies (see Chapter 9).

ASSESSMENT

Clinical evaluation of violent patients must include a detailed exploration of violent acts and impulses, along with thorough psychiatric and medical histories. People rarely exhibit random violence, but become dangerous to others only under specific circumstances. You must therefore pay close attention to the particular social, biologic, and psychological stressors that trigger violent impulses in each patient.

Only by constructing individual "profiles" of violence can you tailor treatment to individual patients' needs. Also, if you can identify specific settings, events, and other factors that trigger violence in your patient, you will improve your ability to predict when he or she may act violently in the future.

Evaluating Violence

The following questions may help you assess a patient's current status after a recent episode of violent behavior or violent threats:

Current crisis
- What happened?
- Who decided that you needed help? (You? A relative? A friend?)
- Do you think your behavior is a problem? Do others think so? If so, in what way?
- What prompted this crisis? (Fears of others, threats from others, etc.)
- Where did it happen? (in a bar, at home, at work)
- Who was involved? (spouse, policeman, passerby)
  In as much detail as possible, reconstruct exactly what was said, what was done, and who was involved. Also note whether drugs or alcohol were involved. What were the patient's thoughts and feelings throughout the episode?

Potential victims
- Who do you feel angry at now?
- Is there anyone you would like to hurt/kill?
- Is there anyone you feel wants to hurt *you*?
- Are you likely to see these people soon?

Available weapons
- How would you carry out your threat/protect yourself?
- Do you have a gun, knife, etc.?

History of violent behavior
- How far back does your trouble with violence (getting into fights) go?
- What is the most violent thing you have ever done?
- How badly have you hurt someone in the past?
- What is the closest you have come to killing someone?
- Do you get into fights (with X) more or less often than you used to?
- Are the fights getting worse?
- Have you ever been arrested? (document dates)

- Have you been convicted of any crimes? (document crimes, sentences)
- Have you ever been hospitalized because of your violent behavior?
- What weapons have you used in the past? Against whom?
- Do you ever hit your spouse/child?
- Where do fights usually occur? With whom? What do you usually fight about?

Try to get a detailed picture of previous situations in which the patient has acted violently—e.g., when intoxicated, upon ending a relationship, when fired from a job, when manic.

Environment

Assess family situation, peer pressure.

- Has anything recently changed at home or with friends? (Is an important relationship suddenly threatened?)

Note that 75 percent of all emergency commitments occur when family members are attacked or threatened. Half of all homicides are committed by family members or lovers.

- Are you the only one at home/at work/among your friends who gets into fights?
- Have you had trouble at work lately?

Judgment

- Can the patient accurately appraise situations and anticipate the consequences of his or her actions?
- Do you think you will need to behave violently again?
- What do you think will happen to you if you do what you have in mind?

Psychiatric Evaluation

A general psychiatric evaluation is part of every assessment of the violent patient. Special attention should be paid to:

Drug and alcohol history.

Childhood history—abuse or neglect, violence in the home, tantrums, frequent fights, school difficulty, delinquency, problems with authority.

Sexual concerns.

Mental status examination—particularly delusions (e.g., thought control, thought broadcasting) and hallucinations (commands or threats from imaginary beings), depersonalization, paranoia, suicidal ideation, and impulsivity.

TREATMENT

When a patient comes to you in an outpatient clinic or emergency room with a history of recent violent or threatening behavior, you must judge whether it is safe to allow that person to return to the community. Obviously, your decision will be based on many factors, including the patient's mental status, the presence of underlying medical or psychiatric illness, and your assessment of the likelihood that the patient will harm someone if released.

If you are concerned that a patient will be violent if allowed to go home, it is safest to hospitalize him or her so that you have more time to thoroughly evaluate the situation. Again, it is better to be safe than sorry.

Hospitalization

Indications for hospitalization include (1) specific homicidal intent with a definite, workable plan and the availability of weapons and intended victims; (2) lack of internal controls—impulsivity, poor judgment, faulty reality testing; (3) lack of social supports—family and friends are unavailable or are themselves in danger; (4) acute psychosis; and (5) toxic states that do not clear rapidly.

Patients who fear their own violent impulses may willingly agree to hospitalization. Involuntary commitment is justified in most states only when there is a substantial risk of physical harm to others or evidence that the patient has placed others in a reasonable fear of harm.

When involuntary commitment is indicated. Involuntary commitment must be presented to the patient in a firm and nonpunitive manner. Staff must remain with the patient at all times to prevent escape, and transportation must be carried out by ambulance and/or by security forces. Hospitalization should not mean rejection—whenever possible, if you do the initial assessment, you should make a follow-up visit once the patient is admitted.

When involuntary commitment is not indicated. You face a dilemma when the patient does not fit the criteria for commitment and refuses voluntary hospitalization, but there is concern that a specific intended victim might be harmed. Recent court rulings (e.g., Tarasoff v. Regents of University of California) have upheld the idea that clinicians are obligated to warn intended victims when patients express homicidal intentions toward specific people. Since it constitutes a breach of confidentiality in the doctor-patient relationship, this concept is under heated debate. Also, given psychiatrists' demonstrated inability to reliably predict their patients' future violent behavior, many feel that the profession has become legally bound to perform a task of which it is incapable. Nevertheless, the physician must contact and warn intended victims if patients are sent home with persistent thoughts of violence focused on particular individuals. A useful therapeutic stance is to inform the patient that the rules of confidentiality do not hold in cases where the patient's or someone else's life is in danger.

When you make judgments about a patient's dangerousness, it is essential that the basis for these judgments and subsequent interventions be carefully documented in the patient's record.

Outpatient Treatment

Patients who reveal no clear violent intention or plan, and who have no history of violence, may be followed up in outpatient treatment if they appear capable of allying themselves with you and seeking help before they act on violent impulses. Before the patient is sent home, it is essential that precise arrangements for follow-up be made, ideally involving you if you performed the initial assessment.

Psychotherapy. Psychotherapy can be helpful to patients who want and can use an ongoing relationship. The therapist should assume an interested but nonintrusive attitude, avoid all physical contact and initially avoid the use of humor, which may be misunderstood by a suspicious patient. The focus of work is on helping the patient recognize violent urges and behavior patterns, and on finding verbal or other means of ventilating these urges without acting them out. Patients must learn to predict the times and situations when they are likely to act violently, and to develop means of preventing such acts.

Clinicians disagree about the best treatment regimen. Some consider regular outpatient appointments with one therapist the treatment of choice. Others recommend treatment on an "as needed" basis at one facility by a variety of treaters, in order to dilute the intense and potentially overwhelming feelings that might develop in a therapy relationship and that could actually promote violence toward the therapist. Most clinicians agree that violent people need access to one institution on an ongoing basis for crisis intervention.

Table 13-3. Some medications that may be indicated in the management of violent behavior.

Medication	Indication
Antipsychotics	Psychosis and overwhelming anxiety
Lithium	Affective disorders and disorders of impulse control (e.g., episodic dyscontrol)
Antidepressants	Depression
Benzodiazepines	Anxiety
Anticonvulsants	Underlying seizure disorders, including psychomotor seizures
Disulfiram (Antabuse)	Alcohol addiction

Pharmacologic treatment. There are no specific medications for the long-term management of violent behavior. Medication should be used only when it is likely to alleviate an underlying mental disorder, and only after a thorough discussion with the patient (see Table 13-3).

In rare cases of intractable violence, psychosurgery has been effective. In violence associated with sexual activity, antiandrogen therapy with drugs like medroxyprogesterone (Depo-provera) has proved useful. However, both treatments raise particular ethical problems for the clinician.

YOUR REACTIONS TO VIOLENCE

Anxiety in dealing with violent patients is real and must be used as data rather than ignored. In the struggle to remain in control of the situation, you may defend against your own uneasiness in a variety of unproductive ways:

Denial. You may overlook important evidence of the patient's dangerousness (e.g., not hearing veiled threats, forgetting to ask about weapons) and see only the patient's nonthreatening qualities.

Reaction formation. "I'm afraid of you" may become "I'm not afraid of you," and your fear may be transformed into an overly warm and solicitous manner that can raise a paranoid patient's level of anxiety.

Withdrawal. If you feel helpless in treating a violent patient, you may avoid or openly reject the patient without being aware of your own emotional withdrawal.

Retaliation. Anger at the patient can be expressed through punitive treatment (e.g., the unnecessary use of restraints). You may find yourself enraged at someone who threatens you, and you may actually find pleasure in the "revenge" involved in restraining a violent patient with medication or by physical force. If this happens, simply step back from the situation and allow others to take over for you. Anger and fear are normal reactions to violence—you need not be ashamed of them. However, you are obliged as a professional to remove yourself (at least temporarily) from the treatment situation if such feelings begin to influence your clinical decisions.

Treatment for the Treaters

Working with people who resort to violence is extremely stressful. Witnessing violent behavior, and fearing for your own safety, are experiences that arouse some of our most primitive emotions. You must have support in doing such work, including:

Group support. Staff members who have been involved in a crisis with a violent patient commonly meet when the crisis has passed to "decompress" and discuss their reactions to what has happened.

Supervision. Supervisors who have experience in working with violent people can help you understand your reactions to threatening patients and improve your therapeutic skills.

Review of security procedures in the facility where you work. This may allay some anxiety and will improve your future efficiency in managing crises with violent patients. Review in detail plans for summoning help and procedures for carrying out physical restraint.

Visit a maximum security psychiatric facility. This is likely to broaden your perspective on how violent behavior can be controlled and treatment facilitated.

Peer support. The most helpful support usually comes from your colleagues, who best understand your reactions as a trainee in a stressful situation.

Violence, perhaps more than any other clinical situation, highlights the fact that you cannot care effectively for others if you do not take care of yourself.

REFERENCES

Benson DF, Blumer D: Temporal lobe epilepsy and its psychiatric significance, in Psychiatric Aspects of Neurological Disease. New York, Grune and Stratton, 1975, pp 119-217.

Drugs that cause psychiatric symptoms. The Medical Letter 23:9-12, Feb 6, 1981.

Lion JR: Evaluation and Management of the Violent Patient. Springfield, IL, Charles C Thomas, 1972.

Monahan J: The Clinical Prediction of Violent Behavior. Washington, DC, National Institute of Mental Health, U.S. Department of Health and Human Services, 1981.

Rada RT: The violent patient: rapid assessment and management. Psychosomatics 22:101-109, 1981.

Report to the President. Washington, DC, President's Commission on Mental Health, 1978.

Rockwell DA: Can you spot potential violence in a patient? Hospital Physician 10:52-56, 1972.

Tupin JP: Management of violent patients, Manual of Psychiatric Therapeutics. Edited by Shader RI. Boston, Little, Brown, 1975, pp 125-136.

Part IV

INTRODUCTION

The two major forms of treatment in modern psychiatry are the psychotherapies and the somatic therapies. No matter what area of health care you choose, you must be familiar with the applications of these treatments to mental disorders, since many of your patients will come to you needing psychiatric care.

Chapter 14 is a discussion of several different types of psychotherapy. The array of psychosocial treatments now used in mental health care is vast. This chapter could not begin to teach you about all of them, and no attempt is made to do so. Instead, the chapter includes an extensive discussion of traditional psychodynamic psychotherapy and a much more cursory description of some of the most important nonpsychodynamic modalities.

Why the emphasis on psychodynamics? First, as a medical practitioner, you will need to have more than a superficial understanding of this approach to mental illness, since it continues to be the major form of psychotherapy used in psychiatry. Second, Freudian psychodynamic theory is the foundation upon which many subsequent theories of the mind were constructed, and it is the school of thought against which many psychological theorists have reacted. Your understanding of the "basics" will greatly enhance your ability to think critically about the many ways in which these principles have been modified in later efforts to understand and treat psychiatric disorders.

Chapter 15 covers the somatic therapies, beginning with a general discussion of the principles of using psychotropic medications. You may want to read this section in its entirety. The subsequent sections on specific classes of medication are there for you to refer to as questions about particular medications arise in the course of your clinical work. Electroconvulsive therapy (ECT) is discussed at the end of the chapter.

14

Psychotherapies

CONTACT WITH OTHER HUMAN BEINGS can relieve distress, change behavior patterns, and alter our views of ourselves and the world. All psychological therapies rely on this fundamental premise. From the infinitely complex ways in which people interact, psychosocial theorists attempt to tease out the factors that promote emotional well-being and those that foster ill health. These studies have yielded a variety of schemes for understanding emotional life and treating psychological impairment.

The term *psychotherapy* includes those means by which a therapist attempts to provide new interpersonal experiences for another human being. These experiences are designed to enhance one's ability to manage subjective distress and to participate in loving relationships and satisfying work.

To be sure, these are ambitious goals. They are, in essence, no different from the goals any physician brings to work with patients, for the aim of all therapeutics is to improve the quality of life. Most medical practitioners rely heavily on the use of concrete aids in their therapeutic interventions—medications, surgical procedures, and an ever-increasing array of tools and machines. Psychosocial therapists, by contrast, rely on themselves as the primary agents of treatment. Yet the medical and psychosocial models of therapy are much closer than they at first appear. Regardless of specialty, experienced medical practitioners invariably attest to the therapeutic power inherent in the doctor-patient relationship.

How Can a Human Relationship Be Therapeutic?

Each type of therapy discussed in this text emphasizes a particular view of mental illness and particular treatment techniques. Yet all therapeutic situations share certain important factors that promote recovery.

The patient brings to therapy an expectation that help is possible. Psychotherapy prescribes that the therapist and the patient work together in specific ways that they both believe will be a means of restoring health. The therapist offers a sincere, interested, attentive, and reliable presence; the patient generally comes to view the therapist as a benign and powerful force. Most patients come to treatment with the hope that the therapist has benevolent powers. This hope underlies the majority of doctor-patient relationships in all areas of medicine.

Where does this hope come from? Human beings spend many years in a dependent relationship to their parents and other caretakers. As children, we learn that needs can be satisfied, fears allayed, and pains eased by the care and attention of adults. This learned expectation of help becomes activated in many situations in our adult lives, e.g., when we consult health care professionals.

These hopes serve as the cornerstone for successful treatment. In psychoanalytic terms, this phenomenon is referred to as *positive transference*, since we transfer positive expectations we had for early caretakers to people we expect to play similar roles in our adult lives. As a rule, people who have not learned to trust in this manner were deprived of care during early infancy. Such people may bring to therapy ingrained attitudes of suspicion and hate that take months or even years to overcome, or their mistrust may be so pervasive that it is impossible to establish a therapeutic relationship.

Psychotherapy gives the patient a conceptual scheme for making sense of bewildering mental phenomena. Each type of psychotherapy provides a set of concepts that patients can use to label and explain confusing subjective states and seemingly inexplicable behaviors. This enhances the patient's sense of control over problems. (This also occurs in other forms of medical treatment.)

The therapist offers the expectation that the patient can make positive life changes. Although this may appear obvious, many people come to therapy believing that they are incapable of self-improvement. Relatives and friends may share this pessimism, and everyone in the patient's life may be quite comfortable with the view that the patient is "disturbed" or "a mental case" or "the one with problems." In such situations, the therapist offers a different perspective and an unwillingness to share these stereotyped views.

The patient adopts certain of the therapist's positive attitudes. This happens through *identification,* a process that occurs in all of us from early childhood onward, as we consciously and unconsciously take on the characteristics of important others (e.g., parents, teachers) we want to be like. The patient in psychotherapy identifies with the therapist's attitude that problems can be faced squarely, and that seemingly unbearable thoughts and feelings can be tolerated and managed. For example, a patient who is brutally self-critical can identify with the therapist's more tolerant and realistic view, thus gaining the ability to be more flexible and less demanding of perfection.

Therapy offers a safe place for taking risks. The patient learns that it is possible to discuss "forbidden" feelings, attitudes, and experiences with another person without being judged or reprimanded. Developing a trusting, confiding, emotional relationship with the therapist is, in and of itself, a considerable achievement for many isolated and inhibited people, and serves as a model for developing more satisfying relations with others. The patient can also use therapy to experiment with new behaviors, in a situation that carries no real threat of punishment.

The safety of therapy lies in its structure: the sessions have clear boundaries of time and space, the therapist is restrained and professional, and the activities that go on between patient and therapist are strictly limited. These limitations are at times frustrating, but also reassuring. For example, a patient who is frightened by sexual impulses can learn that it is possible to talk with the therapist about such feelings without having to act on them.

Therapy expands one's horizons and increases one's options. This occurs in innumerable ways. Many forms of therapy help the patient arrive at a fuller awareness of self, particularly those aspects of the self that were previously disavowed or distorted. Therapy also helps patients see the ways in which they repeatedly distort their perceptions of others. This opens up the possibility of dealing with people in more productive and satisfying ways. Some therapists explicitly teach new behaviors; others attempt to teach new cognitive styles. All therapies offer new possibilities for viewing oneself and dealing with the world—i.e., they reopen the future by facilitating growth.

Psychotherapy cannot alter the problems of the world in which the patient lives. It cannot, for example, eliminate stress or poverty. But therapy can enhance self-acceptance and help the patient cope more effectively with the environment.

Models of Psychotherapy

There are two basic models of psychotherapy. Psychodynamic therapies are based on the idea that people can achieve greater understanding of the psychological forces that motivate their actions, and that insight achieved through psychological exploration opens up possibilities for change in personality and behavior. The classic insight-oriented therapy is *psychoanalysis*, which will serve as a prototype for our discussion of psychodynamic change.

A second model is that of the *behavior therapies*. Behavior therapies do not aim to develop insight or bring about personality change, but instead use directive techniques to remove specific symptoms. Persuasion and learning theories provide the theoretical bases for these therapies.

Behavior therapy and psychoanalysis may be seen as two ends of a broad spectrum of psychological treatments. In fact, most therapies involve some admixture of supportive-directive work and self-exploration.

THE PSYCHODYNAMIC MODEL OF CHANGE

Psychodynamic therapy encompasses a vast array of treatment modalities, including individual, group, couples, and family therapy. Sigmund Freud (1856-1939) is generally acknowledged to be the major figure in the genesis of this approach, for he was the first person to systematize a method of understanding seemingly unintelligible behavior in adult life by relating such behavior to childhood experiences.

All psychodynamic therapies share the assumption that the present is shaped and governed by the past—i.e., that our present attitudes and styles of reacting to the world are, to some extent, carry-overs from our attitudes and reactions to people and events earlier in life. Psychodynamic theorists focus on childhood—particularly on infantile experience—in attempting to understand mental health and mental illness. This is not to say that childhood trauma is invariably the cause of psychological difficulties in adult life. Indeed, human behavior cannot be reduced to simple causal explanations. Nonetheless, how children experience pleasure and pain, punishment and reward, in the context of family and social life prompts the gradual development of personality traits, ideas about oneself, and expectations of others.

Each of us develops along different lines. We have different caretakers as children and different family constellations; we play different roles within those constellations; and we bring different inborn characteristics to our dealings with the world. Each person's "take" on the world is unique, and the psychological traits and forces that develop early in our lives are highly individual, like fingerprints. These forces are modified as life proceeds, but the extent to which early roles and attitudes persist into adulthood and rule our adult lives is considerable.

Many of these psychological forces operate without our being aware of them. They are *unconscious*. The unconscious consists of fantasies, feelings, expectations, memories, attitudes—virtually all types of mental phenomena (see Chapter 2).

Why do some things lie outside our awareness? Material is pushed into the unconscious because it reflects experiences that are unacceptable at the time and in the circumstances in which they first occur. For example, a small boy may be totally unaware that he feels murderous rage toward his abusive mother. The child *represses* his anger—i.e., banishes it from his consciousness—because he cannot resolve the conflict between his wishes to murder his mother and his very real need for mother's care and protection.

The idea of *conflict* is central to the psychodynamic model of mental illness. Conflict refers to the opposition between seemingly irreconcilable forces. Examples include a wish to excel and a wish not to defeat others, or a wish to please someone that can only be fulfilled by doing something that is considered wrong.

Many of those who seek psychological treatment are enmeshed in conflict and are in some way hampered by it. Battles between opposing psychological forces can consume a tremendous amount of energy and leave the individual exhausted and incapable of effective functioning:

> A young man who had unconsciously adopted his parents' strong prohibitions against sexuality found himself caught in a desperate struggle between his own sexual longings and the dictates of a stern conscience. Sexually frustrated and incapable of forming a satisfying sexual relationship, he sought gratification in other, less intimate activities. He turned to auto racing, which, although objectively more dangerous, was emotionally safe. Despite his considerable success in this endeavor, he remained unsatisfied with his life and preoccupied. Moreover, he began to have difficulty completing projects at work and was increasingly unable to concentrate on even the simplest of tasks.

In many cases, such as this one, people who are caught between conflicting intrapsychic demands or desires find themselves unable to derive satisfaction from work or play. They may feel anxious or depressed, or develop discrete symptoms such as phobias or compulsive rituals; but, because the conflict is unconscious, they are not aware of the cause of their distress.

Psychoanalytic theory holds that conflict fosters the development of symptoms in three stages:

- The presence of an unresolvable conflict
- An attempt to repress the conflict
- The return of the repressed conflict to conscious life in a disguised form—as a symptom (e.g., anxiety or compulsive behaviors) or as a pathological character trait (e.g. passive-aggressive characteristics).

Life events and the process of growing up can ease internal conflicts, and many people find their way out of such dilemmas without psychotherapeutic intervention. However, some people become "stuck" and cannot find satisfactory solutions on their own.

Psychological conflict often manifests itself in disturbed relationships with others—a phenomenon that is especially prominent in many personality disorders. People with these disorders characteristically transpose their intrapsychic dilemmas onto a larger interpersonal stage and rely on distorted perceptions of others to ease their internal distress. For example, a man who cannot accept his feelings of murderous rage toward his family may develop the belief that other people are "out to get him." What starts out as danger from *within*—the threat that he may act on unacceptable impulses—is transformed into a danger from *without*, and the patient is able to assume the role of victim instead of victimizer. Not surprisingly, such distortions can upset family, friends, and even entire social institutions. A person enmeshed in such struggles with the world is likely to be brought to treatment when those around him or her become exasperated.

The notion of conflict provides a framework for understanding many symptoms of mental illness. However, some people—particularly those who are more severely impaired—seem to have an absence of certain emotional and intellectual capacities that are normally acquired in the process of growing up. They are thought to have psychological *deficits* that make them incapable of certain activities most of us take for granted. Examples of psychological deficits include a lack of the capacity to control violent or sexual impulses, the inability to anticipate the consequences of one's acts, and the inability to understand the difference between one's own and another person's feelings.

In pursuing the nature of mental illness, psychodynamic theorists and clinicians continue to debate whether certain symptoms and character traits result from conflicts or from deficits. This controversy has important implications for treatment.

Sources of Data in Psychotherapy

Patients come to psychotherapy because they have problems and need help. Their presenting complaints usually involve immediate life events and specific symptoms, but they are generally unaware of the deeper issues that underlie their complaints, as in the following case:

> A 23-year-old woman sought therapy after breaking up with her 45-year-old boyfriend. She reported that she became inexplicably anxious and had to flee the relationship as it became more intimate. She was aware that other relationships, also with older men, had ended in a similar fashion but she did not understand why. In the treatment that followed, the patient and her therapist explored the origins of her need to flee from intimacy, particularly when it involved older men. Eventually she recalled a childhood experience in which an uncle's physical affection had frightened and excited her. She was also able to recall the shame she felt not only because her uncle had caressed her body but also because from time to time, she wished that he would do it again. In her adult life she found herself pursuing older men but, at the same time, unconsciously equated sexual intimacy with her fear of sexual exploitation and with her forbidden interest.

As a therapist, how would you work with a patient to understand the presenting problem? The therapist has several sources of data about how patients' minds work. First, they offer information about their past experiences: their relationships with important people and how they felt and behaved in a variety of situations. Second, as sessions proceed, patients generally bring information about their current lives and relationships. Third, the patient forms a relationship with the therapist. This relationship is a powerful tool, because patients bring the same set of unconscious conflicts and motives to therapy that they bring to their dealings with other people in their lives. Thus, they are bound to recreate in therapy many of the pathological patterns that brought them into treatment in the first place. The therapist can then help the patient step back from the relationship and attempt to understand its unsatisfying and destructive aspects.

This brings us to two of the most important concepts that psychoanalytic theory has contributed to our understanding of the human mind: transference and resistance.

Transference

We are not born knowing how to relate to other people. From the first moment of life, the infant begins to form relationships and, in doing so, learns patterns of dealing with others that are not arbitrary but are determined both by the infant's inherent temperament and by the environment into which he or she is born. The way we learn to form relationships is strongly influenced by the particular people who are important to us early in life—most often, parents or other primary caretakers, and siblings. We carry our feelings for these people with us into adult life, and they serve as templates on which we form later relationships.

Thus, our reactions to new people in our lives are not only based on how we experience them in reality. We also tend to displace onto new people the feelings and attitudes we had toward early significant figures (parents, siblings, etc.)—*transferring* feelings from old relationships to new ones. This happens with particular intensity when someone in the present resembles someone important from the past. The resemblance may be in very particular details (appearance or tone of voice) or it may simply be in the nature of the relationship itself (e.g., to an authority figure). An individual may thus stir up intense feelings of worship or hatred, longing or fear, that are totally inappropriate to one's real knowledge or experience of that person. This is transference, and it is, for the most part, unconscious.

Transference feelings are present to some extent in all of our relationships, and they help determine our choices of friends, lovers, and colleagues. But transference reactions are likely to occur with particular strength toward people who perform functions that were originally carried out by parents—including teachers, lovers, celebrities, bosses, and, of course, therapists.

Patients instinctively reenact their earliest interpersonal patterns and conflicts in the relationship with the psychotherapist. They do this by attempting to coerce the therapist into being something other than a therapist—e.g., a lover, a protector, or a competitor.

> A patient complained that throughout his adult life he had always established highly idealized relationships with women, but the women he went out with always fell short of his expectations. Similarly, in the therapeutic situation, his therapist (who happened to be a woman) always disappointed him in that she "never quite understood what I was driving at," sometimes had to change his appointment time, and occasionally had the temerity to go on a family vacation. Eventually the patient began to realize that what he really wanted in a relationship was the nurturance he wished his mother had provided. Further exploration, however, revealed that in fact his mother had been somewhat cold and ungiving. Thus, what he expected from other people, (especially women) was the perfect "idealized" mother of his fantasy life. Anger at others for continually disappointing him and anger at himself for feeling so dependent colored all his relationships and eventually caused others to become angry at him and to leave, proving that they were in fact as undependable as his mother had been.

Because psychotherapy sessions are unstructured and the therapist remains a relatively neutral, nondisclosing figure, the psychotherapeutic situation encourages transference feelings to blossom. When these feelings become sufficiently intense, the therapist can help patients discover their distortions of the doctor-patient relationship and thereby to discover how they misperceive and misjudge other relationships in their lives. Such revelations can have major therapeutic impact, because they are based on patients' actual experiences in the therapy sessions.

Countertransference

Countertransference is, in essence, the therapist's transference to the patient. Like transference, countertransference feelings are inappropriate to the therapy situation because they belong to a relationship in the therapist's past. For example, a male psychiatry resident may find in talking with an older female patient that he is reluctant to explore the sexual concerns for which the patient has come to him for help. At the root of the difficulty is that fact that the patient reminds him of his mother, and he reacts to her in subtle ways as if she *were* his mother. In this case, the resident must recognize his distortions (e.g., with the help of a supervisor) in order to be of assistance to his patient. Countertransference is for the most part, unconscious. Thus, it is imperative that therapists-in-training have supervision and, if possible, be in psychotherapy themselves, so that they become well enough acquainted with their own countertransference responses to be able to deliver effective treatment without imposing their own distortions onto therapeutic relationships.

Resistance

Patients come to therapy for help, and usually express a desire to cooperate in the hope of getting better. Toward this end, they try to form an alliance with the therapist. Paradoxically, they also try to keep the therapist and themselves at a distance from the sources of their emotional pain. Indeed, people in emotional distress have often spent much time and psychic energy warding off pain, and many have achieved a tenuous, if unsatisfactory, emotional balance. The therapeutic relationship offers the prospect of psychological insight and change, and any change threatens to upset this hard-won emotional balance.

Even patients who suffer distressing symptoms will feel safer holding on to familiar ways of coping with the world than venturing into unknown territory. And they may have "good" reasons for not getting better—increased attention from others, decreased responsibility, a desire to make others feel guilty for their suffering, or an unconscious need to punish themselves. Thus, patients may be aware of wanting to get better, but largely unaware of their fears about change. They are also likely to be unaware of how they attempt to keep themselves and others away from their real feelings and concerns. This distancing process is known as *resistance*.

Resistance can assume innumerable forms, and examples are easy to find in daily clinical work. Patients may arrive late for appointments, leaving less time to do the work, or, once in the therapist's office, find that they have nothing to say. Others discover that they are suddenly well after one visit and need no more help ("flight into health"). Some deliberately withhold information, while others "forget" important data because of conflict over whether to disclose it. Any means of distracting attention from the task of therapy can be seen as resistance—

e.g., when the patient is seductive or amusing, when the patient tries to divert the discussion to talk about the therapist's private life, or when the patient rejects the therapist's efforts to engage in conversation. The use of psychiatric jargon is also a resistance when it is used to ward off genuine understanding.

Resistance may be so strong as to completely undermine the therapy, but such sabotage can often be avoided if the therapist addresses the problem, along with the feelings that prompt resistances. However, resistance is more than just an obstacle that needs to be overcome. Like everything else in therapy, resistance constitutes important data about how the patient's mind works. The ways in which patients keep their true feelings out of the interviews are likely to be the ways in which they avoid them in other areas of their lives. In therapy, people can learn to recognize these defensive maneuvers and understand how they get in the way of forming satisfying relationships.

To facilitate the clear emergence of transference distortions and resistances in the therapy hours, particular therapeutic techniques—free association and dream analysis—are especially helpful. They are used most often in psychoanalysis but also, to a lesser extent, in other types of dynamic therapy.

Free Association

Free association is a process by which patients say whatever comes to mind as they talk with the therapist. They are instructed not to change the sequence of undirected thoughts, and not to withhold feelings or thoughts that seem irrelevant, illogical, or distressing. This sort of uncensored, uninhibited verbalization is not easy to achieve, for the flow of thoughts is interrupted by the patient's various resistances to the work of therapy. Over time, patterns of resistance can be understood and clarified as they emerge to obstruct the free flow of material.

Free association is facilitated in psychoanalysis by the use of the couch, so that the supine patient does not look at the therapist and is at more liberty to pursue his or her own thoughts. Also, the psychoanalyst says relatively little, so that the flow of associations can continue uninterrupted. In face-to-face psychotherapy, free association is not used per se, but the patient's associations and the order in which they occur provide critical information about unconscious mental content.

The reluctance to associate about some matters can be instructive of the unconscious wish to avoid certain feelings or material, and changes from one subject to another can signal an unconscious linkage that can then be illuminated.

> A patient, informed of her therapist's upcoming vacation, suddenly became silent. When asked what was on her mind, she recalled a series of memories about the unexpected death of her father. Subsequently she related this memory to her now acknowledged dread of the forthcoming interruption in her treatment. What remained unspoken, however, was the considerable rage she felt toward the therapist for "leaving her," and her unconscious fear that her rage might be destructive enough to harm the therapist.

Dream Analysis

Dream analysis is another means of discovering unconscious material. Dreams differ from most mental content in that they lack some of the careful censorship the mind exerts over unconscious ideas during waking life. Thus, dreams often reveal underlying motives and yearnings more clearly than consciously directed thoughts. Freud called dreams a "royal road to the unconscious." Carl Jung was among the first to study the symbolic meanings of dreams and to develop a theory of a universal "collective unconscious mind," based on his observation that similar dream symbols occur in many different cultures.

Psychoanalytic theory holds that dreams reveal our childhood wishes in symbolic form. Recent theories have emphasized the role of dreams in our efforts to solve problems from waking life as we sleep. Dreams also provide evidence of feelings for the therapist.

Although the meanings of some dream symbols are widely recognized (e.g., a long slender object is equated with a phallus), it is almost always wise to assume unique and multiple meanings for the content of any dream. Thus, a simple dream reported by a young woman of being chased by a threatening man could be understood on many levels—as a wish to be pursued, a flight from sexual responsibility, or a conflict about being "chaste." Further information from the patient indicated that the man in the dream resembled her employer, an older married man whose first name was the same as that of her father's twin brother. Thus, a deeper analysis of the dream might eventually lead into her repressed wishes to sleep with her employer or even with her uncle or her father.

It should be noted that the interpretation of dreams and their usefulness for understanding hidden motivations or conflicts is a subject of debate. Indeed, there are some who view dreams as simply random neuronal discharges that have little relevance for understanding human behavior. Others suggest that, although dream content itself may be of limited value, the patient's associations to (i.e., thoughts about) the content reveal a great deal about what he or she finds emotionally significant.

THE PROCESS OF PSYCHODYNAMIC CHANGE

Lifting Repression

One of the fundamental assumptions of psychodynamic theory is that we handicap ourselves by banishing certain anxiety-arousing thoughts and feelings from our awareness and relegating them to the realm of the unconscious. This process of *repression* fosters the development of a great many psychological symptoms and irrational behaviors. A primary aim of psychodynamic treatment is to undo the repression that has taken place over many years, in order to give patients access to material buried in the unconscious. When unconscious material is made conscious, decisions become more rational, and we cease to feel like the victims of feelings, thoughts, and behaviors that seem beyond our comprehension and control.

The lifting of repression in treatment occurs gradually. As it happens, patients remember matters that were previously inaccessible to them. Repressed wishes—often the unrealistic pleasure-seeking demands we had as small children—can be examined by our adult minds. By bringing adult reason and logic to bear, patients can lessen some of the anxiety, shame, and guilt connected with them. Patients can also abandon their ways of defending themselves against the recognition of these infantile wishes, freeing up energy to deal with the adult world more creatively and more effectively.

The Role of Regression

Regression (literally "to go backwards") denotes a tendency to return to more infantile or childish ways of thinking, feeling, and behaving. Regression may be quite healthy and productive, as when we engage in various forms of play, or when we allow ourselves to be cared for when we are ill. Regression is easily seen in young children—for example, when the toilet-trained youngster regresses to bed-wetting during a stressful time.

The therapeutic situation encourages regression by its very nature, for it stirs up old longings to be cared for by an all-powerful parent. When regression occurs, patients find themselves experiencing the therapist as they experienced important people during childhood. In fact, the patient who is having a regressive reaction in therapy may literally feel like a small child vis à vis the therapist and may speak in a childlike voice, make unrealistic demands for love and affection, and even insist that he or she is physically small and helpless. How a patient reacts to the therapist during such periods of regression constitutes important data about the person's early experiences. It allows the therapist and the patient to understand how such regressive experiences distort the patient's perceptions of and responses to current life situations.

This requires considerable flexibility on the part of the patient. While genuinely experiencing feelings of being a child, the patient is asked to step back with the therapist and understand those feelings with the mind of an adult. After feeling like a child in the therapy hour, the patient must be able to go back into the world and function as an adult.

Many people are not capable of this sort of flexible, reversible regression. More disturbed patients (e.g., those with psychotic illnesses or severe personality disorders) are "stuck" in infantile modes of functioning in their daily lives. For them, further regression in psychotherapy is unnecessary and often dangerous. Other people, who function well in their daily lives, may have achieved this level of functioning with great difficulty; their tenuous psychological equilibrium might be disrupted by a major regression in psychotherapy. The therapist must therefore constantly assess the patient's capacity to tolerate regression, so that experiencing childhood emotions and behaviors does not overwhelm the patient and interfere with the work of therapy.

Both the patient's capacities to tolerate anxiety and frustration and the strength of the therapist-patient alliance are important indicators of the patient's ability to benefit from the experience of regression in therapy. The question of how much regression is useful, and for whom, continues to be a topic of heated debate among clinicians.

Interpretation and Working Through

Life events (past and present), dreams, associations, and the patient's mode of relating to the therapist are all invaluable sources of data about how the patient's mind works. It is the therapist's job not only to elicit this information, but to help the patient find meaning in it. The therapist perceives connections between various aspects of the patient's mental life and can offer tentative interpretations—the validity of which the therapist and patient can then test out together. Through interpretation, the patient gains some insight into the dynamic motivations that lead to persistent symptoms. Interpretation connects present thoughts, feelings, and behaviors with unconscious wishes and the defensive maneuvers the patient uses to keep from recognizing those wishes.

Interpretations make the unthinkable thinkable. They are therefore bound to stir up anxiety and must be timed so that the patient is more or less receptive to them. This usually involves waiting until the patient has worked on a problem long enough that unconscious material is very close to awareness. Interpretation may also be necessary when the patient's level of frustration is so great that it becomes difficult to continue the work of therapy unless the source of the frustration is clarified.

Ideally, a single interpretation of the origin of a symptom or behavior would bring about change and "cure." However, this is rarely the case. Intellectual understanding is not equivalent to emotional understanding and real integration of a new piece of knowledge. So, for example, a patient might suddenly become aware of the roots of his phobia of horses, yet find that his fear persists.

Single interpretations are not enough to bring about change, because single bits of awareness are intertwined with many other patterns of reacting and thinking. In fact, any new piece of awareness that comes from an interpretation must be relearned and tested in new situations and in association with other experiences—it must be integrated more fully into the patient's self-concept.

This process of rediscovering interpreted material in new contexts is known as *working through*. It involves amassing evidence to support the truth of some new piece of information—evidence that includes recovered memories, present life situations, and the relationship with the therapist. The same issue must be discussed repeatedly in therapy before the sort of insight comes about that involves genuine change. This process of validating new knowledge is one of the rate-limiting steps in psychotherapy and a major reason that psychotherapy takes longer than many people think it should.

Common Misconceptions About
Psychodynamic Therapy

Among the most frequently voiced erroneous ideas about psychodynamic treatment—particularly psychoanalysis—are the following three:

Myth: Treatment uncovers original childhood traumas that are the causes of symptoms in adult life. In fact, there are rarely single original traumatic events underlying psychological problems. People learn to behave as they do over many years by repeating behaviors in similar situations. The goal of treatment is to examine the patient's current experiences in life and in the relationship with the therapist, and to demonstrate how old patterns of thinking, feeling, and behaving are still active in the patient's current relationship to the world. Memories of the past simply confirm the continuity between present and past attitudes. Human behavior cannot be reduced to simple causal explanations. So rather than playing detective and looking for the single childhood trauma that "caused" an adult symptom, the therapist looks for ways in which the patient has repeatedly dealt with stressful experiences in maladaptive ways. We can almost never answer the question of *why* someone developed a symptom, any more than we can know why someone else with similar childhood experiences remains symptom-free in adult life.

Myth: The psychodynamic therapist must be a "blank screen" and not a real person in the therapy. Psychodynamic therapy involves very different degrees of self-disclosure on the part of the therapist, depending on the needs of the patient. But all therapies rely to a considerable degree on the reactions of the therapist as a real person. The patient needs this aspect of the doctor-patient relationship to highlight the ways he or she distorts this (and other) relationships.

Myth: Psychodynamic therapy makes the patient unnecessarily dependent on the therapist. Regression in therapy can make the patient feel as if he or she were a child relating to a powerful parent. However, this is only a temporary phase of treatment that helps the patient see how new relationships become distorted by feelings from the past. In fact, psychodynamic therapy aims to give patients the skills to continue to understand their own mental life long after treatment has ended—i.e., to become *more* autonomous rather than less so.

TYPES OF PSYCHODYNAMIC PSYCHOTHERAPY

The model of psychodynamic change described above serves as the basis for a variety of therapies. The most prominent of these will be described here very briefly.

Individual Psychotherapy

Psychoanalysis. Psychoanalysis was the original mode of treatment developed by Freud and his followers. It aims at a reorganization of character structure, with an emphasis on self-understanding and the correction of developmental lags. Symptom relief usually occurs as a result of this understanding but is not the immediate objective of the treatment. The patient lies on a couch, while the analyst is seated behind the patient and out of view. Free association, dream analysis, and the development and working through of transference distortions in the relationship with the analyst are the most salient features. Sessions are usually held four or five times a week, and a completed analysis generally takes three to five years, but length of treatment varies considerably with the nature of the problems being treated.

Patients in psychoanalysis must be able to tolerate a fair degree of frustration and ambiguity because of the lack of structure in the analytic situation. Analysis is therefore suitable for patients at the healthier end of the spectrum of psychological disorders—people with neurotic conflicts and personality disorders of lesser severity. The usefulness of psychoanalysis in the treatment of severe personality disorders is questionable, and its use in schizophrenia and other psychotic illness is generally contraindicated.

Table 14-1. Types of psychodynamic therapy.

Individual psychotherapy
   Psychoanalysis
   Exploratory psychotherapy
   Supportive psychotherapy
   Time-limited psychotherapy
Group psychotherapy
Couples therapy
Family treatment

Exploratory psychotherapy. Like psychoanalysis, exploratory psychotherapy aims at understanding motivations and unconscious forces that hamper daily living. However, exploratory psychotherapy focuses less on the analysis of infantile wishes and conflicts, and more on current life situations and dynamic patterns of dealing with others in the here and now. Analysis of transference remains a central feature, but transference reactions are often less intense than in analysis, where the therapist's relative inactivity allows such reactions to flower. The sort of temporary regression that is fostered in psychoanalysis is usually avoided in psychotherapy.

The patient does not lie on a couch but sits in a chair, promoting a more "real" face-to-face interaction with the therapist. Sessions are usually held once to three times a week (occasionally more frequently), depending on the patient's motivation and capacity to tolerate the intense feelings that are more likely to be stirred up when sessions are frequent. Treatment may last for several sessions, or several years, depending on the nature of the problem and the extent of the patient's motivation. Medication may be used in combination with exploratory therapy if the patient's symptoms indicate the need.

Exploratory psychotherapy is employed in the treatment of a wide range of psychiatric illnesses, including many psychotic conditions, depression, personality disorders, and neuroses. Patients must be motivated to understand their inner life and its manifestations in their dealings with the world. The major contraindication to exploratory psychotherapy is the inability to tolerate the exploration of feelings without having to act on them in destructive ways (e.g., suicidal behavior or violent acts toward others). The therapist must be alert to such adverse reactions in therapy, adjusting the frequency and intensity of sessions according to what the patient can tolerate.

Supportive psychotherapy. Although all forms of psychodynamic therapy involve some measure of support, supportive therapy is distinct from exploratory work and psychoanalysis because its goal is not the development of insight, but the lessening of anxiety. The therapist does this through reassurance, advice, modification of social factors where possible, and the bolstering of the patient's personal strengths and more adaptive defenses (see Chapter 4). The therapist is generally more active and more directive than in the other modalities.

One potential danger in doing supportive therapy is that it may foster a dependency relationship that is harmful and infantilizing rather than helpful. But some patients who have little interest in or capacity for achieving psychological insight can function much better in the world when "maintained" by a supportive relationship with a therapist. Supportive therapy generally occurs once a week or less, but at times it is carried out more frequently. Supportive treatment is indicated for those in need of temporary emotional support during a crisis, for those who are resistant to or too severely disturbed to respond to insight-oriented treatment, and for those who are not interested in changing their lives but simply in returning to a previous level of adjustment.

Time-limited psychotherapy (also called *brief psychotherapy* and *short-term anxiety-provoking psychotherapy*). Time-limited psychotherapy is a specific form of psychodynamic treatment developed as an alternative to more prolonged and more costly treatments. It is particularly useful when the demand for treatment exceeds available resources. The aim of time-limited therapy is to help the patient understand the roots of and achieve some resolution of a particular emotional problem that is a source of acute distress. Rarely does the therapy touch on transference issues or character problems; instead it focuses on current life situations. Dependence and regression are actively discouraged.

The number of sessions is usually agreed upon at the outset of treatment (from 8 to 20 or more), and there is an emphasis on patient autonomy and independent functioning throughout the course of therapy. The therapist works actively to maintain the focus of the sessions on a central issue that is identified by therapist and patient at the outset of treatment. This often keeps the patient's anxiety level relatively high throughout the treatment.

Patients who do well with this sort of treatment are generally the same ones who would profit from intensive insight-oriented work, i.e., people who function relatively well at work and in relationships, who can think in psychological terms, and who have a clear motivation to change. However, short-term therapy may be more desirable than prolonged work for patients who are in an acute crisis that has an easily identified focal issue, and who are interested in crisis resolution rather than a thorough exploration of themselves with the potential for a deeper restructuring of character.

Group Psychotherapy

The psychodynamic principles used in individual psychotherapy have been applied with much success in working with groups. Group therapy is a powerful treatment modality by itself, and it is also used effectively in conjunction with individual therapy for some patients. Both because of its therapeutic effects and because it is less costly than individual therapy, group therapy has been widely employed in many settings.

Groups vary greatly in structure and in the way meetings are run. Group membership may range from 2 or 3 patients to more than 15, but most groups have 6 to 10 members. Groups of this size are large enough for a sense of group identity to develop and for clear patterns of group interaction to emerge, but not so large as to lose sight of each individual's issues and needs. There is usually one leader, but co-leaders are not uncommon—often male and female co-leaders to help elicit patients' transference feelings for parents. Groups generally meet once a week for 1 1/2 hours, but sessions may be more or less frequent.

The goals of group therapy are primarily the same as those of individual therapy—self-understanding, self-acceptance, and the modification of behavior to enable the patient to form more satisfying relationships. The tools used in group therapy are also similar, including the use of transference interpretations, associations, and even dream material. However, the very fact that several people with emotional difficulties come together with therapists in one room to discuss their lives opens up the possibility for a wider range of interactions than can take place between one patient and one therapist.

Patients can provide each other with mutual validation of experiences, so that individuals feel less isolated by what they think are unique and unacceptable emotional difficulties. Patients also give one another advice, which is often less helpful in its content than in its demonstration of concern and caring. Patients who have felt like burdens to family and friends are able to experience being helpful to other group members as they offer support, insight, and reassurance in group meetings.

Groups are very effective in recapitulating family situations. Patients interact with group leaders and other group members as they once interacted with parents and siblings. Through interpretation, they can come to understand how they are distorting these current relationships. Group members can also learn social skills from one another—how to resolve conflict, how to be responsive to others, and how to be less judgmental of others' behavior. As members come to be more comfortable with one another, they can take risks and try out new behaviors that are too threatening to test out elsewhere (e.g., a patient may begin to experiment with increased assertiveness). The group becomes a microcosm of larger social groups, and patients can learn how they operate in group situations (e.g., family, job) outside therapy.

Group therapy has been used for virtually all types of psychiatric illness. It is particularly useful for patients with personality disorders, whose character problems are obvious to others but not to them. Such patients can often tolerate being confronted by their peers with evidence of their maladaptive behaviors better than they can tolerate confrontation by an authority figure like the group leader. Sociopaths, drug addicts, and alcoholics are among those who have benefited from such treatment. Group treatment is also used for people who are psychotic (e.g., schizophrenics). Group meetings with psychotic patients are usually fairly structured and actively guided by the therapist, often focusing on specific tasks like the improvement of patients' social skills.

Group therapy may be used alone or in conjunction with other forms of treatment (e.g., medication or individual therapy). Patients may be in group therapy for months or years, depending on their motivation. Groups may contain members with many different types of problems, or may be limited to people with a particular illness (e.g., alcoholism, manic-depressive illness). Groups are used for both outpatient therapy and inpatient work, and are useful in such diverse settings as prisons and college health services.

Couples Therapy

Couples therapy deals with a partnership between two people and the problems that arise within this relationship. Formerly called "marital therapy," it is useful not only for married couples, but for heterosexual and homosexual couples who are living together or committed to each other in some other fashion. Its usefulness has certainly extended beyond the bounds of the traditional institution of marriage.

Psychodynamic couples therapy focuses on the intrapsychic conflicts and dynamics of each member of the dyad, but only insofar as these issues affect the relationship. Therapy is aimed at facilitating communication within the couple, clarifying individual goals and resolving conflicts where possible, and helping each member see how he or she distorts the relationship with the partner as a result of earlier life experiences with parents, siblings, and other important people. Couples therapy is *not* necessarily aimed at keeping the couple together, but at helping the couple to understand how the relationship works and does not work, and whether problems can be resolved.

Common issues dealt with in couples therapy are discrepancies in verbal and nonverbal communications between the partners, varying expectations of the relationship, and problems in sexual functioning. Sessions are usually held weekly, but may be more or less frequent. Couples therapy may be done in combination with individual therapy (for one or both partners) or may be used as the only treatment modality. Although treatment by a single therapist is common, couples treatment is also quite effectively carried out by two therapists of different sexes, since this may enable each member of the couple to feel that he or she has a same-sex "ally" to identify with in the therapy. Sessions are usually carried out with both partners present, but there may be individual sessions at the outset or at various times during the course of therapy, as issues arise that need one-to-one attention.

Contraindications to couples treatment are few, but include acute psychosis in one or both partners, obvious psychopathology in one or both partners that requires individual therapy before couples work can proceed, or the harboring of an "unexposable" secret by one partner.

Family Treatment

Family relationships have always been of intense interest to psychodynamic therapists, but the actual direct treatment of entire family units is a relatively new development in psychiatry.

Dynamically oriented family therapy explores how family members interact during sessions with one or more therapists. The therapists observe patterns in styles of communication among family members, family patterns of becoming organized or disorganized in response to specific challenges, and roles and alliances adopted by various members. Families generally do not notice these patterns, because they are caught up in perpetuating them in order to maintain some equilibrium within the family unit. Family therapists not only observe behaviors that create disharmony and dysfunction in the family, but also ask the family to step back and look at themselves as they have been unable to do in the past. Family therapy provides a setting in which the members often become more aware of how other members feel. As family members come to understand more about the consequences of their pathological behavior patterns, they have the possibility of changing behaviors and testing more satisfying ways of dealing with one another.

Like group therapy, family therapy generally requires more activity by the therapist than does individual therapy. It may also require directive techniques aimed at realigning alliances, proposing alternative means of managing problems, and insisting upon the rights or needs of family members to be heard.

Family therapy is often carried out in conjunction with couples therapy and/or individual therapy for one or more family members. Sessions are generally held weekly. As in couples work, many family therapists work in pairs, both to model interactions between the therapists and to check with one another their perceptions of the family's style of behaving.

The Goals of Psychodynamic Treatment

Patients seek psychotherapy for a wide variety of problems. The specific therapeutic modalities and the intensity of their application are determined only after careful assessment of the patient's needs. Each of the dynamic therapies seeks to increase the patient's sense of self-acceptance and well-being, while improving the patient's ability to obtain satisfaction in work and at play.

Two general categories of beneficial effect can be discerned in patients who have undergone psychodynamic psychotherapy. The uncovering of unconscious sources of conflict acts to free patients from the burden of irrational fears and inhibitions carried over from early life experiences. Further, it enables them to handle the stresses and conflicts of everyday life more effectively.

The second benefit is in the gradual shift in the patient's view of self and others. The therapeutic relationship provides a unique opportunity for self-exposure and intimacy in a protected setting. At the same time, heightened awareness of the complexity and ambiguity of human interaction gradually replaces the "tunnel vision" and automatic behavior that often characterize patients who seek this form of treatment. The result is a richer and deeper recognition of life's inherent difficulties and limitations, and the development of a more flexible repertoire of responses to these limitations.

BEHAVIOR THERAPY

Behavior modification, or behavior therapy, is an approach to the treatment of specific behavioral symptoms such as phobias, compul-

Table 14-2. Models of behavior therapy.

Systematic desensitization
   Mastering anxiety-provoking situations by approaching them gradually
      and in a relaxed state that inhibits anxiety
Flooding
   Confronting the feared stimulus for prolonged periods until it is no longer
      frightening
Positive reinforcement
   Strengthening behavior and causing it to occur more frequently by
      rewarding it
Extinction
   Causing a behavior to diminish by not responding to it
Negative reinforcement
   Responding to an undesirable behavior with some means of punishment

sions, anxiety, and speech disorders. Behavior therapy focuses on observable actions rather than inferred mental states, and it aims at eliminating maladaptive behaviors by means of techniques that are based largely on learning theory.

Behavior therapy begins with an analysis of the responses that cause the patient distress or diminish his or her satisfaction and productivity. This analysis outlines the types of situations and reinforcing factors that have fostered and maintained the problematic behavior (e.g., stuttering). The next step consists of developing a detailed schedule of exercises for eliminating these behaviors and replacing them with more desirable ones. Among the most important forms of behavior therapy currently in use are systematic desensitization, flooding, positive reinforcement, extinction, and aversive conditioning.

Systematic Desensitization

Systematic desensitization is widely used in modern psychiatry. It is based on the premise that people can master anxiety-provoking situations by approaching them gradually and in a relaxed state that inhibits anxiety. Patients are first taught the technique of *progressive relaxation*, which consists of tensing major muscle groups and then relaxing them in a fixed order (often beginning at the top of the head and working down). In the next step, the patient and therapist determine which situations produce anxiety and construct a hierarchy of feared situations.

For example, in the case of a man who is afraid to fly in an airplane, the hierarchy would involve 10 to 12 scenes that might include buying a ticket, walking to the gate, entering the plane, taking off, and landing. These scenes are ordered according to how much anxiety they produce. The patient then puts himself into a relaxed state, using progressive relaxation, and he is asked to vividly imagine the first scene while in his deeply relaxed state. He repeats the exercise for the first scene until he experiences only minimal anxiety, at which time he can move on to the next scene. The goal is to be able to imagine the most anxiety-provoking scene (e.g., the plane landing) while remaining calm. This inhibition of anxiety carries over into corresponding real-life situations. It is often helpful for the patient to practice entering actual feared situations between treatment sessions, once the fears have been overcome in therapy.

Systematic densensitization is commonly used with great efficacy in treating phobias. It is also helpful to some people with compulsive behaviors and sexual dysfunctions. It is less useful for more diffuse anxiety that is not specific to particular situations.

Flooding

Flooding is another approach to treating situation-specific anxiety. In flooding, patients confront the feared object or situation (e.g., a spider) at full intensity for prolonged periods of time until it is no longer frightening. The confrontation may be done by having the patient imagine the frightening scene, but results are better when the exposure is to a real-life situation. This technique is less widely used than systematic desensitization, in part because it involves such a high degree of anxiety that many people do not tolerate it well.

Positive Reinforcement, Extinction, and Negative Reinforcement

The basic premise of *positive reinforcement* is that behavior will be strengthened and will occur more frequently if it is rewarded—e.g., with praise, increased attention from others, or the avoidance of pain. The theory behind *extinction* holds that a specific behavior will diminish if it is not responded to at all, and *negative reinforcement* involves responding to an undesirable behavior with some means of punishment.

You may see these principles put into use in constructing treatment programs for severely disturbed patients on hospital wards or in day-care facilities. You may, for example, work on an inpatient unit that has a *token economy*—a system in which patients earn tokens for adaptive, socially sanctioned behaviors and are fined for maladaptive ones. Patients may earn tokens for such activities as grooming themselves properly, cleaning rooms, or helping in group activities. They can then use the tokens to buy snacks, watch television, or take a trip off the hospital grounds (e.g., to a movie). They are fined tokens for such behavior as disrupting meetings, becoming physically abusive, or remaining isolated and uncommunicative. Such a system can be individually tailored to each patient's needs, to help him or her acquire the skills and behaviors that will promote better functioning and more autonomy. Such systems have also been useful in other communities— e.g., in treatment facilities for juvenile delinquents or the mentally retarded.

Aversive conditioning involves applying negative reinforcement to well-established behaviors. A maladaptive behavior is coupled with a noxious stimulus, so that the patient experiences a motivational conflict between the desired behavior and the unpleasant consequences that go with it. For example, aversive conditioning has been used to treat alcoholism, by giving ethanol along with an emetic that produces severe nausea and vomiting. Repeated administration of this treatment suppresses many patients' desire to drink. Critics argue that this approach provides only a temporary solution to what is usually a chronic problem.

Aversive conditioning has also been used to treat people who want to change a homosexual orientation to a heterosexual one. Patients are shown erotic homosexual scenes on film, and concurrently receive either emetics that produce nausea and vomiting or mild electric shocks. The patients are then shown erotic heterosexual films, without concurrent noxious stimuli. This form of treatment has also been used for sexual perversions (see Chapter 10). Its use in changing the choice of sexual object from homosexual to heterosexual is quite controversial, and it has not been clearly demonstrated to be effective in achieving this goal.

In general, behavior therapy is very useful in treating relatively specific symptoms. It does not, however, address deeper psychological problems, such as those encountered among patients with neurotic conflicts or personality disorders, nor is it the primary mode of treatment in any of the psychotic illnesses.

Every clinician should know about behavioral treatments and ideally should be able to practice some simple techniques.

HYPNOSIS

Hypnosis is neither a form of sleep nor a form of therapy. Rather, it is a particular type of concentration that is attentive, receptive, and quite focused. It is accompanied by diminished awareness of peripheral stimuli. You have undoubtedly experienced hypnotic or trance-like states—for example, in being so absorbed in a novel that you ignore what is going on around you and must reorient yourself· to the environment when you stop reading.

In a treatment situation that employs hypnosis, the patient allows the therapist to structure this form of intense concentration in a way that facilitates and accelerates the achievement of particular psychotherapeutic goals. Hypnosis is most often used for the relief of specific symptoms such as anxiety, insomnia, phobias, conversion reactions, and pain. It is also used to control habits—particularly smoking and overeating.

Essentially, treatment involves teaching patients self-hypnosis techniques so that they can put themselves into a trance-like state, and then use hypnotic suggestions that "restructure" their thinking about the problem being treated. For example, patients who want to quit smoking are taught to put themselves into a trance-like state every few hours and at any time they crave a cigarette. In this state, they run through several points that are designed to reorient their thinking, e.g.—"Smoking damages my body/I need to take care of myself/I will not harm myself in this way." Similar suggestions for use under self-hypnosis can be designed by therapists and patients to ease anxiety, curb overeating, help overcome phobias, and lessen the psychological components of chronic pain.

Hypnosis has significant limitations as a therapeutic technique. It cannot, for example, treat more global difficulties, such as neurotic conflicts, psychotic illnesses, or personality disorders. Its usefulness even for the isolated symptoms mentioned above is questioned by some clinicians, who argue that symptom relief resulting from hypnotherapy is only temporary in many cases. Nevertheless, hypnosis continues to be a valuable tool in modern psychiatric practice when applied judiciously.

COGNITIVE THERAPY

Cognitive therapy is a relatively new mode of short-term psychotherapy specifically developed for the treatment of depression and anxiety. It is based on the premise that our moods and feelings are influenced by our thoughts, and that self-defeating and self-deprecating patterns of thinking foster dysphoric moods in many depressed people. By correcting these distorted ways of thinking, the cognitive therapist restructures depressed patients' views of themselves, the world, and the future— substituting more realistic, self-enhancing thoughts that reduce such painful feelings as anxiety, guilt, and hopelessness.

Cognitive therapists identify many common forms of cognitive distortion that foster depression. For example, a student who feels like a failure when she gets an A− instead of an A on an exam is using what cognitive therapists call "all-or-nothing thinking"; the worker who blames himself when the car breaks down and he is late for work is using "personalization." Cognitive distortions involve faulty interpretation of real events—usually in a way that casts the depressed person in a very negative light. These distortions often stem from self-defeating "silent assumptions" that depressed people harbor about themselves, e.g., "I am worthless if I cannot do things perfectly."

Patients in cognitive therapy are asked to identify and write down negative thoughts—at first with the help of the therapist, and subsequently on their own. The therapist can then help the patient identify the distortions in these thoughts and substitute more rational responses. The therapist also helps the patient recognize self-defeating silent assumptions and exchange them for more realistic ones.

Cognitive therapy is a short-term treatment (often 10 to 15 sessions) that has been compared favorably with the use of imipramine in preliminary trials with depressed patients. Its efficacy remains to be proven in large-scale controlled studies that are currently under way. Critics argue that negative thoughts do not cause painful feelings but *result* from them, and that changing one's thinking is not sufficient to bring about a lasting change of mood. These critics also argue that the real therapeutic factors in cognitive therapy are the trust, support, and rapport that are part of any good therapeutic relationship. Nevertheless, cognitive therapy may prove to be an effective, low-cost modality that could be used widely in the treatment of depression.

CLIENT-CENTERED PSYCHOTHERAPY

Client-centered psychotherapy is a form of treatment introduced by Carl Rogers. It is often referred to as "rogerian therapy." It is nondirective and emphasizes the importance of the relationship between patient and therapist, as well as the patient's right to self-determination. The therapist attempts to act as a catalyst to facilitate the patient's emotional growth—ideally without imposing any of the therapist's views on the patient. Patients verbalize their problems, and the client-centered therapist rephrases their words to reflect and clarify the feelings they are trying to express. The therapist must be genuine, must offer the patient unconditional acceptance, and must provide accurate empathic understanding of the patient's problems. When these three conditions are met, client-centered therapists believe that the patient will have increased self-understanding and a greater capacity for adaptive behavior.

However, many clinicians have criticized rogerian therapy as not being useful for certain types of patients, particularly those with personality disorders. They argue that uncritical acceptance of the patient can be undesirable, particularly when patient's behaviors are clearly maladaptive. (For example, the patient with an antisocial personality disorder who steals to buy drugs must be confronted about such behavior.) Client-centered therapy is best suited for people with neurotic disturbances, who can benefit from an empathic and nonjudgmental relationship.

SUMMARY

The types of psychotherapy described above are but a few of the many forms of treatment developed in the past few decades. You have no doubt heard of a great many others—modalities such as gestalt therapy, transactional analysis, and emotive therapy. There are also many different schools of thought besides Freudian psychology within psychodynamic psychotherapy—including Jungian, Adlerian, and Sullivanian theories and techniques. A general survey of all these types of therapy is beyond the scope of this chapter. Rather, this discussion is meant to indicate the range of psychosocial treatments currently in use.

REFERENCES

Childress AR, Burns DD: The basics of cognitive therapy. Psychosomatics 22:1017-1027, 1981.

Frank JD: General Psychotherapy: the restoration of morale, in American Handbook of Psychiatry. Vol. 5. Edited by Arieti S. New York, Basic Books, 1975, pp 117-132.

Frankel FH: Hypnosis: Trance as a Coping Mechanism. New York, Plenum Press, 1976.

Fromm-Reichmann F: Principles of Intensive Psychotherapy. Chicago, University of Chicago Press, 1950.

Greenson RR: The Technique and Practice of Psychoanalysis, Vol. 1. New York, International Universities Press, 1967.

Kolb LC: Psychotherapy, in Modern Clinical Psychiatry. 9th ed. Philadelphia, EB Saunders, 1977, pp 767-804.

Kovacs M: The efficacy of cognitive and behavior therapies for depression. Am J Psychiatry 137:1495-1501, 1980.

Marks IM: Review of behavioral psychotherapy, I: obsessive-compulsive disorders. Am J Psychiatry 138:584-592, 1981.

Marks IM: Review of behavioral psychotherapy, II: sexual disorders. Am J Psychiatry 138:750-756, 1981.

Marmor J: Short-term dynamic psychotherapy. Am J Psychiatry 136:149-155, 1979.

Minuchip SA: Families and Family Therapy. Cambridge, MA, Harvard University Press, 1976.

Strachey J: The nature of the therapeutic action of psychoanalysis. Int J PsychoAnal 15:127-159, 1934.

Wolpe J: Psychotherapy by Reciprocal Inhibition. Stanford, CA, Standford University Press, 1958.

Wynne L: Some indications and contraindications for exploratory family therapy, in Intensive Family Therapy Edited by Boszermonyi-Nagy I, Framo J. Hoeber, 1965.

Yalom ID: The Theory and Practice of Group Psychotherapy, 2nd ed. New York, Basic Books, 1975.

15

Somatic Therapies

THE SOMATIC THERAPIES USED in modern psychiatry consist of psychotropic medications and electroconvulsive therapy (ECT). This chapter covers general principles of the pharmacologic treatment of mental disorders and the use of specific classes of psychotropic drugs. ECT is discussed briefly at the end of the chapter.

PSYCHOTROPIC MEDICATIONS

Psychotropic drugs are chemical agents that have an effect on the mind. Many mind-altering substances are abused in our society for "recreational" purposes. Only a minority of known psychotropic agents are actually useful in the treatment of mental disorders.

Why are psychotropic drugs used in psychiatry? The question is not an idle one. The media and popular literature have, at times, painted a rather gloomy picture of mental institutions in which patients are kept "spaced out" on large doses of medication. A few critics of our mental health care system argue that drugs deprive patients of their right to be psychotic. The mention of major tranquilizers conjures up images of mind control and the repression of freedom.

Yet the advent of modern psychopharmacology in the last three decades has revolutionized the treatment of mental illness, giving millions of people relief from symptoms that are both frightening and crippling. Prior to the 1950s, there were few methods available for treating severely disturbed people. Seclusion behind locked doors and barred windows and the use of physical restraints were more common and more necessary than they are today. Treatment included "hydrotherapy," insulin shock, neurosurgery, and management with narcotics, barbiturates, and bromides. These have virtually disappeared from psychiatry, and for good reason. Mania, florid hallucinations, severe agitation, and life-threatening depression have all proved responsive to modern psychopharmacologic agents. Fewer patients require long-term treatment behind locked doors, and it has been possible to return patients and treatment facilities to the community.

The number of patients hospitalized in psychiatric facilities at any given time has been drastically reduced over the last 20 years. To be sure, this is due in part to our society's increased awareness of the detrimental effects of chronic institutionalization on human behavior, as well as to economic and political considerations. Also, new applications of group therapy techniques in day-care programs and outpatient clinics have proved effective in helping people live outside a structured inpatient setting. But much of the credit for this shift from inpatient to outpatient treatment must go to the use of psychotropic medications. They have not only proved effective in relieving acute psychotic symptoms, but have also been useful in preventing recurrences and stabilizing patients' functioning over long periods of time.

We must temper this praise, however, with some perspective on the limitations of the psychotropic medications. In fact, they only alleviate symptoms—*they do not cure.* In this respect, their efficacy is limited to staving off some of the manifestations of major mental illness, without exerting any clearly definable, lasting effect on the underlying pathology. Also, many patients do not respond to these medications, even when "classic" symptoms would predict a good response. The drugs carry side effects that range in severity from uncomfortable to dangerous, and all can be toxic. Finally, they are generally slow to work in at least one crucial respect—the antipsychotic effect of the major tranquilizers may take days or weeks to be evident, and the antidepressant effects of the tricyclics generally appear many days after the medication is begun.

What do psychotropic medications do? It is useful to

think of these drugs as falling into discrete groups. Each group of psychotropics alleviates a particular set of symptoms. They can generally be grouped as shown in Table 15-1.

The major groups of psychotropics—antipsychotic agents, antidepressants, and antimanic agents—have actions that are directed against specific symptoms of mental illness. Unlike "uppers" or "downers," these drugs do not work through simple arousal or sedation, but through more specific effects. Normal subjects do not experience euphoria when they take antidepressants or depression when they take an antimanic drug, and they do not find their thought processes altered by the antipsychotics. If anything, the major psychotropic medications produce little more than sedation in normal subjects, but they produce specific therapeutic effects in those who are ill.

The other classes of psychotropic medications are less specific in their actions. Antianxiety agents, psychomotor stimulants, and sedative-hypnotics produce similar effects in most people who use them, whether a mental illness is present or not. These drugs are of little value in treating psychosis and mood disorders. They are much more commonly abused than the major psychotropics.

A word about terminology is in order. The term *tranquilizer* is frequently used incorrectly to describe any sedating drug. There are two very different types of medications to which the term is correctly applied. *Major tranquilizers* are also called antipsychotic agents; their effects are both antipsychotic and sedating. This group includes drugs like chlorpromazine (Thorazine), trifluoperazine (Stelazine), and haloperidol (Haldol). *Minor tranquilizers* are the antianxiety agents, such as diazepam (Valium) and chlordiazepoxide (Librium), which alleviate anxiety but do not alleviate psychotic symptoms. Other sedating drugs (e.g., the barbiturates) are more accurately labeled *sedative-hypnotics*.

Table 15-1. The types of psychotropic medications.

The major groups—act against specific symptoms
    Antipsychotic agents
    Antidepressants
    Antimanic agents
Other classes—produce particular effects without regard to presence or
  absence of illness
    Antianxiety agents
    Psychomotor stimulants
    Sedative-hypnotics

Included in Appendix D is a table listing commonly used psycho-tropic medications by trade names, with their corresponding generic names and medication type. When you hear a drug referred to by its brand name, you can use this table to quickly find its chemical name and major use in clinical practice.

PRINCIPLES OF PRESCRIBING PSYCHOTROPIC MEDICATIONS

For every psychiatric patient you see, you must make a judgment as to whether pharmacotherapy is both warranted and prudent. This requires facts.

Clinical Evaluation

First, your clinical evaluation must be thorough. You must arrive at a tentative diagnosis based on the following factors.

A careful history. You should enlist the help of family members in getting a history if the patient's reliability is questionable. In particular, a careful delineation of symptoms, previous treatments and responses, history of drug or alcohol abuse, family psychiatric history, medical history, and current medications are important.

A physical examination. You, or another clinician, must assess the patient's physical health and rule out underlying somatic disorders that might mimic psychiatric illness. For outpatients, a routine examination done by the family physician in recent months will suffice if no medical problems are suspected.

Laboratory tests. These tests should include routine studies to rule out organic causes of psychiatric symptoms (e.g., hypothyroid-ism as the basis for depression) and may include special diagnostic tests to predict response to medication—e.g., measuring urinary 3-methoxy-4-hydroxyphenylethyleneglycol (MHPG) to predict response to various types of antidepressants. The routine laboratory work-up for each type of medication is discussed below.

A period of observation. When there is no acute problem (such as severe agitation or life-threatening behavior) that requires immediate use of medication, it is helpful to observe the patient in a drug-free state for several days (or even several weeks) to see how symptoms change over time. This is particularly useful if there is some question about whether medication is likely to be helpful, or when there is confusion about the diagnosis. For example, a patient admitted to the hospital with a psychotic episode might not reveal to you that he has abused drugs. If you immediately administer an antipsychotic, you may erroneously believe that the medication alleviated a psychosis that would have abated of its own accord when the abused substance was cleared from the patient's body. Or an outpatient's depressive symptoms might improve dramatically after one or two meetings with a con-cerned therapist. If this patient had been given antidepressants immedi-ately, the effect would have been attributed to the medication, and the patient might be maintained on the drug unnecessarily. Another patient's anxiety might mask an underlying psychosis. Such a patient could easily be medicated incorrectly with an antianxiety agent before the disordered thinking became apparent.

Course of the Illness

You must know the expected course of the illness you have diagnosed. Some psychiatric conditions are self-limiting (e.g., drug-induced psycho-sis). When it is safe to do so, it is always preferable to treat such cases conservatively and supportively until the illness runs its course.

Risks of Treatment

You must weigh the risks of not treating your patient against the risks of the various forms of therapy available. Tricyclic antidepressants, for example, are highly lethal when taken in overdose; with suicidal people, this must always be taken into account. Major tranquilizers produce *tardive dyskinesia* (discussed below) in a minority of patients, and this is generally refractory to treatment. Pharmacotherapy should never be undertaken lightly.

Choosing a Drug

Once you decide to prescribe psychotropic medication, you must determine which class of drug you will use. This will depend on your diagnosis and your understanding of the patient's symptoms. But once you have decided to use an antidepressant, or an antipsychotic, or an anxiolytic, you have a wide assortment of specific medications from which to choose. Within the broad groups of medications mentioned above, individual drugs differ very little in their ability to affect constellations of symptoms. Thus, the choice you make about which particular antipsychotic or anxiolytic to use will often be based on factors other than the symptoms you are trying to alleviate:

The patient's previous treatment response is an excellent indicator of what to try and what not to try. If something worked once, it is likely to work again. The converse is, of course, also true. Thus, if a patient tells you that Haldol (haloperidol) was of no help in relieving his psychotic symptoms ten years ago, you would be wise to avoid it now. If, however, he tells you that Loxitane (loxapine) was the only drug that took away his auditory hallucinations, and you are treating the same symptom at present, loxapine is likely to be your best bet. This is, perhaps, stating the obvious. Yet too often we forget that these are chronic conditions, that patients often have considerable prior experience with medication, and that they often know what has worked for them in the past. *Do not forget to ask.*

Medication histories of biological relatives can be invaluable in helping you with your decision. Treatment response and side effects are strongly determined by genetic factors. So, for example, if a depressed patient reports that her father was depressed and got better on imipramine (Tofranil), then imipramine would be a good first drug to use with her.

The patient's history of side effects is equally important. No one is likely to take a medication that produces unbearable side effects. When you are dealing with someone who has been given a variety of antipsychotics in the past, find out which of those drugs were least unpleasant for the patient to take.

Your familiarity with a particular drug is very important. It is best for the beginner to select only a few drugs in each class, and to learn well their effects, side effects, and toxicity.

Cost of the drug may be a factor, particularly if long-term treatment is required. Drug prices vary greatly according to the availability of generic forms and the extent of competition in the market. As a rule, newer drugs are more expensive.

Determining Drug Dosages

Unlike many other medications used in medical practice, there are no precise doses prescribed for most of the psychotropic drugs. Rather, there is a dosage range—often very broad—within which you must determine the amount that best meets your patient's needs. And responses are highly individual. One patient may require two, three, or even four times the amount of medication needed by another patient of similar body weight in order to achieve similar therapeutic effects. Prescribing thus involves a process of fine tuning the therapy according to the symptoms and responses of the individual patient.

There is a high correlation between the severity of the target symptoms at which you aim your treatment and the minimum dosage that produces a favorable response. Severe symptoms will generally require higher dosages of medication, while mild symptoms are more likely to respond to dosages at the lower end of the therapeutic range. The most important considerations in determining drug dosages are *safety* and *therapeutic efficacy*.

Several of the antidepressants have a "therapeutic window"—a dosage range within which a therapeutic response is to be expected. Dosages that are outside the therapeutic window (i.e., too high or too low) are likely to have no effect or even adverse effects on the patient. The antipsychotics have no such window, but they have an unspecified upper limit for safe and effective treatment. In such cases, you cannot rely solely on manufacturers' recommendations but must be particularly diligent about weighing the therapeutic effects against side effects in deciding how much medication is enough.

Administering Psychotropic Drugs

The two major routes of administration are oral and intramuscular. Intravenous administration of psychotropics generally takes place in well-controlled inpatient settings, often for research purposes. Most situations can be managed without intravenous medication.

Doses administered by injection are roughly two to four times as potent as the same doses taken by mouth. This is largely because the liver, which does the bulk of the body's work in metabolizing psychotropics, is bypassed by intravenous injection, so that the medication reaches the circulation directly.

Although the minor tranquilizers and some other sedating drugs are at times given by injection, the drugs most often given intramuscularly are the antipsychotics. Injection is used:

- To produce rapid relief of severe agitation and other symptoms that might pose a danger to the patient or to others.

- If the patient is unable or unwilling to take medication orally.
- When oral absorption of the drug is thought to be poor.

The disadvantages of giving these medicines intramuscularly are that:

- Some of them are painful (e.g., chlorpromazine) and may cause irritation at the site of injection.
- Intramuscular injection may be seen by some severely disturbed patients as an assault.

When used to control agitation, intramuscular medication is a chemical restraint. This raises important issues about the patient's right to refuse treatment. A full discussion of the legal and ethical dilemmas involved in chemical restraint is beyond the scope of this chapter, but it should be noted that chemical restraint must be used only when the need is clear—i.e., to protect the patient or others from harm, when other means of treatment have failed to put the patient and others out of danger. It must *never* be used as punishment.

In addition to chemical restraint, the most common situations in which intramuscular medication is used are (1) in emergency rooms, where patients present in crisis and need rapid relief, and (2) in outpatient programs when people who cannot comply with daily oral regimens are given *depot* forms of antipsychotic medication by injection every two to four weeks.

Advising Your Patients About Medication

How you present the treatment plan to your patient can make a great difference in the amount of cooperation you receive, particularly when you prescribe psychotropic drugs. Not only is compliance important but, in most cases, the patient must *tell* you whether or not the treatment is working. There are few independent laboratory measures of drug response with the psychotropics, so you and your patient must agree on specific target symptoms that you are trying to alleviate, and then together you must evaluate whether, in fact, those symptoms have been affected by the drug.

When your patient is confused, unreliable, or otherwise unable to comply with the regimen on his or her own, you should include a responsible friend or relative in your discussion of how the medicine is to be taken. Assure the patient that you are available to talk about the medication when questions arise.

Especially at the beginning of drug treatment, it is important that you and/or other staff members be available by telephone or in person so that the patient is not left alone with distressing side effects or other unexpected adverse reactions. In explaining your treatment plan to the patient, be sure to include the following information:

What you are trying to treat (target symptoms). Patients will expect medication to help *all* their psychiatric symptoms, and this is almost never the case. Your patient must know which specific symptoms the drug treatment is aimed at and which symptoms the drug cannot be expected to alleviate.

For example, if you prescribe an antidepressant for a recently widowed woman with severe vegetative depression, tell her that the medication could help her sleep better and perhaps increase her appetite, but that she will continue to feel sad about her husband's death and may mourn his loss for some time to come. If a patient is receiving another form of therapy (e.g., psychotherapy) in addition to medication, be sure the patient knows what each treatment is meant to accomplish. Too often, patients assume that drugs are panaceas, that the problem is all "chemical," and that there is no need to cooperate in other forms of therapy. Such assumptions set the stage for disillusionment when the medication fails to cure everything that ails the patient.

Side effects that might occur. This is tricky. You want your patients to have some idea of what to expect when they take medication, but you must not frighten them with an endless list of horrible possibilities. Here, judgment is critical. It is generally useful to describe the most common side effects, and to explain how the patient can handle them if they occur (e.g., "The medicine might make your mouth dry. Many people find that chewing gum or hard candy helps keep the mouth moist").

Possible toxic effects or other dangers. Again, mention only those effects that are common. For example, if drowsiness or dizziness is a common side effect, then the patient must be cautioned about driving a car. If the effects of alcohol are enhanced by the medication, then caution the patient about even social drinking. And the patient must be alerted to the warning signs and symptoms of drug toxicity (e.g., symptoms of lithium toxicity such as nausea, vomiting, diarrhea, and stupor).

Above all, let the patient know that you are available, and that it is important to share questions or problems with you as they arise. If patients feel that they ought not to bother you with their concerns about medication, they may suffer distressing side effects (e.g., impotence) without reporting these, or they may discontinue the medication without discussing their concerns with you first.

Managing the Side Effects

Virtually all psychotropic medications have side effects, but we have little way of predicting which people will be particularly sensitive to which medications. The management of side effects is crucial to the successful drug treatment of mental illness, because treatment is commonly necessary for months or years. Compliance depends upon the patient's willingness and ability to tolerate the medication.

Patients often discontinue their medication without consulting a physician, most commonly because they believe that the drug is not helpful or that they no longer require it, because they cannot bear unpleasant side effects, or because they believe their discomfort is due to side effects when it is in fact due to the symptoms of their illness.

Side effects can be difficult to recognize. Psychotic patients may report bizarre symptoms that are actually manifestations of their illness, or they may be uncommunicative and incapable of reporting side effects at all. In dealing with people who are in emotional distress and who have impaired cognition, the alliance between doctor and patient is particularly important. The following are some effective ways of minimizing or eliminating side effects:

> Monitor the patient's mental and physical status regularly, includ-
> ing frequent meetings with the patient—and, where indicated,
> the family.
>
> Pay careful attention to all the patient's complaints, even when
> they seem trivial.
>
> Work as a team with other people involved in the patient's care—
> nurses, mental health workers, social workers, psychologists,
> and other physicians. Professionals who see the patient in other
> settings may be able to give you much-needed information
> about your patient's reactions to medication.
>
> Prescribe the lowest dosage that produces the desired effect. Many
> side effects are related to dosage.
>
> Advise and reassure the patient. Many patients are capable of
> tolerating a significant amount of discomfort and inconve-
> nience, provided they know it is in their interest to do so, and
> that you are concerned and supportive.
>
> Use adjunctive medication. Particularly in the case of antipsy-
> chotics, side effects can be effectively relieved by
> antiparkinsonian drugs (discussed below).

Discontinue the medication and try another medication if side effects become intolerable.

Frequently reevaluate the patient's need for the medication. If drug regimens are not regularly reevaluated, drug maintenance may be prolonged unnecessarily.

Avoid polypharmacy—the prescribing of many drugs concurrently for a patient in the hope that something will work. Each medication should be carefully chosen and its effect rigorously and frequently evaluated.

Combining Psychotropic Drugs

As a rule, combining two or more drugs of the same type (i.e., two antipsychotics or two antianxiety agents) is not desirable. Rather than enhancing the desired therapeutic effect, such combinations generally result in an increased risk of toxicity and side effects, and little or no therapeutic advantage.

However, combinations of *different* types of drugs are often useful. Antipsychotics, antidepressants, lithium, and anxiolytics are frequently used in combination. Ideally, drug combinations are prescribed as a result of—and not instead of—a careful diagnostic evaluation. When medications are added to a regimen with no rationale and no target symptoms in mind, the result is usually a muddled and sometimes dangerous treatment.

A cardinal rule in drug treatment: Whenever possible, do one thing at a time. Too often, the clinician tries unsuccessfully to make several changes in the treatment regimen concurrently. The results can be quite confusing. For example, if you lower the dosage of a patient's antipsychotic medication and simultaneously increase the dosage of an antidepressant, the patient may take a turn for the better or worse, but you will be unable to assess which medication change made the difference.

If you *make one change in a treatment regimen at a time*, you will have a much better chance of understanding the effects of your interventions. This is true not only for medications, but for other elements in a patient's treatment. For example, if you decide to lower the dosage of your patient's antipsychotic medication just as he or she is about to begin a new job, you may not know whether an increase in psychotic symptoms during the first weeks on the job is due to the lowered dosage of the medication or to the stresses of new employment.

Failure of Drug Treatment

The four most likely possibilities if your drug treatment does not seem to work are:
- You selected the wrong type of drug.
- You selected the correct drug, but the wrong dosage.
- You selected the correct drug and dosage, but the patient has not yet been taking the drug long enough to produce a therapeutic effect.
- You have not obtained your patient's cooperation in taking the medication reliably.

When drug treatment appears to fail, do not give up. Consider the points noted above and try to determine whether any of these factors is responsible for the treatment failure. Also remember that individuals respond quite idiosyncratically to psychotropic medications—a patient who does not benefit from one drug may respond well to a different drug in the same class.

Gather all the information you can from the patient, family members, and other members of the patient's treatment team, and then determine what changes you can make—one at a time and systematically—to try to achieve the therapeutic effect you seek. If it is feasible, get a consultation, for two heads are often better than one.

The Treatment Team

You will often be treating patients in conjunction with others. While you prescribe medication, others may be involved with the patient in psychotherapy, behavior therapy, group work, rehabilitation activities, and a host of other treatment modalities. Speak with these other treaters and enlist their cooperation in your efforts at pharmacologic intervention, preferably *before* you prescribe any new medication.

There are several reasons for this. First, it makes for good patient care. Psychologists, nurses, social workers, and other physicians must know what to expect when a new treatment is introduced. They can be helpful both in ensuring the patient's compliance with the medication regimen and in reporting the effects they notice. Second, the patient must have the sense that members of the treatment team are coordinating their efforts—that the right hand knows what the left hand is doing. If you prescribe a potentially lethal drug for a suicidal patient, everyone involved in the treatment *must* know the risks and benefits involved in this plan, so that the patient's use of the drug and suicidal impulses can be carefully monitored.

Finally, you should include other treaters in your efforts as a matter of professional courtesy. Although you have the power to prescribe and have specialized knowledge about psychotropic drugs, you must show others that you value their input. Otherwise, you may find that the other treaters can undermine your treatment plan, if only through ignorance of what you are trying to accomplish.

These basic guidelines for the use of psychotropic medications apply to each of the specific classes of drugs discussed in the following sections.

ANTIPSYCHOTIC MEDICATIONS

Antipsychotic medications are useful primarily in the treatment of thought disorders and, more acutely, to relieve severe agitation.

How Do They Work?

The mechanism of action of the antipsychotics is not completely understood. The areas of the brain most affected by these drugs are the reticular formation, basal ganglia, hypothalamus, and limbic system. At the cellular level, the drugs inhibit the transmission of nerve impulses in the central nervous system (CNS) by blocking the action of dopamine, a neurotransmitter, at post-synaptic receptor sites. It is not known whether this dopamine-blocking activity is the mechanism by which psychosis is ameliorated.

Whatever their mechanism of action, the antipsychotics have been shown in large-scale studies to be extremely effective against the symptoms of acute psychosis.

What Are the Indications for Using an Antipsychotic?

Several illnesses which may call for the use of an antipsychotic include:

Schizophrenia. This is the major condition for which antipsychotics are indicated. They are used in the following ways:

- Intramuscularly to control acute, severe psychotic agitation or excitement

- Orally in daily doses to control acute episodes of the illness
- As maintenance therapy to prevent recurrent exacerbations, in daily oral doses or in intramuscular doses, of depot fluphenazine every two to four weeks

Manic-depressive illness. Manic excitement is alleviated by antipsychotics, which are often used in combination with lithium in cases of acute mania and then discontinued when mania abates. The efficacy of long-term maintenance therapy of manic-depressive illness with antipsychotics is unproved (see Chapter 6).

Amphetamine psychosis. Antipsychotics are the drugs of choice. They are used only so long as psychosis persists (see Chapter 11).

Drug-induced psychosis. If the drug cannot be identified, it is better in most cases to "talk the patient down" rather than use medication. However, if agitation is life-threatening, antipsychotics can be of great benefit. Do not use antipsychotics to treat atropine-induced psychosis.

Agitated or psychotic depression. Antipsychotics are very effective, often in combination with an antidepressant. The efficacy of antipsychotics in retarded depression is less clear.

Chronic brain syndromes. Syndromes that involve psychosis may be treated symptomatically with antipsychotics.

Anxiety. Antipsychotics are *not* the drugs of choice. They should be used only when antianxiety or antidepressant agents have proved ineffective and anxiety is incapacitating.

If one of the above-mentioned illnesses has been diagnosed, you must still determine whether the symptoms of the illness are likely to

Table 15-2. Responsiveness of symptoms to antipsychotic medications.

Most likely to respond	Less likely to respond
Combativeness	Lack of insight
Hyperactivity	Poor judgment
Tension	Impaired memory
Hostility	Disorientation
Hallucinations	Chronic delusions
Sleeplessness	
Poor hygiene and self-care	
Acute delusions (of recent onset)	
Social isolation	

respond to an antipsychotic. The symptoms that are most likely to respond are combativeness, hyperactivity, tension, hostility, hallucinations, sleeplessness, poor hygiene and self-care, acute delusions (of recent onset), and social isolation. The symptoms that are less likely to respond are lack of insight, poor judgment, impaired memory, disorientation, and chronic delusions.

In considering the use of an antipsychotic, you must first arrive at a clear sense of what has caused the symptoms. Among those patients for whom antipsychotics are indicated diagnostically, you will find that the tense, hyperactive or hypoactive, obviously psychotic patient is likely to improve with the drug. The patient whose level of activity is normal and who simply appears to be in a fog will be less likely to improve. Nevertheless, it is worth giving such people a trial of antipsychotic medication.

Before you start a patient on an antipsychotic the following basic work-up is indicated:

- History and physical examination
- Blood pressure, both standing and reclining, to note baseline postural changes
- Laboratory studies—complete blood count (including white blood cell count), liver function tests, urinalysis
- A baseline electrocardiogram (EKG) for patients with any history of cardiac problems and all patients over 40

Types of Antipsychotic Medications

There are several pharmacologically distinct classes of antipsychotics, but all of them have similar therapeutic actions and all are about equally effective. There is no need to describe here in detail the different pharmacologic properties of these classes. Excellent discussions of the pharmacology of the antipsychotics can be found in the references at the end of this chapter. Clinically, there are three important differences among the groups of antipsychotics:

Potency. Because the antipsychotics are of such different potencies, drug doses vary by a factor of up to 10^3.

Side effects. The side effects, discussed below, vary greatly from one type of drug to another.

Patients' idiosyncratic responses. Some patients who do not respond well to a drug of one class respond satisfactorily to a drug that is chemically quite distinct.

Table 15-3 presents the most commonly used antipsychotic agents. They are listed according to their pharmacologic group. Their potencies are given relative to the potency of chlorpromazine (Thorazine).

Clinical applications of Table 15-3. This table can serve as your "bible" for determining proper dosages of the antipsychotics. Essentially, the table helps you think of the dosage of any antipsychotic in terms of "chlorpromazine equivalents"—i.e., the strength of the dosage relative to an equivalent dosage of chlorpromazine.

Suppose, for example, that you want to treat an acutely psychotic

Table 15-3. Equivalent doses of commonly used antipsychotic agents by chemical type (chlorpromazine = 100).

Generic name	Trade name	Potency relative to chlorpromazine
Phenothiazines		
Aliphatic		
Chlorpromazine	Thorazine	100
Piperidine		
Mesoridazine	Serentil	50
Piperacetazine	Quide	12
Thioridazine	Mellaril	100
Piperazine		
Acetophenazine	Tindal	20
Fluphenazine	Prolixin	2
Perphenazine	Trilafon	10
Trifluoperazine	Stelazine	5
Thioxanthenes		
Aliphatic		
Chlorprothixene	Taractan	65
Piperazine		
Thiothixene	Navane	5
Dibenzazepines		
Loxapine	Loxitane, Daxolin	15
Butyrophenones		
Haloperidol	Haldol	2
Indolones		
Molindone	Moban	10
Rauwolfia alkaloids		
Reserpine	Serpasil, etc. (generic)	1-2

young man with trifluoperazine (Stelazine). It has been determined that the minimum dosage of chlorpromazine that is likely to be effective in treating acute psychosis in a young adult is 400 mg orally per day. How much trifluoperazine (Stelazine) is the daily equivalent of 400 mg of chlorpromazine (CPZ)?

The arithmetic is simple:

$\dfrac{\text{Potency of drug X}}{\text{Potency of CPZ}}$	$\times$	Desired dose in CPZ equivalents	$=$	Desired dose of drug X
$\dfrac{5}{100}$	$\times$	400 mg	$=$	20 mg

As shown above, 400 mg of CPZ equals 20 mg of trifluoperazine. Thus, you would want to give your patient at least 20 mg/day of trifluoperazine to adequately treat his condition.

If this psychotic patient showed no improvement on trifluoperazine, even at increased doses, you would probably try another antipsychotic of a chemically different class, going back to the table to choose a drug like haloperidol or molindone. You would then determine the initial dosage of the new drug on the basis of its potency relative to chlorpromazine.

Side Effects

All antipsychotics carry side effects. You can expect to see side effects in most patients you treat with these drugs.

Sedation. Sedation occurs in 80 percent of patients, and usually lasts about one week. This may be a desired effect (for insomniacs), or it may be a problem (e.g., for students or for those who feel drowsy when driving an automobile). To treat sedation, try lowering the dosage, giving the entire daily dose at bedtime, or using a less sedating drug.

Extrapyramidal side effects (EPS). Extrapyramidal (neurologic) side effects occur in 10 to 30 percent of patients. There are several types:

Dystonia occurs early in treatment, often within the first two days. Manifestations include spasms of the eye, face, neck, and back muscles, which can be quite dramatic and frightening. However, dystonia is more commonly experienced as simple muscle stiffness. Acute

Table 15-4. Side effects of antipsychotic medications.

Sedation	Postural hypotension
Extrapyramidal side effects (EPS)	Allergic or toxic side effects
Dystonia	Agranulocytosis
Parkinsonism	Dermatitis
Akathisia	Allergic hepatitis
Akinesia	Metabolic or endocrine side effects
Tardive dyskinesia	Toxic retinopathy
Lowered seizure threshold	EKG changes
Anticholinergic side effects	Retrograde ejaculation
Dry mouth	
Blurred vision	
Constipation	
Urinary retention	

dystonic reactions are easily and rapidly treated as described below. For recurrent dystonias, lower the dose, switch to another antipsychotic, or use antiparkinsonian medications prophylactically in conjunction with the antipsychotic.

Parkinsonism—i.e., symptoms like those seen in Parkinson's disease—occurs generally within one to four weeks after treatment is begun. Symptoms include bradykinesia (decreased movement), shuffling gait, decreased energy, mask-like facies, and tremor. Parkinsonism is treatable by the same means as dystonias (see below).

Akathisia is very common, and occurs within one to six weeks after treatment is begun. It involves restlessness, pacing, rocking, and an inability to sit still. It is often experienced as "jumpy legs." Akathisia is treatable with antiparkinsonian drugs, but it is easy to mistake for psychotic agitation; do not worsen the situation by raising the dosage of the antipsychotic.

Akinesia is relatively uncommon, but its late and insidious onset make it easy to miss. It involves markedly decreased or absent body activity, which can be mistaken for a symptom of psychosis and wrongly treated by raising the dosage of the antipsychotic. Proper treatment involves lowering the dosage, switching to another drug, or using antiparkinsonian medication.

Tardive dyskinesia is the most ominous of the side effects of the antipsychotics. This syndrome develops late in treatment (after 1 to 20 years of maintenance therapy); it is estimated to occur in from 2 to 50 percent of chronic schizophrenic patients. It involves involuntary kinetic activity, including lip smacking and sucking, jaw movements, "fly-catcher" tongue movements, choreiform and athetoid movements of the extremities, and occasional difficulty swallowing. Although many cases are irreversible, some do remit completely when antipsychotic medication is discontinued. Antiparkinsonian drugs are of no help in treatment and may increase the severity of the movement. The best (and probably the only) treatment for tardive dyskinesia is prevention, by using antipsychotics only when absolutely indicated and in the lowest effective doses, and by monitoring patients on antipsychotics frequently with trials off medication to assess their ongoing need for the drug. Obviously, the occasional discomfort and impairment caused by these involuntary movements (they are often mild and not noticed by the patient) must be weighed against the patient's psychotic illness in determining whether antipsychotic medication is warranted even when symptoms of tardive dyskinesia develop.

Lowered seizure threshold. Chlorpromazine in particular increases the likelihood of seizures in patients who have preexisting seizure disorders. Therapy with antipsychotics must therefore be undertaken with caution (but is not contraindicated) in such patients.

Anticholinergic side effects. These are very common, usually mild, but somewhat annoying; they disappear within days or weeks. Dry mouth, blurred vision, tachycardia, nasal congestion, and constipation are the most frequent of such effects. Occasionally, the side effects are more severe, such as paralytic ileus, or urinary retention. Be careful to screen patients for preexisting narrow-angle glaucoma, since antipsychotics can precipitate acute exacerbations of this condition, which may result in loss of eyesight.

Postural hypotension. This is particularly common in the elderly and must be monitored closely to prevent falling and possible head trauma.

Allergic or toxic side effects. Although these are uncommon, you must be alert to their possible occurrence.

Agranulocystosis occurs in the first three to eight weeks of treatment in roughly 1 in 5,000 patients on chlorpromazine, and somewhat less commonly with other drugs in this class. Early manifestations are fever and sore throat that usually precede altered white blood cell count. Treat it by stopping all medication and working to prevent infection.

Dermatitis of three types is possible: systemic, contact, and phototoxic. Patients must be forewarned to use sun blockers when exposed to the sun.

Allergic hepatitis occurs chiefly in chlorpromazine-treated patients (about 1 in 500 patients) during the first four weeks of treatment. It is manifested by jaundice. This is a benign condition that remits when the drug is stopped.

Metabolic or endocrine side effects. These very un-common effects include weight gain, menstrual irregularity, galactorrhea and gynecomastia, hyperglycemia, and hypothermia or hyperthermia.

Toxic retinopathy. This is caused only by thioridazine (Mellaril) in dosages of more than 800 mg per day.

EKG changes. Arrhythmias, T-wave inversions, and changes in the QRS interval are relatively rare, but they are more common with thioridazine (Mellaril) than with other antipsychotics.

Retrograde ejaculation. Since this is primarily caused by thioridazine (Mellaril), other agents are recommended in treating men for whom this might be a problem.

Treatment of Extrapyramidal Side Effects (EPS)

Dystonias, parkinsonism, akathisia, and akinesia are all responsive to antiparkinsonian drugs. The most commonly used drugs in the treatment of EPS are the following:

Diphenhydramine (Benadryl) is an antihistamine that is very safe, not prone to being abused, and useful in acute dystonias since intravenous administration brings relief within minutes. It can be given orally, intravenously, or intramuscularly. Sedation and pronounced anticholinergic effects make this drug less desirable for treating patients on a long-term basis. The dosage is 25-50 mg intramuscularly or intravenously for acute dystonia, and 25-50 mg orally every four to six hours to prevent recurrent dystonic episodes.

Benztropine mesylate (Cogentin) is an antiparkinsonian drug that is very effective for acute and long-term treatment of EPS. Administer 1-2 mg orally one to three times a day as needed to prevent EPS. It may be used on a long-term basis, and is also available in intramuscular and intravenous forms (in doses of 0.5-2 mg) for treatment of acute reactions.

Trihexyphenidyl (Artane), another antiparkinsonian drug, is quite similar to Cogentin. Many patients find it less sedating than either Cogentin or Benadryl, and therefore more suitable for long-term treatment. The usual dosage is 2 mg orally one to three times a day.

Lorazepam (Ativan) has been found effective in treating akathisia, but at this time it has not been formally approved by the Food and Drug Administration (FDA) for this purpose. Generally, a dosage of 0.5-2 mg orally two or three times a day is sufficient.

If the patient requires an antiparkinsonian drug for side effects, continue the drug for one to three months and then taper it off to determine whether it is still required. A majority of patients will have become "acclimated" to the antipsychotic and will not exhibit their previous side effects when the antiparkinsonian drug is discontinued. However, a significant number of patients require antiparkinsonian therapy for as long as they take the antipsychotic.

Note that some patients experience a "high" from Cogentin and Artane, and will abuse these drugs when the side effects are no longer present.

Use During Pregnancy

The antipsychotics have not been shown to cause an increased incidence of congenital malformations in the fetus when taken by the mother during pregnancy. Nevertheless, it is advisable to avoid administering them if possible, at least during the first trimester, unless psychotic symptoms are clearly evident and require control. The medications are excreted in breast milk, and should therefore be avoided if possible while a patient is breastfeeding a child.

Drug Interactions

Some drugs that interact with the antipsychotics include the following:

The efficacy of *oral anticoagulants* is decreased by phenothiazines.

Antacids may decrease the absorption of antipsychotic medications.

The phenothiazines potentiate the effects of *antihistamines*, *antihypertensives*, *CNS depressants* (e.g., alcohol), *oral hypoglycemics*, and *succinylcholine*.

Scopolamine overdose (e.g., Compoz, Sominex) or *diuretics* in combination with the phenothiazines can cause a hypotensive crisis.

Choosing an Antipsychotic

Since they are all of roughly equal efficacy, how do you decide which antipsychotic to use for a particular patient?

Rely on the patient's history. If your patient has had antipsychotic medication in the past, find out which drugs worked and which did not.

Consider compliance. If you work with an outpatient who cannot reliably take daily oral medication, you must consider using depot fluphenazine intramuscularly every two to four weeks. Fluphenazine is one of the only antipsychotics available in this long-acting form.

Decide which side effects are least likely to be troublesome to the patient. Since all antipsychotics carry side effects, you must weigh one set against another. In most cases, you are choosing between low-potency drugs, which have primarily anticholinergic and sedating effects, and high-potency drugs, which are less sedating but more likely to cause extrapyramidal reactions (dystonias, parkinsonism, and akathisia). For a severely agitated patient who cannot sleep well, you might deliberately choose a more sedating (low-potency) drug like chlorpromazine (Thorazine) because sedation would be desirable. Paranoid patients might be particularly frightened by muscle spasm (dystonia), so a high-potency drug might be avoided, or given along with prophylactic antiparkinsonian medication. For a college student who is studying for examinations, a low-potency antipsychotic might cause too much drowsiness and blurred vision, whereas a high-potency drug like haloperidol (Haldol) would not compromise his or her studying capacity.

Table 15-5 lists some of the most commonly used antipsychotics, showing the degree to which they cause sedation and/or extrapyramidal side effects (EPS).

Prescribing the Antipsychotics

Once you have chosen an antipsychotic, how do you prescribe it?

Emergencies ("rapid neuroleptization"). Severely combative, aggressive, and destructive psychotic patients can be rapidly and effectively treated with repeated intramuscular doses of an antipsychotic to decrease excitement and to protect the patient and others from harm. Before you use such a treatment with a patient who is unknown to you

Table 15-5. Commonly used antipsychotics, their relative potencies, and their sedating and extrapyramidal effects.

Generic name	Trade name	Relative potency	Sedation hypo-tension	EPS
Phenothiazines				
Aliphatic				
Chlorpromazine	Thorazine	100	+++	++
Piperidine				
Thioridazine	Mellaril	100	+++/++	+
Piperazine				
Fluphenazine	Prolixin	2	+	+++
Perphenazine	Trilafon	10	+	+++
Trifluoperazine	Stelazine	5	+	+++
Thioxanthenes				
Aliphatic				
Chlorprothixene	Taractan	65	++	++
Piperazine				
Thiothixene	Navane	5	+	+++
Dibenzazepines				
Loxapine	Loxitane	15	++	+++
Butyrophenones				
Haloperidol	Haldol	2	+	+++
Indolones				
Molindone	Moban	10	+	++

(e.g., in the emergency room), you must *rule out* the following, which might be obscured or worsened by the administration of an antipsychotic:

- Head injuries
- Space-occupying intracranial lesions (e.g., subdural hematoma)
- Epilepsy
- Severe hypotension or hypertension
- Anticholinergic intoxication
- Electrolyte imbalance

If none of these is present, any one of the antipsychotics listed below may be used intramuscularly (initial doses are suggested, along with an acceptable dosage range):

- Haloperidol (Haldol) 2 mg—range 1-10 mg
- Perphenazine (Trilafon) 10 mg—range 4-30 mg

- Fluphenazine HCl (Prolixin HCl) 2.5 mg—range 1-25 mg
- Trifluoperazine (Stelazine) 5 mg—range 1-10 mg
- Thiothixene (Navane) 5 mg—range 4-30 mg

The end point of this *rapid neuroleptization* is a decrease in excitement, and the process is commonly continued until the patient falls asleep. To achieve this, the dose may be repeated every hour (even every 30 minutes if excitement is severe). Intramuscular doses can be safely repeated as long as there is no significant hypotension, so frequent monitoring of blood pressure is essential during this treatment.

There is an ongoing argument in the literature as to whether rapid neuroleptization is more effective than a single intramuscular injection followed by oral medication.

Acute psychosis. For patients who are acutely psychotic but who do not exhibit severe agitation, rapid neuroleptization is not necessary. Instead, begin with oral doses of the medication. Start at a subtherapeutic dosage and increase it gradually until the desired effect is achieved or until the side effects become intolerable and some adjustment must be made. The phases of acute treatment, when effective, are likely to be as follows:

- **1 to 5 days**—Excitement and hyperactivity disappear, and the patient becomes more cooperative
- **2 days to 2 months**—The patient's thought disorder persists but he or she functions better in daily living
- **1 to 6 weeks** (or more)—Amelioration of the patient's thought disorder

Acute psychosis responds to a minimum of 300-400 mg per day of chlorpromazine (or the equivalent dose of another drug) in most healthy patients. The average dosages required for the acutely psychotic patient range from 400 to 900 mg a day orally. How quickly you reach this dosage will depend on the patient's size (larger people often require higher dosages), age (the elderly generally require lower dosages), and history (tolerance of high dosages in the past permits you to increase the dosage rapidly). For young, healthy patients who have had no prior experience with antipsychotics, start with 100 mg per day and increase the dosage over several days as rapidly as it is tolerated.

How high is too high? You can increase the dosage of an antipsychotic quite a bit to achieve the desired result if the side effects are tolerable, but daily dosages above 1,500 mg orally do not often result in additional improvement. (However, a few patients improve on dosages of up to 4,000 mg orally per day).

The antipsychotics have very long half-lives—i.e., they are metabolized slowly and are long-acting. Thus, you may give the entire daily dosage at one time and still achieve the same antipsychotic effects, if the patient can comply more easily with a once-a-day regimen.

Maintenance therapy. Once the patient has been stabilized on an antipsychotic, how long do you continue this treatment? The answer is not clear. Chronic therapy with an antipsychotic carries significant risks, particularly the risk of tardive dyskinesia. Thus, *only use maintenance therapy if there is a clear indication that the patient requires such treatment.*

Acute drug-induced psychoses generally remit rapidly; prolonged antipsychotic treatment is not necessary. Mania is treated acutely with antipsychotics, but most manic-depressive patients need not be continued on antipsychotics once the acute psychosis has cleared and they are stabilized on lithium.

A patient who suffers a first psychotic episode of unknown etiology (particularly an adolescent) must be tapered off the medication after several weeks to several months of successful drug treatment, so that the ongoing need for medication can be assessed. Such a patient may never have a subsequent psychotic break, and should not be medicated indefinitely.

Maintenance therapy is required for *chronic* conditions in which psychosis recurs within weeks or months after treatment is stopped. Most patients who fall into this category are chronic schizophrenics, schizoaffectives, and those manic-depressives who do not remain symptom-free on lithium alone. About 40 to 60 percent of patients who are diagnosed as chronic schizophrenics have relapses within six months after antipsychotic treatment is stopped. For these people, long-term maintenance has been shown to decrease their rates of relapse and rehospitalization.

Even the most chronic patients (i.e., those with a history of multiple psychotic episodes and multiple hospitalizations) should be given occasional closely supervised trials off medication to be sure that treatment is not being prolonged unnecessarily.

Long-term maintenance dosages of antipsychotics can usually be lowered to 20 to 50 percent of the dosage required during the acute psychotic episode. There is no standard maintenance dosage, so you must arrive at it by monitoring your patient's symptoms carefully and determining the lowest dosage at which target symptoms are kept in abeyance.

If treatment seems ineffective, consider whether the dosage is adequate and whether the patient is taking the drug. If the patient shows *no* response to an adequate dosage of medication after two weeks of treatment, try another medication. Lack of response to one antipsychotic does not imply that the patient will not respond to another.

ANTIDEPRESSANTS

Drugs that alleviate and prevent depression have proved invaluable in the treatment of mood disorders. These drugs fall into two major classes—the tricyclic antidepressants (TCAs) and tricyclic-like medications, and the monoamine oxidase inhibitors (MAOIs). These medications, along with electroconvulsive therapy (ECT), are the most effective somatic therapies now available for the treatment of certain types of depression. Stimulants, such as amphetamine, were once widely used in elevating the depressed patient's mood, but since the advent of these more effective and more specific antidepressant agents, mood elevators are no longer the treatment of choice.

As was mentioned in Chapter 6, the causes, symptoms, and clinical courses of various depressive syndromes are quite varied. No one treatment is uniformly effective for all types of depression, and the antidepressants are not panaceas. Nevertheless, a majority of patients with severe depression *do* respond favorably to antidepressants, and many who do not respond to one drug will respond to another or to ECT.

Psychotherapy or Medication?

This choice is *not* an either-or proposition. Many advocates of medication argue that drugs work more rapidly than psychotherapy to alleviate depression, and that they are more cost-effective. Psychotherapists counter that medication interferes with effective treatment since it allows patients to attribute a "chemical" cause to their difficulties and thereby avoid important intrapsychic and interpersonal issues that have fostered the depression.

In fact, *medications and psychotherapy work in complementary ways*—the medication alleviates many of the physiological symptoms of the illness, while psychotherapy helps to ease emotional pain and promote more effective functioning in the world. Outpatient studies of mild depression have shown the combination of psychotherapy and pharmacotherapy to be more effective than either treatment alone.

Which depressed patients are most likely to benefit from an antidepressant? Two factors should be considered in answering this question—the symptoms and the syndromes, as shown in Table 15-6. The depressive *symptoms most likely* to be alleviated by antidepressant medication are *the vegetative signs*: appetite disturbance and weight loss, sleep disturbance (especially early morning awakening), decreased energy, decreased libido, psychomotor agitation or retardation, and diurnal mood variation (depression worse in the morning).

The *symptoms less likely* to respond to antidepressants are those that are more *subjective* and *psychological*: demoralization, low self-esteem, hopelessness, and helplessness. Such feelings are more responsive to psychotherapeutic interventions.

The depressive *syndromes most likely* to respond to antidepressants include vegetative signs and discrete episodes of illness that seem to have a life of their own. Discrete episodes of depression have a clear time of onset, as opposed to more "characterologic" depression, which the patient regards as having always been present. *Major depressive episodes* ("endogenous depression") are not greatly influenced by changes in the

Table 15-6. Responsiveness of symptoms and syndromes to antidepressant medications.

Most likely to respond	Less likely to respond
Symptoms	
Appetite disturbance and weight loss	Demoralization
	Low self-esteem
Sleep disturbance	Hopelessness
Decreased energy	Helplessness
Decreased libido	
Psychomotor agitation or retardation	
Diurnal mood variation	
Syndromes	
Major depressive episodes	Dysthymic disorder
Agitated depression	Personality disorder

patient's environment or by specific social or therapeutic interactions; they generally include vegetative signs. *Agitated depression* ("involutional melancholia") is common in people over 45 and is characterized by pacing, hand-wringing, hair-pulling, and vocal expressions of psychic pain, antipsychotics and ECT are also particularly useful in these cases.

The *syndromes less likely* to respond to antidepressants are those that have no clear onset or discrete episodes, but have a clear relationship to environmental events (i.e., the patient's wife has left him) and minimal vegetative disturbance. These include *dysthymic disorder* that has been present for at least two years in adults and is characterized by longstanding feelings of hopelessness, inadequacy, and low self-esteem without prominent physiologic disturbance, and *personality disorders* in which depression is a concomitant of longstanding interpersonal difficulties and chronically impaired functioning. For example, patients with borderline personality disorder often complain of depression, and may even report sleep and appetite disturbance, but these symptoms are often the direct result of the underlying personality disorder and current life events. Such difficulties are not resolved by pharmacotherapy.

Syndromes that are generally self-limiting do not require antidepressant therapy. *Reactive depression* due to severe environmental stress includes, for example, grief reactions after the death or loss of a loved one. Support, psychotherapy, and brief symptomatic treatment (e.g., with antianxiety agents) usually suffice. *Drug-induced depression* (e.g., by reserpine) is usually resolved when the offending drug is discontinued. *Depression secondary to physical illness* generally resolves when the underlying physical condition improves (e.g., anemia, hypothyroidism).

Syndromes that are not "pure" depressive syndromes are *sometimes responsive* to antidepressant treatment. These include *manic-depressive illness* and *schizoaffective disorders*. Although lithium treatment is more common and generally more effective on a long-term basis, antidepressants can be useful in treating the acute depressive phases of manic-depressive illness. A word of caution however—since antidepressants can precipitate mania, they must be used judiciously with patients who are prone to manic episodes. For schizoaffective disorders, antipsychotics and antidepressants are often used in combination when patients manifest features of both affective illness and schizophrenia. Again, antidepressants must be used with caution since they exacerbate psychosis in some cases.

In cases of depression that are not clear cut, when symptomatology is not clearly vegetative, the decision to medicate or not to medicate remains a matter of clinical judgment. Most clinicians agree that it is best to try antidepressants when there is a reasonable possibility that the drug could be of benefit to the patient, and when a trial of the medication can be carried out safely.

Dexamethasone Suppression Test

As the discussion above suggests, there is disagreement over which patients are likely to respond to antidepressants. In the past few years, much publicity has been given to the dexamethasone suppression test (DST), which promised to be a definitive biochemical test for depression enabling clinicians to reliably sort out those depressed patients who would respond to antidepressant therapy from those who would not. Since you are likely to encounter the DST in your work in psychiatry, a brief discussion of this new laboratory study is provided here.

The development of the DST began with the observation that many depressed patients had elevated serum cortisol levels and poor regulation of adrenocorticotropin (ACTH) production. In normal people who are given a small dose of dexamethasone (a synthetic steroid), the body's production of cortisol (a natural steroid) will automatically be suppressed over the next 24 hours. However, in some depressed patients given the same oral dose of dexamethasone, cortisol production is only partly suppressed or recovers too early, suggesting an abnormality in the regulation of hormone production in the hypothalamic-pituitary-adrenal cortical axis.

The DST is given as follows: 1 mg of dexamethasone is given orally at 11 p.m., and venous blood is drawn for cortisol assays at 8 a.m., 4 p.m., and/or 11 p.m. the following day (in outpatients, the test is usually limited to a 4 p.m. sample). The DST is considered abnormal if any of the samples shows a plasma cortisol level above 4.5-5.0 mg/dl. The test costs $25 to $50 for each blood sample assayed.

Investigators have reported that 90 percent of patients who have abnormal ("positive") DST's have melancholic or endogenous depression—a high rate of specificity for this test. Ideally the DST could help clinicians establish or rule out the presence of endogenous depression if the clinical findings were equivocal. However, the test is not particularly sensitive, for only about 50 percent of patients who are diagnosed clinically as suffering from major depression have abnormal DST responses; the rest are not identified by this screening measure.

To complicate matters, many medical conditions other than depressive illness can give false positive DSTs—including Cushing's disease, liver disease, pregnancy, and drug use (e.g., alcohol, phenytoin, carbamazepine, or sedatives). New research suggests that the DST may not specifically identify people who are endogenously depressed, but may also be positive in some cases of mania, acute psychosis, chronic schizophrenia, stroke, and dementia.

The DST has not been shown to be superior to clinical findings in predicting whether a patient will respond to antidepressant therapy, nor has it proved helpful to clinicians in choosing particular medications for treating depression. Some psychiatrists use serial DSTs to measure the patient's response to treatment, but it has not been shown that this technique for monitoring improvement is more reliable than one's clinical judgment. Therefore, the diagnostic interview continues to be the most accurate tool available for the diagnosis and treatment of depression that is responsive to somatic therapy, and the DST remains of greater research interest than clinical utility.

Clinical Evaluation

Before you begin a patient on an antidepressant you must look for data that might influence your choice of treatment.

History. Pay particular attention to:

Current medications—Drugs like reserpine, methyldopa,

Table 15-7. Medical work-up for antidepressant therapy.

Medical history
  Current medical conditions
  Current medications
  Family history

Physical examination

Baseline laboratory studies
  Complete blood count with differential
  Routine blood chemistry—SMA-12
  Thyroid function tests (T3, T4, TSH)
  Urinalysis

EKG (if patient over 40 or any history of cardiac symptoms)

---

stimulants, oral contraceptives, alcohol, marijuana, and other drugs of abuse can cause depression.

Family history—A family history of depressive episodes that were responsive to medication is a good predictor of response in your patient. Note which drugs alleviated depression in relatives, because drug responsiveness, like depression itself, has genetic determinants, and what worked for grandfather is likely to work for grandchild as well. If there is a family history of mania, proceed with caution in using antidepressants, because they can precipitate mania in those who have an underlying bipolar illness.

Current medical conditions—Cardiac problems are particularly important to elucidate, given the side effects of the antidepressants (discussed below). Question the patient carefully about a history of congestive heart failure, myocardial infarctions, arrhythmias, and postural hypotension. Other problems to screen out include prostatic enlargement (antidepressants can cause urinary retention) and narrow-angle glaucoma (antidepressants can precipitate acute exacerbations and result in loss of eyesight).

Suicidal ideation—This is a tricky problem, since many depressed patients are prone to suicidal ideation and attempts. Tricyclics are highly lethal in overdose, and the lethal dose is only 10 to 30 times the daily therapeutic dosage. MAOIs can interact with certain tyramine-containing foods (discussed below) to cause severe hypertension, resulting in stroke and death. For suicidal patients, prescribing must be done with care. Prescriptions for outpatients can be written weekly or even every few days if necessary as a sign to the patient of your concern and attention. Severely suicidal patients can be treated in the hospital to prevent overdose in the initial phases of treatment.

Physical examination

Baseline laboratory studies. The following laboratory studies are useful in ruling out possible metabolic and hematologic causes of depression:

- CBC with differential
- Routine blood chemistries
- Thyroid function tests (T_3, T_4 and TSH)
- Urinalysis

Tricyclics and Related Drugs

The tricyclic antidepressants (TCAs) and tricyclic-like compounds constitute the treatment of choice for most depressions. Except in a limited number of cases for which ECT is more clearly indicated, the tricyclics should be the first treatment you consider when you think about somatic therapy for depressed patients.

Despite considerable research, we do not know how these drugs alleviate depression. As was discussed in Chapter 6 (Affective Disorders), some depressed patients have been found to have low CNS levels of the neurotransmitters *serotonin* and *norepinephrine*. The tricyclics affect the concentration of these neurotransmitters at synapses in the CNS by blocking their re-uptake by presynaptic neurons, thus increasing their availability at the junctions between neurons. It has been hypothesized that this *neurotransmitter effect* is the mechanism by which the drugs alleviate depression, but the data supporting this theory are equivocal.

Clinically, it is useful to know which TCAs are serotonergic and which are noradrenergic, because a patient whose depressive symptoms do not respond to one drug may respond to a drug of the other type; see Table 15-8 for the characteristics of the commonly used antidepressants.

The Tricyclics. *Imipramine* (Tofranil) and *amitriptyline* (Elavil) are the oldest and best studied of the tricyclic antidepressants. They are still the most widely prescribed TCAs, but newer drugs with fewer side effects are beginning to be used extensively in clinical practice. Amitriptyline is quite sedating and has predominantly serotonergic effects; it is therefore useful in treating patients who have sleep difficulties. Imipramine is less sedating and primarily noradrenergic in its effects.

Desipramine (Norpramin) is a demethylated metabolite of imipramine; it is thus "purer" in its noradrenergic effect. It has fewer anticholinergic side effects (dry mouth, blurred vision, constipation) than the other TCAs and is therefore quite useful for sensitive patients. *Nortriptyline* (Aventyl) is another demethylated metabolite of amitriptyline. *Protriptyline* (Vivactyl) has little in the way of sedative properties, and is therefore useful for patients who would find sedation unpleasant. *Doxepin* (Sinequan) has two major advantages: few anticholinergic side effects and very little cardiotoxicity. It is useful for patients whose rhythm disturbances and other cardiac abnormalities necessitate caution in prescribing an antidepressant.

Tricyclic-like compounds. Many new antidepressant

Table 15-8. The commonly used tricyclic and related antidepressants and their characteristics.

Generic name	Trade name	Chemical group	Noradrenergic or serotonergic	Daily dosage range (mg)	Comments
Dibenzocycloheptadienes					
Amitriptyline	Elavil and others	Tricyclic	Mostly serotonergic	75-300	Sedating
Nortriptyline	Aventyl	Tricyclic	Both	40-100	Demethylated metabolite of amitriptyline
Protriptyline	Vivactyl	Tricyclic	Both	15-60	Least sedating tricyclic
Dibenzazepines					
Imipramine	Tofranil and others	Tricyclic	Mostly noradrenergic	75-300	Oldest, most widely studied
Desipramine	Norpramin, Pertofrane	Tricyclic	Noradrenergic	75-300	Demethylated metabolite of imipramine; least anticholinergic
Dibenzoxepines					
Doxepin	Sinequan, Adapin	Tricyclic	Both	75-300	Very sedating; least cardiotoxic
Dibenzoxazepines					
Amoxapine	Asendin	Tricyclic	Both	200-300	Rapid onset of action
Dibenzo-bicyclo-octadienes					
Maprotiline	Ludiomil	Tetracyclic	Noradrenergic	150-250	May have more rapid onset of action
Triazolopyridines					
Trazodone	Desyrel	Triazole	Serotonergic	200-300	Little cardiotoxicity, some antianxiety effects

agents that are related to the tricyclics have recently come onto the market or are under investigation. *Amoxapine* (Asendin) is related both to the tricyclics and to the dibenzazepine group of antipsychotics. It has both antidepressant and sedating properties, and its onset of action is more rapid than that of the tricyclics (often as little as four to seven days). There is some concern that amoxapine carries a risk of tardive dyskinesia because of its chemical similarities to the antipsychotics. *Maprotiline* (Ludiomil) is a tetracyclic antidepressant that has mild anticholinergic and sedating side effects. Its antianxiety properties are questionable. *Trazodone* (Desyrel) is chemically distinct from all other available antidepressants. It has proved quite effective in alleviating depressive symptoms. It has very few anticholinergic and cardiovascular side effects, and suicide by trazodone overdose has been relatively uncommon.

Side effects of TCAs and related compounds

Autonomic, primarily anticholinergic effects are quite common and are to be expected in most patients. They include *dry mouth, blurred vision,* and *constipation*—all of which resolve spontaneously or with symptomatic treatment. *Sweating* may also occur. *Postural hypotension* may be more serious than the effects mentioned above. The patient may have to make slower changes in posture or wear elastic stockings. Less common anticholinergic effects include *urinary retention, paralytic ileus,* and the acute exacerbation of *narrow-angle glaucoma.*

CNS effects include *agitation, fine tremor, angry states, mania, schizophrenic excitement,* and the *exacerbation of latent psychosis.* Some patients report sudden falls and balance problems. *Sedation* is a property of many of the TCAs. TCA-induced drowsiness may be unpleasant or welcome, depending on the patient's symptomatology.

Cardiovascular effects are more common in overdose than at therapeutic levels, but the TCAs can cause *palpitations and direct depression of the myocardium.* Since the TCAs exert a quinidine-like effect on the heart, they must be used with great caution in patients who have rhythm disturbances or a history of recent myocardial infarction. TCAs cause flattening of T-waves on EKG, and can exacerbate preexisting conduction blocks. A thorough cardiac evaluation is essential for patients who have cardiac symptoms or a history of cardiac illness.

Drug interactions include potentiation of the effects of quini-
dine and antagonism of the antihypertensive effects of guanethi-
dine. TCAs can also cause severe toxic reactions when given in
combination with MAOIs, although this is questioned by some
clinicians. If you shift a patient from TCA treatment to an
MAOI, wait one to three weeks after the TCA is discontinued
before beginning the MAOI.

Overdose results in cardiac arrhythmias, convulsions,
hyperreflexia, confusion, coma, and death. The lethal dose of
most TCAs is relatively low—roughly 10 to 30 times the daily
therapeutic dosage.

Prescribing regimen for TCAs and related compounds
  • Begin with a low dose.
  • Raise the dosage slowly to within the recommended effective
dosage range or until side effects prohibit further dosage increases. A
typical daily dosage for a patient starting on imipramine would be as
follows:

Day 1	50 mg
Days 2-4	75 mg
Days 5-10	100 mg
Days 11-16	150 mg

Similar regimens are suitable for most of the other TCAs. Doses may be
divided (often two or three times per day) to lessen side effects, but a single daily dose is acceptable and may make the patient's compliance
easier to obtain.
  • Obtain a serum drug level if possible to help you adjust medication to a proper therapeutic dosage. The plasma levels shown in Table
15-9 have been associated with maximum therapeutic response. For

Table 15-9. Plasma levels associated with maximal therapeutic response to
tricyclic antidepressants.

Drug	Plasma level (ng/ml)
Nortriptyline	50-170
Imipramine (+ desipramine)	>200
Desipramine	40-160
Amitriptyline (+ nortriptyline)	>160
Doxepin (+ desmethyldoxepin)	>100

drugs whose therapeutic levels have not been established, raise the dosage to within the limits of the recommended therapeutic range, as long as no intolerable side effects develop.

• Wait at least three weeks after the patient is receiving an adequate dosage to evaluate therapeutic effects. If no therapeutic response occurs after three to four weeks, raise the dosage of the TCA or switch to a TCA of a different chemical group.

Continuing therapy. Once the initial depressive symptoms have remitted, how long do you continue antidepressant therapy? Studies have demonstrated that patients are least likely to have a relapse of depressive symptoms if they are treated continuously for seven to eight months after an acute depressive episode. Medication can then be tapered off and discontinued over a week to ten days. If depressive symptoms recur, the drug is then reinstated.

Maintenance therapy. Which patients need long-term maintenance on an antidepressant? This is not an easy question to answer. Some patients have one episode of depression and never experience a recurrence. For such people, maintenance therapy is unnecessary. Other patients have recurrent depressive episodes, but so infrequently (e.g., every ten years) that maintenance therapy is not warranted. On the basis of large follow-up studies, it appears that people who have two depressive episodes within five years are likely to experience recurrences. For such people, prophylaxis of depressive episodes is recommended.

Monoamine Oxidase Inhibitors

The MAO inhibitors block the action of the enzyme monoamine oxidase (MAO), which breaks down norepinephrine within neurons. By inhibiting the action of MAO, the MAOIs increase the concentration of norepinephrine at receptor sites, and this is believed to be related to their antidepressant action.

MAOIs are clearly second-line drugs in treating depression for two major reasons: (1) their clinical efficacy is less than (or at best equal to) that of the TCAs in most controlled trials and (2) their side effects are particularly dangerous. They are clearly not to be used by nonspecialists and, as a rule, they should only be used when other treatment modalities (ECT, TCAs) have failed or are contraindicated. The available MAOIs are shown in Table 15-10.

Some clinicians report that MAOIs are more effective than TCAs

Table 15-10. Available MAOIs and their average dosages.

Generic name	Trade name	Avg. daily dosage (mg)
Hydrazides		
Isocarboxazid	Marplan	10-30
Phenelzine	Nardil	45-75
Nonhydrazide		
Tranylcypromine	Parnate	20-40

in atypical depressions—e.g., for patients who are more depressed in the evening, patients with multiple somatic complaints, and patients with phobic anxiety states. However, the TCAs remain the drugs of first choice for most forms of depression.

Side effects and adverse effects. The major side effects of the MAOIs are *hypertensive crisis* and *synergism with other drugs*.

Hypertensive crisis is perhaps the most widely known side effect of the MAOIs. It occurs primarily when the patient on an MAOI eats foods that contain tyramine. Such foods are numerous, and include certain types of cheese, wine, beer, pickled herring, chicken livers, cream, chocolate, and yogurt. Hypertensive crisis can result in severe headache, stroke, and death. A patient taking an MAOI must be able to comply with a diet that involves the strict avoidance of many foods.

The drug interactions are too numerous to list here, but the major ones include interactions with cold and sinus remedies, analgesics, amphetamines, alcohol, narcotics, diuretics, antihypertensives, and hypoglycemics. The combination of these drugs with an MAOI can cause severe hypertension, hypotension, or CNS depression.

The lethal dose of an MAOI is relatively low—six to ten times the average daily dosage. Thus, the potential for suicide by means of overdose or by the abuse of tyramine-containing foods is high.

These drugs are not to be used in combination with TCAs, except in special cases under the close supervision of a psychopharmacologist.

LITHIUM

As early as 1949, the antimanic properties of the lithium ion were described in the literature (Cade, 1949). By 1970, lithium carbonate was approved for clinical use in the United States. It has been a mainstay in the treatment of manic-depressive illness ever since. Lithium has been shown to be effective against the symptoms of acute mania, as well as in preventing recurrent episodes of affective illness during long-term maintenance.

We do not know how lithium works, nor have we located its site of action. Its physical, chemical, and biological properties are similar to those of sodium. However, it crosses cell membranes slowly, and a therapeutic response is not generally achieved until five to ten days after treatment is begun.

Uses

Acute manic episodes. Lithium has been shown to be effective in controlling acute mania in roughly 80 percent of patients within one to two weeks after treatment is begun. During the "lag period" between the start of treatment and the beginning of the therapeutic effect of the drug, clinicians usually "cover" the patient with an antipsychotic to control agitation and diminish psychosis.

Bipolar illness (maintenance therapy). Lithium has proved effective in preventing severe relapses of both manic and depressive episodes in bipolar patients. It appears to diminish both the severity of the episodes and the frequency of recurrence.

Recurrent unipolar depression (maintenance therapy). Studies have shown lithium to be as effective as imipramine in preventing recurrent depressive episodes in unipolar depressive patients. Although the TCAs are currently the treatment of choice for prophylaxis of depressive episodes, increasing attention is being paid to the benefits of lithium for this purpose. However, the FDA has not yet approved the use of lithium in unipolar depression. There is no conclusive evidence supporting the efficacy of lithium in relieving *acute* depressive episodes.

Schizoaffective disorder. Lithium is of limited use in treating this illness, since the affective features are atypical and mixed with features that are more characteristic of schizophrenia. Antipsychotics are the treatment of choice in schizoaffective disorder, but lithium is often added to the regimen when an antipsychotic alone does not sufficiently ameliorate the symptoms or prevent recurrent exacerbations.

Other uses. Much research is being done on other psychiatric conditions that may be responsive to lithium. Various cyclic mood disturbances are under consideration, along with impulse disorders, other aggressive states, and unstable personality disorders. It appears that a family history of affective illness and/or a favorable response to lithium in some family member favors a therapeutic response in patients with a variety of atypical mood disorders.

Effects

Although lithium takes away the subjective experience of being "high" and ameliorates manic psychosis and excitement, it has almost no effect on normal people. Many patients liken taking lithium to the experience of taking an aspirin. There is little or no sedation, and no appreciable effect on cognition or motor activities in the nonmanic person. Nevertheless, patients who have manic-depressive illness often dislike the drug because it takes away the euphoria that is a subjectively pleasant aspect of mania.

Lithium is given orally, and is rapidly absorbed into the blood stream. It reaches peak levels in one to three hours after ingestion. It is distributed throughout the total body water and is eliminated by the kidneys. Normal kidney function is essential, and renal functioning must be monitored throughout treatment. In normal adults, the half-life of lithium is 24 hours, but the rate of excretion by the kidney may vary as a result of several factors. Most notably, as sodium intake decreases, lithium retention by the kidney increases. Thus, such variables as diet, the use of diuretics, and the rate of perspiration can significantly affect blood levels of lithium and even result in lithium toxicity.

Side Effects

The *early side effects* of lithium treatment, which are very common and usually subside within a few days, include

Gastrointestinal distress, including nausea, vomiting, diarrhea, stomach pain.

Muscle weakness and the subjective experience of being dazed or tired.

Hand tremor—a fine tremor, in contrast to the more coarse tremor of parkinsonism.

Increased thirst and **frequency of urination.**

The *later side effects* include

Persistent hand tremor.

Polyuria and **polydipsia** that may be severe and persistent; treat by stopping the drug, or by careful adding concurrent treatment with a thiazide diuretic (paradoxical effect).

Weight gain and/or **edema.**

Precipitation of latent **hypothyroidism** or induction of non-toxic goiter.

Leukocytosis($\sim$15,000/m³)—frequent and relatively benign.

EKG changes (common), including T-wave depression and widened QRS complexes.

Renal pathology—A small proportion of patients develop renal pathology that is characteristic of interstitial nephritis, often with polydipsia and polyuria, difficulty in concentrating their urine, and reduced creatinine clearance. To prevent such irreversible kidney damage, it is wise to monitor patients on lithium maintenance by measuring their serum creatinine levels at three- to six-month intervals; any severe polyuria should be carefully evaluated.

Lithium Poisoning

Lithium toxicity is common. It occurs when the amount of lithium in the bloodstream is as little as 50 percent above therapeutic levels. Mild lithium toxicity can be reversed simply by omitting several doses and then beginning again at a lower dosage when the serum lithium level has fallen to within a nontoxic range and toxic symptoms have remitted. Severe toxicity must be managed in the hospital, usually by osmotic diuresis.

Common causes of an elevated serum lithium level are:

- **Overdose**
- **Sodium or fluid loss** (e.g., sweating, vomiting, diarrhea)
- **Concurrent medical illnesses**

A patient who contracts even a minor illness should let you know immediately and refrain from taking lithium if he or she experiences vomiting or diarrhea. The level of lithium in the blood should be measured at such times to reassess the dosage.

It is important that both you and your patient be aware of the signs of lithium toxicity: see Table 15-11.

Table 15-11. The signs of lithium toxicity.

Early signs	Late signs
Slurred speech	Impaired consciousness— somnolence, confusion, stupor
Drowsiness	
Muscle weakness	Hypertonic muscles and fasciculations
Coarse tremor and muscle twitching	
	Increased deep tendon reflexes
Anorexia	Hyperextension of arms and legs
Vomiting and diarrhea	Seizures
Ataxia	Coma
Confusion	Death

Clinical Evaluation

Before you start a patient on lithium, you must complete the following evaluations:

History and physical examination. Be sure to elicit any history of renal, cardiovascular, or thyroid disease. Other possible contraindications include the need for a low-salt diet, the use of diuretics, chronic diarrhea, organic brain syndromes, and old age or severe debilitation. Any of these require caution in prescribing lithium. During the physical examination, be sure to palpate the patient's thyroid.

Baseline laboratory tests. These should include:

• **Blood urea nitrogen** (BUN), **creatinine**, and **urinalysis** to assess kidney function. The usefulness of other baseline renal function tests (e.g., 24-hour creatinine clearance) is debatable.

• **White blood count** (WBC), since leukocytosis is common in the course of therapy.

• **Thyroid function tests** (T_3, T_4, and TSH)—Decreased thyroid functioning can occur during treatment.

• **Electrolytes**, especially sodium—Most useful if the patient's hydration status is in question.

• **EKG**—for patients with cardiac symptoms, men over age 35, and women who are postmenopausal.

• **Liver function tests, serum glucose**—for patients who may have liver ailments or who have a history of alcoholism or hypoglycemia.

Follow-up laboratory studies for lithium mainte-nance.

- Every 1-2 months—lithium level
- Every 3 months—serum creatinine
- Every 6-12 months—WBC, T_4, T_3, TSH, urinalysis

Any unexplained change in the patient's lithium level should prompt you to retest the serum lithium level and serum sodium level and to repeat any other studies that seem indicated.

Administration

Lithium comes in three oral forms: regular lithium carbonate (Eskalith, Lithane), a slow-release form of lithium carbonate (Lithobid), and a liquid form, lithium citrate (Cibalith-S). The first is the most commonly used preparation; it comes in 300 mg capsules. Lithium is always given in divided doses, generally two or three times daily (the slow-release form can be given twice a day). Dosages are individually determined for each patient according to his or her serum level of lithium. Therapeutic blood levels are generally 1.2 to 1.5 mEq/l in acute mania, and 0.8 to 1.2 mEq/l for long-term maintenance. *Note* that samples for determining blood levels are drawn about 12 hours after the last dose of medication (usually before the first dose in the morning), because blood levels are artificially high in the hours immediately following ingestion.

Acute mania. Begin with a dose of 900 to 1200 mg of lithium carbonate per day (less in small or elderly people) and measure serum levels every two to three days, raising the dosage until serum levels reach 1.5 mEq/l or until signs of toxicity develop. Some patients require as little as 300 mg per day to reach a therapeutic level, while others require as much as 3600 mg per day. After one to two weeks, when mania subsides, lower the dosage since the patient will no longer require as much medication and may become toxic. A level of 0.8-1.2 mEq/l will usually suffice for maintenance beyond the acute manic phase.

Maintenance. Many clinicians believe lithium is more effective in the prophylaxis of manic and depressive episodes than in the acute treatment of mania. Lithium has been clearly demonstrated to decrease both the severity and the frequency with which mania and depression recur.

Who is a candidate for lithium maintenance? Only those patients who have a history of *recurrent* manic and depressive episodes. Those who have suffered a first episode may be taken off lithium and observed, since subsequent attacks may never occur, or may not recur for many years.

Lithium maintenance involves careful monitoring of blood levels (monthly, or at least bimonthly) to prevent toxicity. Most patients can be maintained on 600-1800 mg per day to achieve a blood level of 0.8-1.2 mEq/l.

Toxic blood levels range from mild toxicity at 1.5 to 2.0 mEq/l, to a potentially lethal condition at 4.0 mEq/l or greater. *Blood levels should be checked immediately whenever the dosage is adjusted, when signs of toxicity develop, when hypomanic symptoms occur, and when any but the most trivial illness develops.*

ANTIANXIETY AGENTS

Anxiety is everywhere. It is a symptom we have all experienced. In many cases, it is quite adaptive to the situations in which we find ourselves. However, anxiety can become so overwhelming that it is incapacitating and leaves people unable to carry on with their daily lives. This has prompted an age-old search for drugs that alleviate anxiety.

Virtually any sedating drug will diminish the effects of acute anxiety, but many sedatives (e.g., the barbiturates) significantly impair a person's ability to think, to perceive and react to stimuli rapidly, and to exercise normal motor skills. Many sedatives are also highly addictive, are widely abused, and have such low lethal doses that suicide with these agents is common.

The antianxiety agents are among the most frequently prescribed drugs in medicine, primarily because the demand for relief from anxiety is great, and because antianxiety agents are safer than sedative-hypnotics. They cause less impairment of cognitive and motor functioning, addiction is relatively uncommon, and they are much less lethal when taken in overdose.

The two major classes of antianxiety agents are the *benzodiazepines* and the *glycerol derivatives*. The benzodiazepines are the safer and more commonly used of these two classes.

Antianxiety agents do not cure anxiety, they only alleviate it temporarily. Thus, these agents are not the primary treatment of choice for any psychiatric disorder. They are most clearly indicated for *short-term* treatment of transient forms of anxiety. Since most people tolerate anxiety without becoming dysfunctional, antianxiety agents are indicated only when the patient becomes in some way *disabled* by his or her distress.

Why the emphasis on short-term treatment, and only when the anxiety is disabling? First, because the drugs are not without hazards, especially when given for long periods of time. Patients soon become tolerant to the antianxiety, euphoriant, and disinhibiting effects of the drugs, and are likely to abuse them to achieve the desired effects as tolerance develops. Psychological dependency and physical addiction thus become hazards in long-term treatment.

Second, antianxiety agents mask the symptom instead of treating the disease. Physicians who prescribe these medications as substitutes for time, concern, and support, do their patients a disservice. Particularly in the case of neurotic and personality-disordered patients, psychotherapy is generally more useful than antianxiety medication.

Uses

The following are the major psychiatric disorders for which treatment with antianxiety agents is indicated:

Acute situational anxiety. Particularly when anxiety lies in the anticipation of some dreaded situation, these agents provide temporary relief. An important use is in relieving anxiety secondary to physical illness and prior to surgical procedures.

Phobic disorders and panic attacks. Antianxiety agents do not treat the primary problem in either of these cases, but they do alleviate the concomitant anxiety and are useful in conjunction with other types of therapy, such as antidepressants and behavior modification (see Chapter 8).

Dysthymic disorder. Antianxiety agents are of limited usefulness on a short-term basis when acute anxiety temporarily impairs functioning. Their use can, however, impede the progress of psychotherapy by masking symptoms and allowing the patient to assume that medication will cure everything.

Drug withdrawal syndromes. The substitution of benzodiazepines for the abused drug is an effective means of withdrawal from some agents, particularly alcohol.

Organic brain syndromes. Antianxiety agents can reduce dangerous hyperactivity and excitement, e.g., in LSD hallucinosis and Alzheimer's disease.

Extrapyramidal side effects. Antianxiety agents are useful in treating EPS, particularly akathisia, caused by antipsychotics.

Antianxiety agents are less useful in somatoform disorders (they are of no use in conversion hysteria), personality disorders, and severe primary affective disorders. They are of little use in schizophrenia and other psychoses.

The Benzodiazepines

The benzodiazepines are the most commonly used antianxiety agents—so common, in fact, that Valium and Librium have become household words. The benzodiazepines have been shown to be effective against acute anxiety, to have relatively few adverse effects, to have few interactions with other drugs, and to be freer from serious dependency problems than other sedating agents. The nine benzodiazepines currently licensed for use in the United States for the treatment of anxiety and insomnia are shown in Table 15-12.

All the benzodiazepines have similar effects:

Disinhibition. The benzodiazepines block conditioned fear and avoidance responses. This may be why the benzodiazepines cause increased hostility and aggressive behavior in some patients.

Sedation. All the benzodiazepines are sedating. Although flurazepam (Dalmane) is highly touted for its usefulness as a hypnotic, studies have shown flurazepam to have no significant advantage over other benzodiazepines in producing sleep. *Patients on benzodiazepines must be cautioned about driving and about the use of alcohol* (the sedative effects of the benzodiazepines are potentiated by alcohol).

Anticonvulsant activity. Some benzodiazepines are used effectively in the treatment (diazepam) and prevention (clonazepam) of seizures.

Muscle relaxant. The efficacy of the benzodiazepines in relieving muscle spasm and tension has been the subject of debate, and the results of controlled studies are equivocal.

Because their effects are essentially the same, the major clinical difference among these drugs is in their duration of action. Long-acting compounds (see Table 15-12) are cleared more slowly, and can build up to high levels in the bloodstream when taken over days or weeks. Since the antianxiety effects of long-acting agents last about as long as those of the short-acting compounds, the long-acting agents must be given in frequent divided doses, despite their long half-lives. Long-acting agents

Table 15-12. Characteristics of the benzodiazepines.

Generic name	Trade name	Duration of action	Average daily dosage (mg)	Comments
Chlordiazepoxide	Librium and others	Long acting	15-100	Muscle-relaxant properties
Diazepam	Valium	Long acting	6-30	
Clorazepate	Tranxene, Azene	Long acting	15-60	
Prazepam	Centrax, Verstran	Long acting	20-60	
Flurazepam	Dalmane	Long acting	15-30	Used primarily at bedtime for sleep
Halazepam	Paxipam	Long acting	60-160	
Lorazepam	Ativan	Short acting	2-6	Used to treat akathisia
Oxazepam	Serax	Short acting	30-120	
Alprazolam	Xanax	Short acting	0.75-1.5	Possible antidepressant effect and efficacy in panic disorders
Clonazepam	Clonopin	Long acting	1.5-20	Prevention of petit mal, akinetic, and minor motor seizures

are metabolized and eliminated particularly slowly in patients who have liver disease and in elderly men. Short-acting agents may have the advantage over long-acting ones in that, since they are more rapidly cleared from the body, they do not exert effects on the CNS much beyond the period of desired sedation and disinhibition.

Administering Benzodiazepines

Benzodiazepines may be given orally, intramuscularly, or intravenously. Most medication is given in oral form, often in an outpatient population. However, the medication can be given intramuscularly for agitation when indicated. Diazepam (Valium) and chlordiazepoxide (Librium) are slowly and sometimes incompletely absorbed when given intramuscularly. Intravenous administration is usually reserved for acute seizure activity because one complication of this route of administration is respiratory compromise or arrest.

Oral benzodiazepines are very safe, since it is virtually impossible to commit suicide by using one of these drugs alone. However, they can be lethal when taken in combination with alcohol or other CNS depressants.

Benzodiazepines versus antipsychotics. Both types of medication are given for excitement and agitation. However, benzodiazepines have no antipsychotic effect and may at times worsen psychosis. Antipsychotics are generally used when psychosis is present, or when panic is overwhelming and unmanageable by other means. Benzodiazepines are indicated for most nonpsychotic forms of anxiety, since they do not cause extrapyramidal side effects and carry no risk of tardive dyskinesia. In this respect they are safer than antipsychotics. Most nonpsychotic anxious-patients find antipsychotics overly sedating and subjectively unpleasant.

Benzodiazepines versus barbiturates. Both are sedatives, but benzodiazepines are safer because they are (1) less addictive; (2) less sedating, causing less drowsiness and ataxia; (3) less lethal in overdose; and (4) less disinhibiting. Although barbiturates are still prescribed by some physicians to treat agitation and anxiety, they are clearly not as desirable as the benzodiazepines for this purpose and ought to be avoided if possible.

Glycerol Derivatives

Glycerol derivatives are a class of minor tranquilizers that were devel-

Table 15-13. The glycerol derivatives.

Generic name	Trade name	Duration of action	Average daily dosage (mg)
Meprobamate	Equanil, Miltown	Long acting	800-3200
Tybamate	Solacen, Tybatran	Short acting	500-1500

oped prior to the advent of the benzodiazepines. They are as effective against anxiety, but they are much less safe than the benzodiazepines. Like the barbiturates, the glycerol derivatives cause excessive drowsiness and ataxia, produce tolerance more rapidly, have greater potential for addiction, and are lethal at relatively low doses.

Meprobamate is particularly lethal in relatively low doses. Its use in suicide attempts is therefore a hazard of treatment. Tybamate has a shorter duration of action and causes fewer side effects than meprobamate. The most common side effects of these drugs are *hypotension* and *allergic reactions* (particularly skin rashes).

The glycerol derivatives are generally less desirable agents in the treatment of anxiety than the benzodiazepines. One exception may be in pregnancy, since meprobamate is thought to be safer for use by pregnant women than the benzodiazepines.

ELECTROCONVULSIVE THERAPY

Electroconvulsive therapy (also known as ECT or "shock therapy") may well be the most wrongly maligned treatment in medicine. Popular literature has depicted ECT as a repressive and cruel procedure. In one state, groups have even worked to outlaw it. Oddly enough, ECT is one of the most humane and most efficacious treatments available to the psychiatrist. Its "bad press" stems largely from outdated information about how ECT is administered, and public concerns about the authoritarian aspects of the mental health system.

ECT involves the induction of a gramd mal seizure by means of an electrical pulse through the brain. Each treatment consists of the induction of one seizure while the patient is under anesthesia, and a course of ECT consists of several such treatments.

Uses

Endogenous depression (major depressive episodes). ECT is a uniquely advantageous treatment for major depressive episodes, since it works much more quickly than antidepressants to relieve symptoms (often within a few days); it is safer for many frail, elderly people who have histories of cardiac illness; and it is probably more effective than TCAs in depression that is accompanied by paranoid or somatic delusions. Major depressive episodes accompanied by severe vegetative disturbances respond remarkably well, with an improvement rate of 80-90 percent. ECT is effective for many severely depressed patients who do not respond to medication. However, it is contraindicated in "neurotic" or "characterologic" depression (i.e., dysthymic disorder), which can be worsened by such treatment.

Acute mania. ECT has been shown to be as effective in treating acute mania as in treating severe depression. Particularly for manic patients who are at risk of harming or exhausting themselves, ECT can give rapid relief.

Schizophrenia. The efficacy of ECT in schizophrenia is a matter of controversy, but acutely ill nonchronic schizophrenics tend to respond to ECT as well as they do to antipsychotics, while chronic schizophrenics tend to do less well with either ECT or antipsychotics. ECT is often used when other treatments have failed with schizophrenics.

Other disorders have not responded well to ECT, although the treatment has been tried in a wide variety of illnesses.

How Does ECT Work?

As with the other somatic therapies in psychiatry, we do not know the mechanism by which ECT exerts its therapeutic effects. The hypotheses put forward to explain its mode of action are too numerous to list here, but one interesting observation is that ECT increases the rate of norepinephrine turnover in the CNS.

Administration

ECT was initially given to patients who were awake and not premedicated. This made the patients quite fearful prior to the procedure and created an increased risk of fractures and dislocations during the seizure itself. Most ECT is now given with three types of medication prior to the treatment: (1) *atropine* to block vagal stimulation caused by ECT and to reduce secretions, (2) *general anesthesia* with a short-acting barbiturate (e.g., methohexital sodium) to reduce the patient's discomfort, and (3) *a depolarizing muscle relaxant* (e.g., succinylcholine) to eliminate complications of the convulsion itself.

ECT is either *bilateral* or *unilateral*. That is, the two scalp electrodes that deliver the seizure-inducing electrical stimulus are either placed over separate cerebral hemispheres or over the same (usually the nondominant) cerebral hemisphere. Although there is some evidence that unilateral ECT causes less subsequent memory loss than bilateral ECT, unilateral ECT may not be as effective as bilateral ECT.

When the patient is fully anesthetized, the electrical stimulus is applied, usually as 70 to 110 volts for 0.1 to 0.5 seconds at an amperage ranging from 200 to 1600 milliamperes (ma). The tonic phase of the seizure begins immediately and lasts for about 10 seconds. Respiration returns to normal within a minute or two, and the patient gradually recovers from the postconvulsive coma. The anesthetist administers oxygen to the patient during the procedure to prevent brain anoxia.

The number of ECT treatments needed for each patient is gauged individually according to the therapeutic response. Depressed patients usually require an average of 6 to 10 treatments, while schizophrenic patients often require between 10 and 20 treatments. Treatments are commonly given three or four times a week (roughly every other day); however, some clinicians have used ECT seven days per week, and others have experimented with giving more than one treatment in the same day.

When the patient has apparently achieved a maximal response— i.e., when successive treatments yield no further beneficial effect—it is prudent to give two or three additional treatments to help prevent early relapse.

Preparing the patient for ECT.

Obtain the patient's informed consent. Explain your reasons for selecting this treatment, as well as the anticipated benefits and potential risks of ECT.

Medical history and physical examination. Pay particular attention to any history of cardiovascular disease, which may increase the risks involved in ECT. Severe hypertension may require increased medication to minimize the possibility of a cerebrovascular accident during ECT. Patients with musculo-skeletal injuries may require additional muscle relaxants during the procedure. The only *absolute contraindication* to ECT is a *CNS neoplasm* that causes increased intracranial pressure, since ECT also causes a transient increase in intracranial pressure and might cause herniation. A history of *recent treatment with catecholamine-depleting drugs* (e.g., reserpine) is also a contrain-dication. ECT is particularly useful for elderly patients, who frequently have cardiac and other major medical problems. You must judge whether the risks of ECT are greater than the risks of allowing severe depression and agitation to go untreated. Often, ECT carries the lesser risk, and the patient's response to treat-ment can be life-saving.

Laboratory work-up. Routine blood chemistries (SMA-12), CBC, urinalysis, chest X-ray, spinal X-ray, EKG, and electroen-cephalograph (EEG).

Pretreatment regimen. If possible, all medications should be discontinued shortly before and during the course of ECT. If this is impossible, the dosages should be reduced as much as possible, particularly for drugs that have cardiovascular effects or side effects. Lithium should not be used concurrently with ECT, since there is evidence of increased neurotoxicity with this combination. The patient should take nothing by mouth for eight hours before treatment, to reduce the risk of vomiting and aspiration.

Side Effects

The most common side effects of ECT are shown in Table 15-14 and de-scribed below.

Memory loss. The acute brain syndrome that follows ECT is the most common and most widely publicized of its side effects. This syndrome consists of a confused state, variable intellectual impairment, and amnesia that may persist for several months following a course of treatment. The amnesia involves both memory for recent events (retrograde) and difficulty in retaining newly learned information (anterograde). The amnesia gradually lessens over the weeks following treatment and resolves completely in six to nine months. Patients who have received unilateral ECT tend to complain less of memory impair-

Table 15-14. Common side effects of ECT.

Most common
  Memory loss
  Headaches
  Muscle aches
Less common
  Weight gain
  Amenorrhea
  Increase in permeability of the blood-brain barrier
  Systemic hypertension
  Apnea
  Cardiac arrhythmias

---

ment than those who received bilateral ECT. The question of whether memory impairment persists beyond a few months is unresolved, but controlled studies have failed to show any permanent memory loss or cognitive impairment in patients who receive a normal course of ECT.

Headaches, which are responsive to aspirin.

Muscle aches, which are transient.

The less common side effects of ECT include the following:

Weight gain, possibly due to treatment of anorexia.

Amenorrhea or other menstrual changes, lasting up to several months.

Transient **increased permeability of the blood-brain barrier**, which may alter the effects of certain drugs.

Marked **systemic hypertension**, which occurs as a part of the generalized seizure.

Apnea following treatments (respiratory support should always be available).

Cardiac arrhythmias, primarily premature ventricular contractions mediated through vagal hyperactivity that can occur during the brief period of bradycardia that normally follows the seizure. This should be prevented by the use of atropine, but cardiac arrests do very rarely occur during treatment, and resuscitation equipment must be on hand.

Risks versus Benefits

Obviously, ECT is not an innocuous procedure, if only because of the risks inherent in the use of general anesthesia. Although death due to cardiac arrest occurs in fewer than 1 in 10,000 treatments, it also constitutes an important risk. And memory impairment can be disconcerting and even frightening to patients.

Yet ECT is the most effective treatment available for serious endogenous depression, and its onset of action is much more rapid than that of any of the antidepressants or lithium. Large-scale studies have shown (1) that the risks of ECT are significantly lower than the risks of untreated severe depression and (2) that ECT is particularly effective in lowering the rates of death from suicide and the total number of deaths among severely depressed patients.

ECT is most clearly indicated:

- In certain types of severe depression, e.g., depression accompanied by somatic delusions.
- When other treatments for depression are likely to be more toxic to the patient, e.g., in frail, elderly patients who have severe cardiac disease.
- When depression is life-threatening—as with actively suicidal patients—and rapid remission is of the utmost importance.

The risks of *not* using this relatively safe treatment must be weighed carefully. Unfortunately, ECT's bad press has at times made patient acceptance of the procedure a problem. In such cases, other forms of treatment (e.g., TCAs) may be tried first, and ECT used as a last resort.

REFERENCES

Abramowicz M (ed): Medical Letter on Drugs and Therapeutics. New Rochelle, NY, Medical Letter, Inc. (A bimonthly publication of new information on all aspects of medication.)

Appleton WS, Davis JM: Practical Clinical Psychopharmacology, 2nd ed. Baltimore, Williams and Wilkins, 1980.

Ayd FJ Jr (ed): International Drug Therapy Newsletter. Baltimore, Ayd Medical Communications. (A monthly newsletter containing information on new research and use of psychotropic drugs.)

Baldessarini RJ: Chemotherapy in Psychiatry. Cambridge, MA, Harvard University Press, 1977.

Bassuk E, Schoonover S, Gelenberg A (eds): The Practitioner's Guide to Psychoactive Drugs. New York, Plenum Press, 1983.

Cade JFJ: Lithium salts in the treatment of psychotic excitement. Med J Aust 2:349-352, 1949.

Crook T, Cohen GD (eds): Physicians' Handbook on Psychotherapeutic Drug Use in the Aged. New Canaan, CT, Mark Powley Associates, 1981.

Goodman LS, Gilman A (eds): The Pharmacological Basis of Therapeutics, 6th ed. New York, Macmillan, 1980.

Shader RI (ed): Manual of Psychiatric Therapeutics. Boston, MA, Little, Brown, 1975.

Shader RI, Greenblatt D, Ciraulo DA: Benzodiazepine treatment of specific anxiety states. Psychiatr Annals 11:16-20, 1981.

Squire LP, Chace PM: Memory function six to nine months after electroconvulsive therapy. Arch Gen Psychiatry 32:1557-1564, 1975.

Weiner RD: The psychiatric use of electrically induced seizures. Am J Psychiatry 136:1507-1517, 1979.

Appendix A

Sample Psychiatric Evaluation

The following is an example of an initial psychiatric evaluation summary of the kind described in Chapter 3. Each psychiatric facility has its own format for such write-ups, and you should follow the form used in the particular institution in which you work. This sample will give you a general idea of how these summaries are done. It is an outpatient evaluation; you may find that inpatient write-ups are more detailed.

HOSPITAL OUTPATIENT CLINIC EVALUATION SUMMARY AND TREATMENT PLAN

Patient: Doe, John

Evaluator: Mary Smith, MS III

Date: October 20, 1983

Identifying Data:

Mr. Doe is a 25-year-old single man who is a third-year law student at Eastern University. He lives by himself in an apartment in Boston and was referred to the Clinic by a friend who had been in treatment here two years ago.

Chief Complaint:

"I feel all screwed up. . . . I've got so many decisions to make in the next few months and all I'm doing is getting high."

History of Present Problem:

Mr. Doe dates his current difficulties as beginning three months ago, when he broke up with the woman with whom he had been living for the past year. The woman, Joan, moved out, and "had been dissatisfied with me because she said I wasn't giving her enough." In addition, in the last eight weeks he has had increased distress from a duodenal ulcer (first diagnosed in 1977). He is being treated for this medical problem by Dr. Michael Jones, internist.

The patient is "worried and indecisive" about his future. He expects to graduate from law school this May but is pessimistic about finding a job. He is also indecisive about what legal area he would like to work in. He worries that he won't pass his bar exams this summer.

Mr. Doe reports awakening at 4:00 a.m. after four hours of sleep most every day for the past two months and is unable to get back to sleep. He feels more depressed in the early morning. He has been smoking two or three marijuana joints per day over the past eight months, and states he feels more able to handle day-to-day responsibilities when he is high. Mr. Doe reports not feeling hungry in recent weeks, and he has lost 12 pounds in two months. At times he has had vague thoughts of suicide but has no plans to hurt himself and no history of self-destructive behavior. He reports frequent periods of weeping when he is alone and thinks of the loss of Joan. He notes a loss of interest in his schoolwork and in sports, and a general feeling of lethargy when he is not high. He is unable to reduce his use of marijuana, even though he states he wishes to do so. He denies any previous history of depressive symptoms, and denies any history of euphoria, increased activity, or disordered thinking. He has no previous psychiatric treatment.

Past History:

Mr. Doe is the only child born to parents of Scottish descent. Father, age 52, is a high school graduate and a machinist at a firm in Boston where he has been employed for the past 28 years. Mother, age 50, is employed as a part-time secretary, and has been working on a part-time basis since the patient was 12 years old. Both mother and father are "hard workers." He continues to see parents at their home for dinner about once a month.

His earliest memory is at age four, when he felt "very frightened and alone" during a hospitalization for a tonsillectomy. During preschool and latency years, patient and father often went on camping trips together and he reports feeling closer to father. As a child, Mr. Doe received some instruction in the Presbyterian Church, but says religion was never that important in his life.

In elementary school and high school, Mr. Doe always received above-average grades. He paid great attention to detail in all his school assignments and at times was ridiculed by his peers for his overzealousness. In elementary school he was friendly with several boys, and was very active in Little League baseball and Boy Scouts. Mr. Doe began to date girls at age 16. He had several brief heterosexual relationships that ended as a result of his being "overbearing, demanding, and too controlling." He notes that he relates to women in this way when he finds himself getting "too close."

In college, he remained very devoted to his studies, often preferring to study rather than to take part in social activities. He received his B.A. in English from Boston University in 1976 and hoped to gain admission to a prestigious law school. In college he received only average grades despite considerable effort, and was "disappointed" that he was unable to gain admission to a more prestigious law school. Both parents, especially father, always took great pride in Mr. Doe's academic achievements. Mr. Doe is the first college graduate in his extended family.

Family Psychiatric History:

Positive for depression: maternal grandfather suffered one episode of depression at age 65, which the patient believes resolved during a brief psychiatric hospitalization that included "shock treatments".

No other family history of affective illness, psychosis, or drug or alcohol abuse.

Medical History:

Negative except for duodenal ulcer (see above). Internist's report has been requested and will be forthcoming. Patient currently takes antacids infrequently, as needed for gastrointestinal discomfort, but no other prescribed or over-the-counter medications.

Drug and Alcohol History:

Marijuana use as noted above. Also drinks four or five beers per week. No other current drug use. Experimented with LSD and "mushrooms" on several occasions in college.

Mental Status:

Mr. Doe presented as a neatly dressed man who looked his stated age of 25. He made little eye contact throughout the interview, and appeared mildly anxious. Speech was clear, normal in rate, and somewhat monotonous in tone. He reported feeling "down in the dumps" and appeared sad, but affect varied little with thought content. He showed no evidence of a thought disorder, and no perceptual distortions. He reported vague suicidal ideation without any plan for harming himself, and denied any homicidal ideation. He was alert and oriented to time, place, and person. Concentration (digit span), memory, and judgment appeared to be within normal limits, as was his ability to interpret proverbs abstractly. He related to the interviewer in a formal and deferential manner.

Formulation:

Mr. Doe presents with a history of depression including anhedonia, lethargy, early morning awakening, and anorexia with weight loss over the past two months. He also reports continuous heavy marijuana use over the past eight months. In recent weeks he has experienced difficulty doing his schoolwork and has lost interest in his usual social and recreational activities. All of this has occurred subsequent to losing his girlfriend and as he faces graduation from law school.

His clear depressive symptomatology over the past two months is complicated by marijuana abuse, and the extent to which cannabis has exacerbated his loss of motivation is unclear. A positive family history of affective disorder, as well as the presence of vegetative signs, suggest a significant biological component to this depressive episode and possible responsiveness to antidepressant medication.

His current symptoms occur in the context of more chronic emotional difficulties, particularly indecisiveness, difficulties with intimacy, and concerns about his own adequacy and self-worth. He is accustomed to being an achiever, and sees himself as falling short of his high standards for performance. The loss of his girlfriend and his fears about finding employment as graduation nears seem to have precipitated the present crisis. His usual obsessional defenses (intellectualization, isolation of affect), "self-medication" with cannabis, and his highly organized and somewhat rigid style of dealing with the world have not been successful in warding off his current depression.

Mr. Doe suffers from vegetative symptoms of depression, apparently precipitated by recent environmental stresses. He also reports long-standing emotional difficulties that impair his work and social life. Given this picture, a combination of psychotherapy and pharmacotherapy may be an effective treatment plan. Career counseling might help to alleviate some of his anxiety about future employment. It will be important to keep Dr. Jones informed of the patient's treatment, in order to coordinate Mr. Doe's medical and psychiatric care.

Diagnosis:

Axis I   296.20   Major depression, Single Episode
             304.31   Cannabis dependence, continuous

Axis II   Obsessive-compulsive traits

Axis III   Duodenal ulcer

Axis IV   Psychosocial stressors
                    a. recent loss of girlfriend
                    b. increased academic pressures
                    c. fear of being unable to find employment as an attorney after graduation

         Severity: 4-moderate

Axis V   Highest level of adaptive functioning past year: 3–Good

Treatment Plan:

1. Once weekly individual psychotherapy to focus on patient's substance abuse, career and adacemic concerns, and difficulty in maintaining gratifying interpersonal relationships.

2. Referral for psychopharmacology consultation to assess suitability for treatment with antidepressant medication.

3. Referral to counselor at Career Planning Bureau at Eastern University to assist him in his job search.

4. Obtain patient's written permission to speak with Michael Jones, M.D., regarding psychiatric and medical treatment.

Mary Smith, MSIII

John Ford, M.D., Chief Resident

Frieda Mason, M.D., Senior Psychiatrist

Appendix B

Table of Commonly Abused Drugs

Class	Trade Name* (or Source)	Street Names
Narcotic analgesics		
morphine	morphine sulfate	dope, M, Miss Emma, morpho, white stuff
heroin	none	H, hard stuff, horse, junk, skag, smack
hydromorphone	Dilaudid	lords
oxymorphone	Numorphan	blues
meperidine	Demerol	
methadone hydrochloride	Dolophine	dollys, amidone
pentazocine	Talwin	
tincture of opium	paregoric	PG, licorice
cough preparations with codeine	elixir Terpin Hydrate	schoolboy, blue velvet
	Robitussin A-C	Robby
hydrocodone	Hycodan	
oxycodone	Percodan	

*Many of these drugs are sold under a variety of trade names; only one or two popular examples are used for each.

Source: *A Psychiatric Glossary*, 5th ed. Washington, D.C., American Psychiatric Association, 1980, pp. 58-62.

Class	Trade Name* (or Source)	Street Names
Nonnarcotic analgesics (continued)		
propoxyphene	Darvon	
Barbiturates		barbs, candy, dolls, goofers, peanuts, sleeping pill
amobarbital	Amytal	blue angels, bluebirds, blue devils, blues, lily
pentobarbital	Nembutal	nebbies, yellow bullets, yellow dolls
secobarbital	Seconal	pink lady, red devils, reds, seccy, pinks
phenobarbital	Luminal	phennies, purple hearts
amobarbital/secobarbital	Tuinal	Christmas trees, double trouble, rainbows, tooies
Other Sedative Hypnotics		
chloral hydrate	Noctec	
ethchlorvynol	Placidyl	
flurazepam	Dalmane	
glutethimide	Doriden	CIBA's
methaqualone	Quaalude	sopors
methyprylon	Noludar	
paraldehyde	Paral	
scopolamine	Sominex	truth serum
Muscle relaxants		
meprobamate	Miltown	
Anxiolytics	Librium	
chlordiazepoxide		
diazepam	Valium	
oxazepam	Serax	
chlorprothixene	Taractan	

*Many of these drugs are sold under a variety of trade names; only a single popular example is used for each.

Class	Trade Name* (or Source)	Street Names
Central nervous system stimulants		
d, di amphetamine amphetamine sulfate	Biphetamine Benzedrine	black beauties A's, beans, bennies, cartwheels, cross-roads, jelly beans, hearts, peaches, whites
amphetamine sulfate/ amobarbital	Dexamyl	greenies
dextroamphetamine sulfate	Dexedrine	brownies, Christmas trees, dexies, hearts, wakeups
methamphetamine hydrochloride	Methedrine	bombit, crank, crystal, meth, speed methyl-phenidate
methylphenidate hydrochloride	Ritalin	
cocaine	cocaine	bernies, big C, coke, flake, happy dust, ice, snow
Drugs with hallucinogenic properties		
d lysergic acid diethylamide (LSD)	synthetic derivative (ergot fungus)	acid, pink wedges, sandos, sugar cubes, LSD
psilocin/psilocybin	mushroom (psilocybe mexicana)	business man's acid, magic, mushroom
dimethyltryptamine (DMT)	synthetic	DMT, DET, DPT
morning glory seeds	bindweed (rivea corymbosa)	flower power, heavenly blue, pearly gates
mescaline	peyote cactus	barf tea, big chief, buttons, cactus, mesc

*Many of these drugs are sold under a variety of trade names; only a single popular example is used for each.

Class	Trade Name* (or Source)	Street Names
Drugs with hallucinogenic properties (continued)		
methyldimethoxy- amphetamine (DOM)	synthetic (derivative)	STP
myristicin	nutmeg	MMDA
muscarine	mushroom (amanita muscaria)	fly
phencyclidine	Sernyl	angel dust, dust, PCP, peace pills
Tetrahydrocannabinols		
marijuana	cannabis sativa (leaves, flowers)	grass, hay, joints, Mary Jane, pot, reefer, rope, smoke, tea, weed, Acapulco gold, Panama red
hashish	cannabis sativa, resin	
Volatile Solvents and Gases		
benzine	gasoline	
toluol	glue vapor	
carbon tetrachloride	cleaning fluid	
naphtha	cleaning fluid	scrubwoman's kick
amyl nitrite	amyl nitrite	amys, pears, snapper, poppers
nitrous oxide	nitrous oxide	laughing gas, nitrous

*Many of these drugs are sold under a variety of trade names; only a single popular example is used for each.

Appendix C

Some Common
Psychotropic Medications
(Classified by type)

Type of Medication	Generic Name	Trade Name*
Antianxiety	lorazepam	Ativan
	clorazepate	Azene, Tranxene
	prazepam	Centrax, Verstran
	clonazepam	Clonopin
	flurazepam	Dalmane
	meprobamate	Equanil, Miltown
	chlordiazepoxide	Librium
	halazepam	Paxipam
	oxazepam	Serax
	tybamate	Solacen, Tybatran
	diazepam	Valium
	alprazolam	Xanax
Antidepressant	doxepin	Adapin, Sinequan
	amoxapine	Asendin
	nortriptyline	Aventyl
	trazodone	Desyrel
	amitriptyline	Elavil

*Many of these drugs are sold under a variety of trade names; only one or two popular examples are used for each.

Type of Medication	Generic Name	Trade Name*
Antidepressant *(continued)*	maprotiline	Ludiomil
	isocarboxazid	Marplan
	phenelzine	Nardil
	desipramine	Norpramin, Pertofrane
	tranylcypromine	Parnate
	imipramine	Tofranil
	protriptyline	Vivactil
Antimanic	lithium citrate	Cibalith-S
	lithium carbonate	Eskalith, Lithane
Antipsychotic	loxapine	Loxitane
	haloperidol	Haldol
	thioridazine	Mellaril
	molindone	Moban
	thiothixene	Navane
	fluphenazine	Prolixin
	piperacetazine	Quide
	mesoridazine	Serentil
	reserpine	Serpasil
	trifluoperazine	Stelazine
	chlorprothixene	Taractan
	chlorpromazine	Thorazine
	acetophenazine	Tindal
	perphenazine	Trilafon
Anticonvulsant	carbamezepine	Tegretol

*Many of these drugs are sold under a variety of trade names; only one or two popular examples are used for each.

Appendix D

Some Common Trade Names of Psychotropic Medications

Trade Name	Generic Name	Type of Medication
Adapin	doxepin	Antidepressant
Asendin	amoxapine	Antidepressant
Ativan	lorazepam	Antianxiety
Aventyl	nortriptyline	Antidepressant
Azene	clorazepate	Antianxiety
Centrax	prazepam	Antianxiety
Cibalith-S	lithium citrate	Antimanic
Clonopin	clonazepam	Antianxiety
Dalmane	flurazepam	Antianxiety
Daxolin	loxapine	Antipsychotic
Desyrel	trazodone	Antidepressant
Elavil	amitriptyline	Antidepressant
Equanil	meprobamate	Antianxiety
Eskalith	lithium carbonate	Antimanic
Haldol	haloperidol	Antipsychotic
Librium	chlordiazepoxide	Antianxiety
Lithane	lithium carbonate	Antimanic
Loxitane	loxapine	Antipsychotic

Trade Name	Generic Name	Type of Medication
Ludiomil	maprotiline	Antidepressant
Marplan	isocarboxazid	Antidepressant
Mellaril	thioridazine	Antipsychotic
Miltown	meprobamate	Antianxiety
Moban	molindone	Antipsychotic
Nardil	phenelzine	Antidepressant
Navane	thiothixene	Antipsychotic
Norpramin	desipramine	Antidepressant
Parnate	tranylcypromine	Antidepressant
Paxipam	halazepam	Antianxiety
Pertofrane	desipramine	Antidepressant
Prolixin	fluphenazine	Antipsychotic
Quide	piperacetazine	Antipsychotic
Serax	oxazepam	Antianxiety
Serentil	mesoridazine	Antipsychotic
Serpasil	reserpine	Antipsychotic
Sinequan	doxepin	Antidepressant
Solacen	tybamate	Antianxiety
Stelazine	trifluoperazine	Antipsychotic
Taractan	chlorprothixene	Antipsychotic
Tegretol	carbamezepine	Anticonvulsant
Thorazine	chlorpromazine	Antipsychotic
Tindal	acetophenazine	Antipsychotic
Tofranil	imipramine	Antidepressant
Tranxene	clorazepate	Antianxiety
Trilafon	perphenazine	Antipsychotic
Tybatran	tybamate	Antianxiety
Valium	diazepam	Antianxiety
Verstran	prazepam	Antianxiety
Vivactyl	protriptyline	Antidepressant
Xanax	alprazolam	Antianxiety

Index

All page numbers in **bold** type
refer to tables in the text.

X-Z